HELICOBACTER PYLORI AND
GASTRODUODENAL DISEASE

Helicobacter pylori and Gastroduodenal Disease

EDITED BY

B.J.RATHBONE MD, MRCP

Consultant Physician and Gastroenterologist,
Leicester Royal Infirmary

AND

R.V.HEATLEY MD, FRCP

Senior Lecturer in Medicine,
University of Leeds;
Consultant Physician,
St James's University Hospital,
Leeds

SECOND EDITION

OXFORD

BLACKWELL SCIENTIFIC PUBLICATIONS

LONDON EDINBURGH BOSTON

MELBOURNE PARIS BERLIN VIENNA

© 1989, 1992 by
Blackwell Scientific Publications
Editorial Offices:
Osney Mead, Oxford OX2 oEL
25 John Street, London WC1N 2BL
23 Ainslie Place, Edinburgh EH3 6AJ
3 Cambridge Center, Cambridge
 Massachusetts 02142, USA
54 University Street, Carlton
 Victoria 3053, Australia

Other Editorial Offices:
Librairie Arnette SA
2, rue Casimir-Delavigne
75006 Paris
France

Blackwell Wissenschafts-Verlag
Meinekestrasse 4
D-1000 Berlin 15
Germany

Blackwell MZV
Feldgasse 13
A-1238 Wien
Austria

First published 1989 as *Campylobacter pylori
 and Gastroduodenal Disease*
Reprinted 1989
Second edition 1992

Set by Alden Multimedia Ltd, Northampton
Printed in Great Britain at the
Alden Press, Oxford

DISTRIBUTORS

Marston Book Services Ltd
PO Box 87
Oxford OX2 oDT
(*Orders*: Tel: 0865 791155
 Fax: 0865 791927
 Telex: 837515)

USA
Blackwell Scientific Publications, Inc.
3 Cambridge Center
Cambridge, MA 02142
(*Orders*: Tel: 800 759-6102)

Canada
Times Mirror Professional Publishing, Ltd
5240 Finch Avenue East
Scarborough, Ontario M1S 5A2
(*Orders*: Tel: 416 298-1588)

Australia
Blackwell Scientific Publications
(Australia) Pty Ltd
54 University Street
Carlton, Victoria 3053
(*Orders*: Tel: 03 347-0300)

A catalogue record for this book
is available from the British Library

ISBN 0-632-03346-0

Contents

List of Contributors

A.T.R.AXON MD FRCP *Consultant Physician, The General Infirmary, Great George Street, Leeds LS1 3EX, UK*

G.D.BELL MD MSc FRCP *Consultant Physician, Department of Medicine, The Ipswich Hospital, Heath Road Wing, Ipswich, Suffolk IP10 0QU, UK*

M.J.BLASER MD *Addison B Scoville Professor of Medicine, Director, Division of Infectious Diseases, Vanderbilt University School of Medicine, Nashville, Tennessee 37232, USA*

E.J.S.BOYD MD MRCP *Ninewells, Hospital and Medical School, Dundee DD1 9SY, UK*

J.G.COGHLAN MRCPI *Research Registrar, Department of Cardiology, Harefield Hospital, Middlesex, UK*

R.COLLINS MB *Research Registrar, Department of Gastroenterology, The Meath/Adelaide Hospitals, Dublin 8, Ireland*

P.CORREA *Professor of Pathology, Louisiana State University Medical Center, 1901 Perdido Street, New Orleans, LA 70112-1393, USA*

A.CURRY BSc PhD *Top Grade Microbiologist, Public Health Laboratory Service, Withington Hospital, Manchester M20 8LR, UK*

M.F.DIXON MD FRCPath *Reader in Gastrointestinal Pathology and Consultant Pathologist, University of Leeds, Leeds LS2 9JT, UK*

C.S.GOODWIN MD FRCPath FRCPA *Professor of Bacteriology, United Arab Emirates University, PO Box 17666, Al Ain, United Arab Emirates*

S.F.GRAY BSc FIMLS *Department of Pathology, St James's University Hospital, Leeds LS9 7TF, UK*

R.V.HEATLEY MD FRCP *Senior Lecturer in Medicine, Department of Medicine, St James's University Hospital, Leeds LS9 7TF, UK*

R.H.HUNT FRCP FRCPC FRCP(Edin) FACG *Professor, Department of Medicine, and Director, Division of Gastroenterology, McMaster University Medical Center, 1200 Main Street West, Hamilton, Ontario L8N 3Z5, Canada*

D.M.JONES MD FRCPath *Director, Public Health Laboratory Service, Withington Hospital, Manchester, M20 8LR, UK*

A.LEE PhD *Professor of Medical Microbiology, University of New South Wales, PO Box 1, Kensington, Sydney 2033, Australia*

J.M.LITTLEWOOD MD FRCP FRCPE DCH *Consultant Paediatrician, St James's University Hospital, Leeds LS9 7TF, UK*

R.P.H.LOGAN MBBS MRCP *Research Fellow, Central Middlesex Hospital, Acton Lane, Park Royal, London NW10 7NS, UK*

M.J.MAHONY MB MRCPI MRCP DCH *Consultant Paediatrician, Paediatric Department, Limerick Regional Hospital, Dooradoyle, Limerick, Ireland*

K.E.L.McCOLL MD FRCP, *Reader in Gastroenterology, University Department of Medicine and Therapeutics, Western Infirmary, Glasgow G11 6NT, UK*

C.A.M.McNULTY MRCPath *Consultant Microbiologist, Public Health Laboratory Service, Gloucestershire Royal Hospital, Southgate Street, Gloucester GL1 1UD, UK*

F.MEGRAUD MD *Professor of Bacteriology, University of Bordeaux and Children's Hospital, 168 Cours de L'Argonne, 33077 Bordeaux, France*

A.MORRIS BSc FRCPA *Microbiology Laboratory, Duke University Medical Center, PO Box 3879, Durham NC 27710, USA*

D.G.NEWELL PhD *Head of Applied Molecular Immunology Unit, Central Veterinary Laboratory, New Haw, Weybridge, Surrey KT15 3NB, UK*

G.NICHOLSON FRCP FRACP *Gastroenterologist, Auckland Hospital, Auckland 1, New Zealand*

C.O'MORAIN MD MSc FRCPI *Consultant Gastroenterologist, Department of Gastroenterology, The Meath/ Adelaide Hospitals, Dublin 8, Ireland*

R.J.OWEN MPhil PhD MRCPath *Deputy Curator, National Collection of Type Cultures, Central Public Health Laboratory, 61 Colindale Avenue, London NW9 5HT, UK*

B.J.RATHBONE MD MRCP *Consultant Physician and Gastroenterologist, Leicester Royal Infirmary, Leicester LE1 5WW, UK*

E.A.J.RAUWS MD PhD *Department of Gastroenterology and Hepatology, Academic Medical Centre, University of Amsterdam, Meibergdreef 9, 1105 AZ Amsterdam, The Netherlands*

B.RUIZ *Department of Pathology, Louisiana State University Medical Center, 1901 Perdido Street, New Orleans, Louisiana 70112, USA*

T.M.SHALLCROSS BSc MRCP *Consultant Physician, Caithness General Hospital, Wick, Caithness, KW1 5LA, UK*

G.M.SOBALA MA MRCP *Senior Registrar in Gastroenterology, The General Infirmary, Great George Street, Leeds LS1 3EX, UK*

A.R.STACEY BFc *Biologics Division, ECACC, PHLS Centre for Applied Microbiology and Research, Porton Down, Salisbury SP4 0JG, UK*

H.W.STEER BSc PhD FRCS *Consultant Surgeon, Department of General Surgery, Southampton General Hospital, Southampton SO9 4XY, UK*

D.S.TOMPKINS MB ChB MRCPath *Consultant Microbiologist, Bradford Royal Infirmary, Duckworth Lane, Bradford BD9 6RJ, UK*

G.N.J.TYTGAT MD *Head of Department of Gastroenterology and Hepatology, Academic Medical Centre, University of Amsterdam, Meibergdreef 9, 1105 AZ Amsterdam, The Netherlands*

J.WEIL MB MRCP *Medical Registrar, Department of Medicine, The Ipswich Hospital, Heath Road Wing, Ipswich, Suffolk IP10 0QU, UK*

K.G.WORMSLEY DSc MD FRCP *Consultant Physician, Ninewells Hospital and Medical School, Dundee DD1 9SY, UK*

J.I.WYATT MB ChB MRCPath *Consultant Pathologist, St James's University Hospital, Beckett Street, Leeds LS9 7TF, UK*

Preface

Since the first edition of this book was published in 1989, as predicted, much has changed in our knowledge about the spiral organism involved in the pathogenicity of gastritis and peptic ulceration. As we were all becoming aware as the first edition went to press, evidence has now confirmed suspicions that the organism is not a member of the genus *Campylobacter*. This revelation has culminated in the reclassification of the spiral bacteria into an entirely new genus – *Helicobacter*. Although this has been relatively recent, the continuing increase in publications and interest has made the new terminology seemingly almost part of current everyday language.

Our knowledge about this organism continues to grow in general and many now believe it is a pathogen responsible for causing chronic active gastritis and probably playing a major part in the pathogenicity of peptic ulceration. Indeed, so great has been the interest in these areas that this has prompted attempts to reclassify the pathology of gastritis, and some now believe that eradication of the organism may, for the first time, alter the natural history of peptic ulcer disease. Evidence also continues to accumulate to implicate *H. pylori* in the pathogenesis of some gastric cancers and undoubtedly this will be a further stimulus for even greater research endeavours in the future. However, not all are impressed by the potential role of this organism in ulcer disease and we have tried to redress this balance in the current volume. The continuing widespread interest in

H. pylori has encouraged the development and ready availability of new diagnostic tests and we are now witnessing new applications for the identification of this organism and the involvement of further disciplines, including medical physicists and immunologists. The developments within the therapeutic arena have stimulated participation in the field by pharmacists, nursing staff and toxicologists. Our increased understanding of the effects of colonization upon gastric physiology has interested biochemists and pharmacologists and the field can now be truly described as having multidisciplinary interest.

The considerable success of our first edition and the continued scientific progress in knowledge concerning *H. pylori* has encouraged us to produce this second edition.

We have been fortunate once again in being joined by a leading international group of experts who all have unsurpassed expertise in *H. pylori* investigational studies and we are most grateful for this continuing support and involvement. We are also indebted to Peter Saugman and his colleagues at Blackwell Scientific Publications for their continued professional expertise and encouragement, which has brought these editions to fruition and success. We hope the second edition of this volume will provide a concise and up-to-date account of our current understanding of the involvement of *H. pylori* in human gastroduodenal disease.

B.J.R., R.V.H.

1 The Historical Associations between Bacteria and Peptic-ulcer Disease

B.J.RATHBONE AND R.V.HEATLEY

Bizzozero [1] in 1893 has been credited with the first demonstration of bacterial colonization of mammalian stomachs with spiral organisms. Studying the microscopic appearance of the gastrointestinal epithelium of various animals, he noted the presence of spirochaetes in the gastric glands and parietal cells of six dogs he examined. Salomon [2] in 1896 confirmed the presence of spiral organisms in the dog and reported similar organisms in the gastric mucosa of cats and rats. He also examined human tissue, apes, monkeys, cattle, pigs and mice without finding similar organisms. Balfour [3] demonstrated spirochaetes in gastric and intestinal ulcers of dogs and monkeys. Lucet [4] observed similar organisms in a dog suffering from haemorrhagic gastroenteritis. The transmission of spiral organism from dog or cat to mouse was demonstrated by Salomon [2] and Kasai & Kobayashi [5].

Human gastric spirochaetes were first reported in necrotic material at the surface of ulcerating carcinomas and in gastric secretions by Krienitz [6] and Luger [7]. Although little attention was paid to the gastric spirals at this time, considerable interest and research were directed to the possible role of non-spiral bacteria in peptic ulceration. In 1888, Letulle [8] reported that the oral or parenteral administration of *Staphylococcus pyogenes* to guinea-pigs resulted in gastric ulcers. Similar results were reported with other bacteria, including dysentery organisms, pyogenic streptococci and lactobacilli. The implication from these reports was that infection may be an occasional or accessory cause of ulceration. The subsequent work mainly concentrated on two organisms, a colonic bacillus and a specific strain of *Streptococcus*.

Whereas the above work reported acute lesions, Turck [9] claimed that chronic ulcers could be produced in 100% of dogs after they had been fed colonic bacilli daily for several months. The photographs illustrating these lesions, however, showed only non-specific gastric and duodenal changes [10]. Completely negative results were obtained when these experiments were repeated [11]. When rabbits were injected with the bacillus, gastric and duodenal lesions occurred within 24 hours but histological examination demonstrated them to have an embolic aetiology. The role of streptococci in ulceration was championed by Rosenow [12–15], who demonstrated that streptococci isolated from humans, especially those with ulceration, produced gastric ulcers when injected into laboratory animals. Rosenow maintained that the *Streptococcus* initiating gastric ulceration had a selective affinity for gastric mucosa, where it produced local destruction of the glandular tissue. This was then digested by the acid gastric juice. He postulated that an acute lesion so produced may be made chronic by the constant discharge into the blood of the specific organisms lurking in distant foci. That injection of streptococci produced ulcers and that organisms isolated from ulcer patients appeared to selectively localize in the stomach when injected were confirmed by other workers [16–18]. In 1930 Saunders [19] isolated an α-streptococcus from human peptic ulcers and demonstrated specific agglutinins to this organism which were present in higher titres in ulcer patients compared with controls with other streptococcal infection. Attempts to produce ulcers in animals by injection of the specific organism, however, were unsuccessful. Saunders suggested that the lesions produced by Rosenow were due to an anaphylactic shock-type reaction, due to foreign protein present in the broths injected into the animals. Celler & Thalhimer [20] isolated a non-haemolytic streptococcus from human ulcers and like Saunders [19] failed to produce ulcers when they injected it into animals. Streptococci can thus be isolated from many ulcers in the stomach and duodenum and when injected into animals have often been associated with acute lesions of the gastric mucosa. These short-lived lesions, however, bear little relation to the ulcer crater seen in human peptic-ulcer disease.

No further work was published concerning human gastric spiral organisms until 1939, when Doenges [21] in a histological study of 242 autopsy stomachs, using haematoxylin and eosin staining of sections, found spirochaetes present in 43% of cases. The organisms occurred predominantly in the glandular lumen but were seen also in the parietal cells. Autolysis made detailed assessment of the gastric histology impossible. To avoid this problem Freedberg & Barron [22] studied gastric resection specimens using haematoxylin and eosin, and a silver stain, which they found best for identifying the bacteria. Overall, 37.1% of their 35 patients were positive for spirochaetes. However, in many cases bacteria were seen only after examining multiple sections. The organisms were mostly associated with gastric ulcers and gastric carcinoma. In 13 duodenal ulcer patients with associated chronic gastritis, only two were positive. In an attempt to confirm the presence of spirochaetes in gastric mucosa, Palmer [23] studied 1180 suction biopsies (mostly from the gastric body) from 1000 patients using haematoxylin and eosin stains. This author reported no spirochaetes or any structure which could reasonably be of a spirochaetal nature.

An indirect clue to the possible presence of gastric epithelial bacteria came in 1924 when Luck & Seth [24] described the presence of considerable urease activity in the stomach. That the urease might be bacterial in origin was suggested in 1959 by Lieber & Lefevre [25], who demonstrated that the hypoacidity found in many patients with uraemia could be reversed with antibiotic therapy. This view was opposed by Mossberg et al. [26]. However, studies using conventional and germ-free animals confirmed that the gastric urease activity in animals was bacterial in origin [27]. No link was made between this urease activity and the presence of gastric spiral bacteria until 1984 [28].

Following the observations by Palmer in 1954 [23], no further reports of gastric spiral bacteria occurred until 1975, when bacteria were described on the lumenal surface of epithelial cells of gastric-ulcer patients [29, 30]. The bacteria were seen to have at least one filum and to be deep to the mucus layer, with the gastric epithelial cells having a diminished mucus content compared with those from a normal stomach. Electron micrographs illustrated phagocytosed bacteria within polymorphonuclear leucocytes and the absence of the bacteria from areas of intestinal metaplasia was noted. Attempted culture of gastric biopsies resulted in the growth of *Pseudomonas aeruginosa*, which was almost certainly a contaminant from the endoscope.

Fung et al. [31] in 1979, correlating endoscopic, histological and ultrastructural appearances of chronic gastritis, described and illustrated bacteria in the crevices between surface mucus cells and in gastric pits. It was noted that many of these bacteria abutted directly on to the plasmalemma of the epithelial cell, but were never seen within the cell and were thus assumed to be of little significance.

Working in the same institution, Warren [32] noted that the majority of endoscopic biopsies from patients with chronic gastritis and peptic ulceration were colonized with curved *Campylobacter*-like orgnaisms. These organisms were poorly stained by haematoxylin and eosin, but seen easily with the Warthin–Starry silver stain. A prospective study was set up and attempts were made to culture the organisms from gastric biopsies, using non-selective and standard *Campylobacter* media for 48 hours. No growth was observed until the 35th biopsy was incubated during an Easter holiday and was thus examined after 5 days' incubation. A heavy growth of *Campylobacter*-like organism was found on the non-selective media. When other biopsies were also incubated for 3–4 days, a similar growth of Gram-negative bacteria was seen [33–35].

Independently, Rollason *et al.* [36], in a retrospective study of endoscopic gastric biopsies, described sprial bacteria in association with chronic superficial and chronic atrophic gastritis. Steer [37], continuing his morphological studies of gastroduodenal mucosa in peptic ulceration, described the scanning electron microscopy appearance of bacteria in patients with ulcer-associated chronic gastritis. The three groups of workers thus independently recognized and reported the association of the gastric spiral bacteria with chronic gastritis.

Although the recent interest in *C. pylori* has certainly focused attention on bacteria and the gastroduodenal mucosa, research has in fact been conducted into these associations over much of the past 100 years [38]. However, the role of bacteria in gastroduodenal disease has never been so close as that between *C. pylori* and active chronic gastritis.

Many of the biochemical and ultrastructural characteristics of *C. pylori* were perhaps more in keeping with the genus *Spirillum* and perhaps also *Wolinella* than with the genus *Campylobacter*, although these features were not typical of either genus [39]. For this reason, in an attempt to resolve this dilemma, Goodwin and his colleagues [40] proposed the transfer of *C. pylori* to an entirely new genus with the name *Helicobacter*. This proposal has achieved rapid international appearance. Thus, it appears that *Helicobacter pylori* has, in a very short time indeed, made a very significant impact on the world of gastroenterology and will probably, in the very near future, have a great influence on the practice of medicine and surgery in this field.

References

1 Bizzozero, G. Über die Schlauchformigen Drüsen des Magendarmkanals und die Bezienhungren ihres Epithels zu dem Oberflächenepithel der Schleimhaut. *Arch. Mikrobiol. Anat.* 1893, **42**, 82–152.

2 Salomon, H. Über das spirillum des Saugetiermagens und sein Verhalten zu den Belegzellen. *Centralbl. Bakt.* 1896, **19**, 433–42.

3 Balfour, A. A haemogregarine of mammals and some notes on trypanosomiasis in the Anglo-Egyptian Sudan. *J. Trop. Med*, 1906, **9**, 81–92.

4 Lucet, M. Sur la presence de spirochètes dans un cas de gastro-entérite hémorragique chez le chien. *Bull. Soc. Centre Med. Vet. Par.* 1910, **64**, 376–9.

5 Kasai, K. & Kobayashi, R. The stomach spirochete occurring in mammals *J. Parasitol.* 1919, **6**, 1–10.

6 Krienitz, W. Über das Aufreten von Mageninhalt bei Carcinoma Ventriculi. *Dtsch. Med. Wochenschr.* 1906, **22**, 872.

7 Luger, A. Über Spirochäten und fusiforme Bazillen im darm, mit einem Beitrag zur Frage der lamblienenteritis. *Wein Klin. Wochenschr.* 1917, **52**, 1643–7.

8 Letulle, M. Origine infectieuse de cetains ulcères simples de l'estomac ou du duodenum. *Soc. Med. D. Hôp. Paris* 1888, **5**, 360–87.

9 Turck, F.B. Ulcer of the stomach: pathogenesis and pathology. Experiments in producing artificial gastric ulcer and genuine induced peptic ulcer. *JAMA* 1906, **46**, 1753–63.

10 Ivy, A.C., Grossman, M.I. & Bachrach, W.H. 1950. *Peptic Ulcer*, 1st edn. The Blakiston Company, Philadelphia, p. 267.

11 Gibelli, C. Contributo critico sperimentale alleziologia dellulcera gastrica in rapporto coi traumi. *Arch. Internat. Chir.* 1908–10, **4**, 127–71.

12 Rosenow, E.C. The production of ulcer of the stomach by injection of streptococci. *JAMA* 1913, **61**, 1947–50.

13 Rosenow, E.C. the causation of gastric and duodenal ulcer by streptococci. *J. Infect. Dis.* 1916, **19**, 333–63.

14 Rosenow, E.C. Etiology of spontaneous ulcer of stomach in domestic animals. *J. Infect. Dis.* 1923, **32**, 384–99.

15 Rosenow, E.C. The specificity of the *Streptococcus* of gastroduodenal ulcer and certain factors determining its localization. *J. Infect. Dis.* 1923, **33**, 248–68.

16 Hardt, L.L.J. Contributions to the physiology of the stomach: XXXIII. The secretion of gastric juice in cases of gastric and duodenal ulcers. *Am. J. Physiol.* 1916, **40**, 314–31.

17 Haden, R.L. The elective localization of bacteria in peptic ulcer. *Arch. Int. Med.* 1925, **35**, 457–71.

18 Nickel, A.C. & Hufford, A.R. Elective localization of streptococci isolated from cases of peptic ulcer. *Arch. Int. Med.* 1928, **41**, 210–30.

19 Saunders, E.W. The serologic and etiologic specificity of the alpha-streptococcus of gastric ulcer. *Arch. Int. Med.* 1930, **45**, 347–82.

20 Celler, H.L. & Thalhimer, W. Experimental studies of the etiology of gastric and duodenal ulcer. *Med. Record* 1916, **90**, 389.

21 Doenges, J.L. Spirochaetes in the gastric glands of *Macacus rhesus* and of man without related disease. *Arch. Pathol.* 1939, **27**, 469–77.

22 Freedberg, A.S. & Barron, L.E. The presence of spirochaetes in human gastric mucosa. *Am. J. Dig. Dis.* 1940, **7**, 443–5.

23 Palmer, E.D. Investigation of the gastric mucosa spirochetes of the human. *Gastroenterology* 1954, **27**, 218–20.

24 Luck, J.M. & Seth, T.N. Gastric urease. *Biochem. J.* 1924, **18**, 1227–31.

25 Lieber, C.S. & Lefevre, A. Ammonia as a source of gastric hypoacidity in patients with uremia. *J. Clin. Invest.* 1959, **38**, 1271–7.

26 Mossberg, S.M., Thayer, W.R. & Spiro, H.M. Azotemia and gastric acidity: the effect of intravenous urea on gastric acid and gastric ammonium production in man. *J. Lab. Clin. Med.* 1963, **61**, 469–75.

27 Delluva, A.M., Markley, K. & Davies, R.E. The absence of gastric urease in germ-free animals. *Biochim. Biophys. Acta* 1968, **151**, 646–50.

28 Langenberg, M.-L., Tytgat, G.N.J., Schipper, M.E.I., Rietra, P.J.G.M. & Zanen, H.C. *Campylobacter*-like organisms in the stomach of patients and healthy individuals. *Lancet*, 1984, **i**, 1348.

29 Steer, H.W. & Colin-Jones, D.G. Mucosal changes in gastric ulceration and their response to carbenoxolone sodium. *Gut* 1975, **16**, 590–7.

30 Steer, H.W. Ultrastructure of cell migration through the gastric epithelium and its relationship to bacteria. *J. Clin. Pathol.* 1975, **28**, 639–46.

31 Fung, W.P., Papadimitriou, J.M. & Matz, L.R. Endoscopic, histological and ultrastructural correlations in chronic gastritis. *Am. J. Gastroenterol.* 1979, **71**, 269–79.

32 Warren, J.R. Unidentified curved bacilli on gastric epithelium in active chronic gastritis. *Lancet* 1983, **i**, 1273.

33 Marshall, B. Unidentified curved bacilli on gastric epithelium in active chronic gastritis. *Lancet* 1983, **i**, 1273–5.

34 Marshall, B.J. & Warren, J.R. Unidentified curved bacilli in the stomach of patients with gastritis and peptic ulceration. *Lancet* 1984, **i**, 1311–15.

35 Marshall, B.J., Royce, H., Annear, D.I., Goodwin, C.S., Pearman, J.W., Warren, J.R. & Armstrong, J.A. Original isolation of *Campylobacter pyloridis* from human gastric mucosa. *Microbios Lett.* 1984, **25**, 83–8.

36 Rollason, T.P., Stone, J. & Rhodes, J.M. Spiral organisms in endoscopic biopsies of the human stomach. *J. Clin. Pathol.* 1984, **37**, 23–6.

37 Steer, H.W. Surface morphology of the gastroduodenal mucosa in duodenal ulceration. *Gut* 1984, **25**, 1203–10.

38 Rathbone, B.J., Wyatt, J.I. & Heatley, R.V. 1988. Bacteria and gastroduodenal inflammation. In Rees, W.D.W. (ed.) *Advances in Peptic Ulcer Pathogenesis*. MTP Press, Lancaster, pp. 101–19.

39 Hudson, M.J. 1989 *Campylobacter pylori*: biochemical characteristics. In Rathbone, B.J. & Heatley, R.V. (eds) *Campylobacter pylori and Gastroduodenal Disease*. Blackwell Scientific Publications, Oxford, ch. 5, pp. 31–38.

40 Goodwin, C.S., Armstrong, J.A., Chilvers, T., Peters, M., Collins, M.D., Sly, L., McConnell, W. & Harper, W.E.S. Transfer of *Campylobacter pylori* and *Campylobacter mustelae* to *Helicobacter* gen. nov. as *Helicobacter pylori* comb. nov., and *Helicobacter mustelae* comb. nov., respectively. *Int. J. Systematic Bacteriol.* 1989, **39**, 397–405.

2 Taxonomy of Helicobacter pylori

R.J.OWEN

The genus *Campylobacter* provided a convenient home for the unidentified gastric spiral bacteria observed and first cultured in 1982 by Warren [1] and Marshall [2] and subsequently named *C. pylori* [3]. However, doubts existed about the correct classification of these bacteria because ultrastructure details pointed to greater affinities to *Spirillum* than to *Campylobacter*. The original difficulty of classifying Marshall and Warren's bacteria is mainly attributable to the fact that *Campylobacter* and other allied genera of Gram-negative spiral bacteria such as *Spirillum* and *Wolinella* are defined on a relatively limited number of positive traditional test characteristics, and their taxonomic affinities are not clearly established. The confusion was largely resolved in 1989, by the proposal of Goodwin and colleagues [4] to transfer *C. pylori* to a new genus with the name *Helicobacter*.

The aim of this chapter is to review the taxonomic development of *C. pylori* with its culmination in the creation of the genus *Helicobacter* comprising six species. The affinities of this new genus to other spirals and *Helicobacter*-like organisms, which colonize the gastric mucosa of a number of animal species and represent a novel and expanding group of bacteria, will be discussed. Only the key taxonomically important characters of *Helicobacter* and *Campylobacter* will be considered as the more traditional characters relevant in clinical microbiology will be dealt with elsewhere.

Development of a classification for gastric spiral campylobacters

Spiral bacteria or 'spirochaetes' have been observed from time to time over the past 100 years or so in gastric specimens of the dog [5] and humans [6–9]. But it was not until Marshall [2] successfully cultured the small curved S-shaped bacilli observed by Warren [1] in the biopsy material from patients with gastritis that any attempt at identification was possible. Warren [1] commented that the bacteria resembled *C. jejuni* by light microscopy but more detailed electron microscopy revealed they were quite different. *Campylobacter* strains characteristically have one polar unsheathed flagellum whereas the gastric isolates have four or five polar sheathed flagella, which according to Marshall [2] suggested affinities to the genus *Spirillum*. Further studies by Marshall & Warren [10] revealed closer similarities to campylobacters as the gastric isolates were microaerophilic and non-saccharolytic and had a deoxyribonucleic acid (DNA) base composition of 36 mol% guanosine plus cytosine (G + C). Skirrow [11] argued that multiple polar flagella were not an exclusive feature of *Spirillum* because some strains of *C. fetus* subsp. *venerealis* had such an arrangement, and he concluded: 'their specific location and association makes the provisional name of "pyloric campylobacter" particularly apt; *pylorus* is Greek for gatekeeper – one who looks both ways. Should these bacteria prove to be campylobacters then *Campylobacter pyloridis* would be an appropriate name.' Marshall & Warren [12] cautiously concluded that their bacilli appeared to be a new species closely resembling the campylobacters although the flagella morphology was not that of the genus *Campylobacter*. They suggested that it was premature to talk of '*C. pyloridis*' and better to use the term 'pyloric campylo-bacter'.

Nevertheless, the name 'Campylobacter pyloridis' was proposed by Marshall et al. [13] and the culture Royal Perth Hospital 13487 (= National Collection of Type Cultures (NCTC) 11637) was designated as the type strain. It should be noted that they described the new species as negative in the ability to hydrolyse urease. However, this reported characteristic was incorrect because the ability to produce an active urease was later shown to be a distinctive diagnostic feature of C. pyloridis [14, 15]. The unusual flagellar arrangement of C. pyloridis was the principal feature that first conflicted with its inclusion in Campylobacter. However, Marshall et al. [13] argued that other multi-flagellate forms of Campylobacter had been observed [16]. Furthermore, there was evidence that a specific antiserum against the Campylo-bacter group antigen fluoresced with C. pyloridis [17]. The new name C. pyloridis was subse-quently validated [18] as required by the Inter-national Code of Nomenclature of Bacteria [19]. However, 2 years later Hartmann & von Graevenitz [20] pointed out that the specific epithet pyloridis was grammatically incorrect and should be pylori (the genitive of the noun pylorus). The species name was subsequently revised to C. pylori by Marshall & Goodwin [3].

Various alternative names or acronyms of C. pylori have appeared in the literature. For example, Owen et al. [15] used the designation GCLO-1 (gastric Campylobacter-like organisms) to distinguish them from a different type of gastric campylobacter (GCLO-2) described by Kasper & Dickgiesse [21] and now identified as a new subspecies of C. jejuni [22]. The name C. pyloridi has also been used [23] although the reason for this variation of the name was not explained.

The results of an ultrastructure study of C. pylori by Jones et al. [24] led them to conclude that the species had greater affinities to Spirillum, in particular Aquaspirillum, than to the genus Campylobacter. However, they observed that there were insufficient data to place these spiral bacteria in their exact taxonomic position and it was suggested that they and other spiral organ-isms noted earlier this century 'might represent a previously unrecognised taxonomic group of organisms'.

Relationships to Campylobacter

The classification of the genus Campylobacter has always been problematic. Member species are relatively inert in most traditional biochemical tests, of which only a small number are suitable for identification and classification purposes. Until recently, the relationships between species within the genus were uncertain and relation-ships to other genera of allied spiral bacteria were highly speculative. Consequently the assignment of a new species to the genus has proved to be a difficult task, particularly if the prospective species had any aberrant charac-teristics.

Development of the genus

Microaerophilic vibrios were first recognized about 80 years ago as a cause of abortion in pregnant ewes [25]. Apparently similar organ-isms were recovered from aborted calves [26] and were subsequently named Vibrio fetus [27]. This classification was generally unsatisfactory as V. fetus differed phenotypically from V. cholerae, the type species of Vibrio. No attempt was made to improve the classification for almost 40 years until Sebald & Véron [28] proposed a new genus, Campylobacter, with C. fetus as the type species. The genus was defined as comprising Gram-negative, slender and curved bacteria which were motile by means of a single, polar flagellum, miroaerophilic with a strictly respir-atory metabolism, produced no acid in media with carbohydrates, and had DNA with G + C contents between 29 and 36 mol%.

The taxonomic concept of the genus was later broadened by Véron & Chatelain [29] who pro-posed that the species described under the names V. coli Doyle, V. jejuni Jones et al., V. sputorum Prevot, and V. bubulus Florent should be transferred to Campylobacter. These workers also suggested that C. fetus, the type of the species, should be divided into two subspecies (subsp. *fetus* and subsp. *venerealis*), and they designated a neotype strain (NCTC 10842) for *C. fetus* subsp. *fetus*.

These studies formed the basis of the genus *Campylobacter* as it is now recognized and provided the official nomenclature used in the Approved Lists of Bacterial Names [30]. There are several excellent reviews of the historical development of the genus [31, 32] and of the significance and features of the present species [32]. Prior to 1980, considerable confusion was caused by the use of a nomenclatural scheme based on the work of Smibert [33] and adopted in the eighth edition of *Bergey's Manual of Determinative Bacteriology*. Smibert [33] speculated, incorrectly as it transpired, that the original strains of *V. fetus* were more likely to have been *V. fetus* var. *venerealis* (Florent). He designated the latter variety as the type species and renamed it *C. fetus* subsp. *fetus*. He also gave the name *C. fetus* subsp. *jejuni* to strains that Véron & Chatelain [29] called *C. jejuni* and *C. coli* respectively.

The definition of *Campylobacter* given subsequently by Smibert [34] was based on the nomenclature of Véron & Chatelain [29] and it is now widely adopted. The genus included species with essentially the same primary characteristics as those in the original description of Sebald & Véron [28] except it also included strains that were motile by means of a flagellum at one or both ends of the cell. The number of species in the genus gradually increased and by 1990 12 names were validly published [32, 34]. Until recently, little was known about the taxonomic diversity or interrelationships between these species or between *Campylobacter* and other bacterial genera. Primary interest has concentrated on species differentiation and strain identification because of the medical importance of *C. jejuni*. However, the use of 16S ribosomal ribonucleic acid (rRNA) sequence analysis to examine the phylogenetic position and structure of the genus has heralded a new era in the taxonomy of *Campylobacter*. The significance of this development and others based on chemical analysis of key cellular macromolecules will be discussed below in relation to *C. pylori* and latterly *H. pylori*.

Relationships between C. pylori and other Campylobacter species

Conventional bacteriological tests. The general morphological and primary characteristics of *C. pylori* conformed with the description of the genus *Campylobacter*. The species comprised curved rod-shaped bacteria that were Gram-negative, motile, microaerophilic, and grew at 37 °C, on conventional culture media with moist chocolate or blood agar as the preferred medium. They exhibited coccoid non-culturable forms and produced catalase and oxidase but were non-saccharolytic. The principal conventional test differences between *C. pylori* and other campylobacters were in flagella arrangement and cell morphology. Strains also differed from the description of *Campylobacter* [34] as they hydrolysed urea and did not reduce nitrate. However, these latter tests are not exclusive for *C. pylori* as proved members of *C. jejuni* and *C. lari* exhibit such features [22, 35].

Ultrastructure. *C. pylori* possesses four to six unipolar, sheathed flagella whereas other campylobacters have a single polar unsheathed flagellum at one or both ends of the cell [12, 24, 36]. These detailed ultrastructure studies on *C. pylori* also revealed a number of other unique features: (i) the ends of the bacteria do not taper; (ii) there is no terminal concavity at the location of the flagella; (iii) cells possess flagella discs without radial structures; (iv) terminal structures internal to the plasma membrane are present; (v) the cell wall is smooth; and (vi) flagella sheaths are in continuity with the unit membrane of the cell wall.

Fatty acid content. The cellular fatty acid (FA) contents of bacteria are very useful taxonomic markers as they are reproducible and relatively unaffected by the growth conditions or medium [37]. Species of *Campylobacter* have been thoroughly investigated by the analysis of FA-methyl esters (FAME) and FA-picolinyl esters

characteristics which provide the basis for concluding that *C. pylori* is not a *Campylobacter sensu stricto*. The 16S rRNA homology data show without question that *C. pylori* is the most divergent of all the species of *Campylobacter* and is sufficiently distinct to warrant exclusion from the genus. Other proven chemotaxonomic generic markers such as cellular FA profiles and MK contents provide further evidence that *C. pylori* is not a *Campylobacter*. These features correlate with the unusual ultrastructure (cell and flagella morphology) of the species, which provides more readily observable features for identification purposes. The value of total protein patterns as generic markers for *Campylobacter* are unclear as there is considerable variation between species and there are no particular bands which are consistently different. However, the protein profile of *C. pylori* is quite distinct from those of all other *Campylobacter* species. The differences at the species level are also reflected in low DNA–DNA sequence homologies between *C. pylori* and other species. Another feature of *C. pylori*, which possibly reflects basic structural and physiological differences from other species of *Campylobacter* and *Wolinella*, is its marked susceptibility to damage during the freeze-drying process [64].

Taxonomic relationships between C. pylori and Wolinella

The various 16S rRNA phylogenetic analyses published between 1987 and 1990 showed that *C. pylori* had the closest affinities to *Wolinella succinogenes*, which is the type species of the genus *Wolinella*, but the two other species in the genus, *Wolinella recta* and *W. curva*, were clustered with *Campylobacter sensu stricto*. This was a surprising discovery because the genus *Wolinella*, the name proposed for a group of curved motile bacteria from the bovine rumen and human buccal cavity, was clearly distinguished from *Campylobacter* in having G + C contents of 42–48 mol% and in growing anaerobically [65, 66].

Similarities to W. succinogenes

Conventional test characters. *W. succinogenes* like *C. pylori* is a Gram-negative, curved, rod-shaped bacterium. It is rapidly motile, grows optimally on blood-containing media and is non-saccharolytic. Table 2.2 lists differences in key taxonomic features. Tanner & Socransky [65] described *Wolinella* as anaerobic but noted that strains would grow on the surface of blood agar plates in an atmosphere including 5% oxygen when a heavy cell suspension was used. Another metabolic feature of *W. succinogenes* was an ability to grow in broth stimulated by a combination of formate and fumarate. Thus, Thompson *et al.* [54] argued that the species was not an anaerobe but an H_2-requiring micro-aerophile.

Chemotaxonomic characters. *W. succinogenes* has a DNA base composition of 47 mol% G + C, which is significantly different from the 36–37% G + C value of *C. pylori*. A difference of 10% indicates a significant amount of genomic diversity. The G + C differences were also reflected in marked differences between the two species in their major and minor FA, which led Hudson *et al.* [41] to conclude that *C. pylori* did not have a close affinity to *W. succinogenes*. Both species contained MK-6 as the main respiratory quinone but *W. succinogenes* also contained TPQ-6 [67]. The 16S rRNA homology data available before 1990 do not, however, provide a clear-cut answer to the relationships between *C. pylori* and *W. succinogenes*. Although Thompson *et al.* [54] proposed that the two species should be included in the genus *Wolinella* with *C. fennelliae* and *C. cinaedi*, the results obtained in the other analyses [51–53] were less conclusive. The details of these analyses were summarized previously [68]. Romaniuk *et al.* [51] suggested that, even though *C. pylori* was more closely related to *W. succinogenes* than to other campylobacters in the RNA dendrogram, the differences between the two species were probably sufficient to warrant separate genera. Likewise, Lau *et al.* [53] suggested on a more limited set of sequences that *C. pylori* should be assigned to a new genus, whereas Paster & Dewhirst [52] concluded that the taxonomic relationships between the two species needed further examination. Even though precise classification may depend on the computation methods used and on subjective interpretation of the phylogenetic dendrograms, the four groups of workers agreed remarkably well in the levels of sequence homology calculated between *C. pylori* and *W. succinogenes* and between *C. fetus*, *C. pylori* and *C. jejuni*.

Phylogenetic position of C. pylori and Wolinella

About 10 major taxonomic groups have been recognized within the eubacteria by analysis of 16S rRNA sequence data [49]. It is not clear, however, from the above phylogenetic studies on *C. pylori* and other campylobacters and wolinellas where they belong exactly among the eubacteria although it has been established that they belong on the same phylogenetic branch [51, 52, 54]. The campylobacters and wolinellas are apparently only distantly related to representatives of the alpha, beta and gamma branches of the purple photosynthetic bacteria now named the Proteobacteria [69] and do not belong to any previously defined branch of that class. Studies of 5S rRNA sequences and semiconserved secondary structural features (signature sequences), which also reflect phylogenetic history, have failed to clarify the position of these bacteria [53] but it is likely they may eventually be accommodated in an expanded version of the Proteobacteria.

An interesting but unexpected result of these rRNA sequence analyses was that *C. pylori* and *Wolinella succinogenes* were found to be as closely related to the genus *Thiovulum* as they were to *Campylobacter* [51, 52]. Little is known about *Thiovulum*, however, except that it is a sulphide-dependent marine bacterium. Although it was initially suggested that *C. pylori* might have affinities to *Spirillum* and *Aquaspirillum* [2, 24], there are no chemotaxonomic data supporting such relationships. Likewise the relationships of *C. pylori* and *Wolinella succinogenes* to other genera of aerobic/microaerophilic/anaerobic motile, helical, Gram-negative bacteria, which include genera such as *Oceanospirillum*, *Azospirillum* and *Anaerobiospirillum*, remain uncertain and require further phylogenetic studies.

C. pylori becomes Helicobacter pylori

In 1989, Goodwin and colleagues [4] proposed the establishment of a new genus called *Helicobacter* and that *C. pylori* should be transferred to that genus as *H. pylori*. The name *Helicobacter* refers to the morphology of the organisms, which are helical *in vivo* but often rod-like *in vitro*. The creation of a new genus was argued on the basis of: (i) the low degree of relatedness between *H. pylori* and any previously described genus except the genus *Wolinella* as represented by *W. succinogenes*; and (ii) the possession of a set of chemotaxonomic properties – namely ultrastructure and morphology, cellular FA, MK, growth characteristics and enzyme capabilities – different from those of the genus *Wolinella* and neighbouring taxa.

Intraspecific variation of H. pylori

H. pylori is a remarkably homogeneous species in traditional test characteristics but strain differences have been observed in cytotoxin production and motility [70], and in preformed enzyme activity [71], which has been suggested as the basis of a biotyping scheme. However, the scope of biotyping within *H. pylori* is limited as strains isolated worldwide from human gastric mucosa exhibit few differences. Some negative variants have been reported in catalase and urease production [72] but *H. pylori* isolated from various animal sources to date appears to be identical to the human isolates. However, there is evidence of considerable strain variation at the molecular level in plasmid profiles [23, 73], in chromosomal DNA restriction digest patterns [72–74], in ribopatterns [74], and in 1D-electrophoretic protein profiles [63]. Various strains of *H. pylori* are deposited in international culture collections and Table 2.3 lists some examples from different animal hosts that are available for reference purposes.

Table 2.3 Species and reference strains of *Helicobacter* and phylogenetically related organisms.

Species	Strain[a]	Host
Helicobacter pylori	NCTC 11637[T]; ATCC 43504	Human, gastric mucosa
	NCTC 11961	Pig, gastric mucosa
	NCTC 12199 (= 82008)	Rhesus monkey, gastric mucosa
Helicobacter mustelae	NCTC 12198[T]; ATCC 43772	Ferret, gastric mucosa
Helicobacter felis	NCTC 12432[T]; ATCC 49179 (= CS1)	Cat, gastric mucosa
Helicobacter nemestrinae	ATCC 49396[T]	Pigtailed macaque, gastric mucosa
Helicobacter (Campylobacter) cinaedi	NCTC 12423[T]; ATCC 35683	Human, rectal swab
Helicobacter (Campylobacter) fennelliae	NCTC 11612[T]; ATCC 35684	Human, rectal swab
Wolinella succinogenes	NCTC 11488[T]; ATCC 29543	Cow, rumen
'Flexispira rappini'	ATCC 49308	Dog, faeces
'Gastrospirillum hominis'	(Non-culturable)	Human, gastric mucosa

[a] Abbreviations used: T, type strain: NCTC, National Collection of Type Cultures, London; ATCC, American Type Culture Collection, Rockville, Md.

Relationships to other gastric spiral bacteria

The discovery of *H. pylori* has lead to a widening interest in the microbiology of other spiral bacteria, particularly the GCLO in the antrum of man and of laboratory and zoo animals. Helical bacteria have been observed to date in the stomachs of man, cats including captive cheetahs, dogs, ferrets, pig, baboons and monkeys (Table 2.3). Further discussion and more detailed descriptions of these spiral organisms, which colonize the mucus layer of the gastric epithelium and have often proved difficult to culture *in vitro*, may be found elsewhere [75, 76]. A feature common to gastric spirals is their rapid production of ureases, and the taxonomy of the best characterized is considered here in relation to *H. pylori*.

H. pylori from animal sources

Baboon and pig gastric organisms. Spiral organisms have been isolated in the UK from the gastric mucosa of baboon and pig stomachs [77, 78] and their similarities to *C. pylori* were confirmed in conventional tests and 1D SDS-PAGE protein patterns [79]. The FAME profile of the baboon strain, however, apparently resembled those of the *C. jejuni* group and the ferret GCLO [41]. Numerical analysis of 1D SDS-PAGE protein patterns of the pig strain also revealed it had close similarities to *C. pylori* [80], and so these strains can be considered to belong to *H. pylori*.

Monkey gastric organisms. In a study of experimental and natural *C. pylori* infections in the rhesus monkey, Newell & Baskerville [81] isolated *Campylobacter*-like organisms (CLO) from the gastric epithelium of 4/7 monkeys. These bacteria were identical to *C. pylori* in urease activity, in flagella and cell morphology [78], in 1D SDS-PAGE protein profiles [80] and in FA content [41], as well as in their immunological characteristics. Apparently similar bacteria were also observed in the gastric mucosa of rhesus monkeys in the USA [80]. Under present nomenclature these organisms can be classified as *H. pylori*.

Cheetah gastric organisms. Epizootic gastritis in

captive cheetahs was recently described in the USA [82] and two kinds of bacteria were identified in the stomachs of infected animals. One type resembled 'Gastrospirillum' (see below) whereas the second type was a short Gram-negative motile spiral bacterium which was urease-, catalase- and oxidase-producing. Ultra-structure examination and SDS-PAGE of bacterial proteins suggested that this organism was closely related to *H. pylori*.

Helicobacter mustelae

Organisms resembling *H. pylori* have been isolated from normal and inflamed gastric mucosa of ferrets in the USA [83] and UK [84]. These bacteria were unlike human *H. pylori* as they were able to reduce nitrate, produced little or no leucine arylamidase, were susceptible to nalidixic acid and were resistant to cephalothin [77, 85]. The human and ferret strains also differed in SDS-PAGE electrophoretic protein patterns [79, 85], in isoelectric points of ureases [79, 85] and in cellular FA content, notably in the relative amounts of $14:0$ and $16:0$ acids [41, 85]. The DNA–DNA hybridizations of Fox *et al.* [58] showed that the ferret and human strains were 72% related at the optimum reassociation temperature but only 55% related at the stringent temperature. Subsequently, the name *C. pylori* subsp. *mustelae* was adopted for those strains [86]. Phylogenetic studies based on 16S rRNA sequences confirmed that the ferret organisms were members of the *W. succinogenes–C. pylori* cluster [52].

Further studies by Fox *et al.* [87] revealed an error in the original DNA–DNA hybridization data and it was confirmed that strains isolated from ferrets in the USA, UK and Australia were members of a single species substantially different from *C. pylori*. The precise level of DNA relatedness, however, differed according to the method and reassociation conditions used. The ferret strains were therefore elevated from *C. pylori* subsp. *mustelae* to species status as *Campylobacter mustelae* [87]. Subsequently, the species was renamed *Helicobacter mustelae* [4].

Helicobacter felis

In 1988, Lee *et al.* [88] described the isolation of a microaerobic spiral or helix-shaped bacterium that colonized the stomach of a cat (cat spiral 1 (CS1)). The organism was tightly coiled with tufts of 10–17 sheathed flagella positioned slightly off-centre at the end of the cell. The body of the cell was entwined with unique periplasmic fibrils that usually occurred in pairs. The organism was strongly urease-, catalase- and oxidase-positive. Recent phylogenetic analyses using 16S rRNA sequences revealed the CS organism to be closely related to *Helicobacter* and it has been proposed that it should be classified in a new species named *H. felis* [89]. Additional strains were isolated from the gastric mucosa of cats and dogs; the health status of these animals was not known. This new species differed from *H. pylori* in a number of characteristics, including ultrastructure, nitrate reduction, growth at $42\,°C$ and mol% G + C content.

Helicobacter nemestrinae

In 1991, Bronsdon [90] proposed the name *H. nemestrinae* for a spirally curved bacterium isolated from the gastric mucosa of a pigtailed macaque (*Macaca nemestrina*). It resembled *H. pylori* in conventional bacteriological features except that its colourless colonies were flat and had irregular edges. The new species exhibited less than 10% DNA–DNA homology to previously described *Helicobacter* species, its G + C content was distinctive (24 mol%), and it had a unique cellular FA composition. The new species was based on a single isolate recovered from a gastric biopsy of a 6-year-old healthy animal.

Helicobacter cinaedi and H. fennelliae

Phylogenetic studies based on 16S rRNA sequences first revealed that *C. cinaedi* and *C. fennelliae* were related to *H. pylori* [54] and this was confirmed in recent studies using DNA–23S rRNA hybridization and immunotyping analysis [91], and numerical analysis of electrophoretic protein patterns [92]. Vandamme *et al.* [91]

believed the genotypic and phenotypic similarities of the species outweighed their differences and justified inclusion in an emended genus *Helicobacter* (see below). Strains of the species were isolated from blood, faeces and rectal swabs of humans with gastrointestinal symptoms.

'Flexispira rappini'

Bryner [93] proposed the name '*Flexispira rappini*' for a group of microaerophilic, Gram-negative, motile, urease-producing bacteria first isolated from aborted ovine fetuses and subsequently from the gastrointestinal mucosa of man and lower mammals (dog, pig and sheep). Members of the species had a G + C content of 43 mol% and possessed seven sheathed polar flagella. They were distinguished from *C. pylori* by the unique coilin fibres found in the periplasmic space, by the flexibility of the cell wall and by the ability to grow at 43 °C. The phylogenetic position of this new taxonomic group was not established but recent phylogenetic studies based on 16S rRNA sequences suggest '*F. rappini*' should be included in the same phylogeny group as the genus *Helicobacter* although its exact position is unclear [89]. However, in a recent DNA–rRNA hybridization analysis, Vandamme *et al.* [91] included '*Flexispira*' in the rRNA cluster III, which also contained *Helicobacter*, *Wolinella* and strain CLO-3 of Fennell *et al.* [94]. Relatedness of '*F. rappini*' to *H. pylori* was also shown by numerical analysis of electrophoretic protein profiles [92].

'Gastrospirillum hominis'

In 1989, NcNulty *et al.* [95] described a new Gram-negative spiral bacterium associated with chronic gastritis, which they provisionally named '*Gastrospirillum hominis*'. The organism has not been cultured but microscopy revealed it was helical (tightly spiralled), 3.5–7.5 μm long and 0.9 μm in diameter with truncated ends flattened at the tips and up to 12 sheathed flagella, 28 nm in diameter, at each pole. It was not thought to be a spirochaete as it had no axial filament. McNulty *et al.* [95] described this organism as 'probably producing urease'. The uncertainty about urease activity was due to the presence of other organisms or low numbers of cells of '*G. hominis*' in tissue samples tested. In a serological study, they found that serum from three patients with spiral bacteria reacted with the antigen prepared from the CS organism of Lee *et al.* [88] (*H. felis*), suggesting an antigenic relatedness. Even though the organism was not cultured by McNulty *et al.* [95] or by other investigators [96] who observed it in human gastric mucosa, rule 18 of the *International Code of Nomenclature of Bacteria* [19] permits classification based on electron microscopy. Its true phylogenetic position, however, remains unclear.

Comments and conclusions

Phylogenetic analyses based on 16S and 23S rRNA sequences and various other forms of chemotaxonomic data as well as ultrastructural features provide incontrovertible evidence that *C. pylori* is not a 'true' member of *Campylobacter* or of *Wolinella*. Such data formed the basis for reclassification of *C. pylori* in a new genus, *Helicobacter* – a decision which has been generally accepted as a rational solution to the taxonomic uncertainties of the past 7 years. Although *H. pylori* and *W. succinogenes*, which are both type species of their respective genera, belong in the same phylogenetic rRNA homology group (see rRNA group II, Table 2.1), they are clearly morphologically, metabolically and genetically distinct organisms and warrant retention in separate genera. The recent molecular studies [89, 91] show that the gastric spiral organism '*F. rappini*' is also a member of this phylogeny group, which now comprises several associated taxa of spiral micro-organisms. The concept of *Helicobacter* expanded with the inclusion of *H. pylori* strains from a wider host range and the recognition of new species, which now include *H. mustelae*, *H. felis*, *H. fennelliae*, *H. cinaedi* and *H. nemestrinae*. The most important consequence of the recent taxonomic developments is the proposal [91] to emend the description of the genus *Helicobacter* originally given by Goodwin *et al.* [4]. The new description, for instance, includes strains that have a single polar flagellum and reduce nitrate but do not hydrolyse urea. Furthermore, the inclusion of *H. nemestrinae* necessitates widening the DNA base composition range for the genus to include low G + C content values of 24 mol%. More detailed descriptions of these new species and bacteriological test characteristics for their identification can be obtained elsewhere [89, 90, 91]. The merits of these latest proposals need to be critically assessed but worldwide interest in gastric spiral bacteria will undoubtedly provide the basis for continuing taxonomic research in this area.

References

1 Warren, J.R. Unidentified curved bacilli on gastric epithelium in active chronic gastritis. *Lancet* 1983, i, 1273.

2 Marshall, B. Unidentified curved bacilli on gastric epithelium in active chronic gastritis. *Lancet* 1983, i, 1273–5.

3 Marshall, B.J. & Goodwin, C.S. Revised nomenclature of *Campylobacter pyloridis*. *Int. J. Systematic Bacteriol.* 1987, **37**, 68.

4 Goodwin, C.S., Armstrong, J.A., Chilvers, T., Peters, M., Collins, M.D., Sly, L., McConnell, W. & Harper, W.E.S. Transfer of *Campylobacter pylori* and *Campylobacter mustelae* to *Helicobacter* gen. nov. and *Helicobacter pylori* comb. nov., as *Helicobacter mustelae* comb. nov., respectively. *Int. J. Systematic Bacteriol.* 1989, **39**, 397–405.

5 Bizzozero, G. Über die Schlauchformigen drüsen des Magendarmkanals und die Beziehungen ihres Epithels zu dem Obserflächenepithel der Schleimahut. *Arch. Mikrobiol. Anat.* 1893, **42**, 82–94.

6 Krienitz, W. Über das Auftreten von Spirochäten verschiedener Form im Mageninhalt bei Carcinoma ventriculi. *Dtsch. Med. Wochenschr.* 1906, **28**, 872–90.

7 Doenges, J.L. Spirochaetes in the gastric glands of *Macacus rhesus* and humans without definite history of related disease. *Arch. Pathol.* 1938, **27**, 469–77.

8 Freedburgh, A.S. & Barron, L.E. The presence of spirochaetes in human gastric mucosa. *Am. J. Dig. Dis.* 1947, **7**, 443–5.

9 Steer, H.W. & Colin-Jones, D.G. Mucosal changes in gastric ulceration and their response to carbenoxolone sodium. *Gut* 1975, **16**, 590–7.

10 Marshall, B.M. & Warren, J.R. 1983. Spiral bacteria in the human stomach: a common finding in patients with gastritis and duodenal ulcer. In Pearson, A.D., Skirrow, M.B., Row, B., Davies, J. & Jones, D.M. (eds) *Campylobacter II. Proceedings of the Second International Workshop on Campylobacter Infections.* Public Health Laboratory Service, London, pp. 11–12.

11 Skirrow, M., 1983. Report on the session: taxonomy and biotyping. In Pearson, D.A., Skirrow, M.B., Rowe, B., Davies, J. & Jones, D.M. (eds) *Campylobacter II. Proceedings of the Second International Workshop on Campylobacter Infections.* Public Health Laboratory Service, London, pp. 33–8.

12 Marshall, B.J. & Warren, J.R. Unidentified curved bacilli in the stomach of patients with gastritis and peptic ulceration. *Lancet* 1984, i, 1311–14.

13 Marshall, B.J., Joyce, H., Anwar, D.I., Goodwin, C.S., Pearmans, J.W., Warren, J.R. & Armstrong, J.A. Original isolation of *Campylobacter pyloridis* from human gastric mucosa. *Microbios Lett.* 1984, **25**, 83–8.

14 Langenberg, M.L., Tytgat, G.N.J., Schipper, M.E.I., Rietra, P.J.G.M. & Zanen, H.C. *Campylobacter*-like organisms in the stomachs of patients and healthy individuals. *Lancet* 1984, i, 1348.

15 Owen, R.J., Martin, S.R. & Borman, P. Rapid urea hydrolysis by gastric campylobacters. *Lancet* 1985, i, 111.

16 Ritchie, A.E., Keller, R.F. & Bryner, J.H. Anatomical features of *Vibrio fetus*: electron microscopic survey. *J. Gen. Microbiol.* 1966, **43**, 427–38.

17 Price, A.B., Dolby, J.M., Dunscombe, P.R. & Stirling, Detection of *Campylobacter* by immunofluorescence in stools and rectal biopsies of patients with diarrhoea. *J. Clin. Pathol.* 1984, **37**, 1007–13.

18 International Union of Microbiological Societies. Validation of the publication of new names and new combinations previously effectively published outside the IJSB. List no. 17. *Int. J. Systematic Bacteriol.* 1985, **35**, 223–5.

19 Lapage, S.P., Sneath, P.H.A., Lessel, E.F., Skerman, V.B.D., Seeliger, H.P.R. & Clark, W.A. (eds) 1975. *International Code of Nomenclature of Bacteria. 1976 Revision.* American Society for Microbiology, Washington, DC.

20 Hartmann, D. & von Graevenitz, A. A note on name, viability and urease tests of *Campylobacter pylori*. *Eur. J. Clin. Microbiol.* 1987, **6**, 82–3.

21 Kasper, G. & Dickgiesser, N. Isolation from gastric epithelium of *Campylobacter*-like bacteria that are distinct from '*Campylobacter pyloridis*'. *Lancet* 1985, i, 111–12.

22 Steele, T.W. & Owen, R.J. *Campylobacter jejuni* subsp. *doylei* subsp. nov., a subspecies of nitrate-negative campylobacters isolated from human clinical specimens. *Int. J. Systematic Bacteriol.* 1988, **38**, 316–18.

23 Tjia, T.N., Hooper, W.E.S., Goodwin, C.S. & Grubb, W.B. Plasmids in *Campylobacter pyloridi*. *Microbios Lett.* 1987, **36**, 7–11.

24 Jones, D.N., Curry, A. & Fox, A.J. An ultrastructure study of the gastric *Campylobacter*-like organism

'Campylobacter pyloridis'. J. Gen. Microbiol. 1985, 131, 2335–41.

25 McFadyean, J. & Stockman, S. 1913. Great Britain Board of Agriculture and Fisheries, Dept. Comm. Epiz. Abortion, London, p. 22 and Appendix, part III.

26 Smith, T. Spirilla associated with disease of the fetal membranes in cattle (injections abortion). J. Exp. Med. 1918, 28, 701–19.

27 Smith, T. & Taylor, M.S. Some morphological and biological characters of the spirilla (Vibrio fetus n. sp.) associated with disease of the fetal membranes of cattle. J. Exp. Med. 1919, 30, 299–311.

28 Sebald, M. & Véron, M. Teneur en bases de l'ADN et classification des vibrions. Ann. Inst. Pasteur 1963, 105, 897–910.

29 Véron, M. & Chatelain, R. Taxonomic study of the genus Campylobacter Sebald and Véron and designation of the neotype strain for the type species Campylobacter fetus (Smith and Taylor) Sebald and Véron. Int. J. Systematic Bacteriol. 1973, 23, 122–34.

30 Skerman, V.B.D., McGowan, V. & Sneath, P.H.A. (eds). Approved Lists of Bacterial Names. Int. J. Systematic Bacteriol. 1980, 30, 225–420.

31 Karmali, M.A. & Skirrow, M.B. 1984. Taxonomy of the genus Campylobacter. In Butzler, J.P. (ed). Campylobacter infection in man and animals. CRC Press, Inc., Boca Raton, pp. 1–20.

32 Penner, J.L. The genus Campylobacter: a decade of progress. Clin. Microbiol. Rev. 1988, 1, 157–72.

33 Smibert, R.M. 1974. Genus Campylobacter. In Buchanan, R.E. & Gibbons, N.E. (eds) Bergey's Manual of Determinative Bacteriology, 8th edn. Williams & Wilkins, Baltimore, pp. 207–12.

34 Smibert, R.M. 1984. Genus Campylobacter. In Krieg, N.R. & Holt, H.G. (eds) Bergey's Manual of Systematic Bacteriology, vol. I. Williams & Wilkins, Baltimore, pp. 111–18.

35 Owen, R.J., Costas, M., Sloss, L. & Bolton, F.J. Numerical analysis of electrophoretic protein patterns of Campylobacter laridis and allied thermophilic campylobacters from the natural environment. J. Appl. Bacteriol. 1988, 65, 69–78.

36 Goodwin, C.S., McCulloch, R.K., Armstrong, J.A. & Wee, S.H. Unusual cellular fatty acids, and distinctive ultrastructure in a new spiral bacterium (Campylobacter pyloridis). J. Med. Microbiol. 1985, 19, 257–67.

37 Jantzen, E. & Bryn, K. 1985. Whole cell and lipopolysaccharide fatty acids and sugars of Gram-negative bacteria. In Goodfellow, M. & Minnikin, D.E. (eds) Chemical Methods in Bacterial Systematics. Academic Press, London, pp. 145–71.

38 Leaper, S. & Owen, R.J. Identification of catalase producing Campylobacter species based on biochemical characteristics and on cellular fatty acid composition. Curr. Microbiol. 1981, 31, 31–5.

39 Wait, R. & Hudson, M.J. The use of picolinyl esters for the characterization of microbial lipids: application to

40 Lambert, M.A., Patton, C.M., Barret, T.J. & Moss, C.W. Differentiation of Campylobacter and Campylobacter-like organisms by cellular fatty acid composition. J. Clin. Microbiol. 1987, 25, 706–13.

41 Hudson, M.J., Bhavsor, P. & Wait, R. 1988. Chemotaxonomy of campylobacters. In Kaijser, B. & Falsen, E. (eds) Campylobacter IV. Goterna, Kungälv, pp. 34–5.

42 Goodwin, G.S., Blincow, E., Armstrong, J., McCulloch, R.K. & Collins, D. Campylobacter pyloridis is unique: GCLO-2 is an ordinary campylobacter. Lancet 1985, i, 38–9.

43 Itoh, T., Yassagawa, Y., Shingaki, M., Takohashi, M., Kai, A., Ohashi, M. & Hamana, G. Isolation of Campylobacter pyloridis from human gastric mucosa and characterisation of the isolates. Microbiol. Immunol. 1987, 31, 603–14.

44 Bartolomé, R., Balado, C., Crespo, E., Fernandez, F. & Abelló, A. A survey of cellular fatty acids composition of Helicobacter pylori. Rev. Esp. Enf. Dig. 1990, 78, Suppl. I, 40–1.

45 Collins, M.D. & Jones, D. Distribution of isoprenoid quinone structural types in bacteria and their taxonomic implications. Microbiol. Rev. 1981, 45, 314–54.

46 Collins, M.D., Costas, M. & Owen, R.J. Isoprenoid quinone composition of representatives of the genus Campylobacter. Arch. Microbiol. 1984, 137, 168–70.

47 Carlone, G.M. & Anet, F.A.L. Detection of menaquinone-6 and a novel methyl substituted menaquinone-6 in Campylobacter jejuni and Campylobacter fetus subsp. fetus. J. Gen. Microbiol. 1983, 129, 3385–93.

48 Moss, C.W., Kai, A., Lambert, M.A. & Patton, C. Isoprenoid quinone content and cellular fatty acid composition of Campylobacter species. J. Clin. Microbiol. 1984, 19, 772–6.

49 Woese, C.R. Bacterial evolution. Microbiol. Rev. 1987, 51, 221–7.

50 Lane, D.J., Pace, B., Olsen, G.J., Stahl, D.A., Sogin, M.L. & Pace, N.R. Rapid determination of 16S ribosomal RNA sequences for phylogenetic analysis. Proc. Nat. Acad. Sci. USA 1985, 82, 6955–9.

51 Romaniuk, P.J., Zoltouska, B., Trust, T.J., Lane, D.J., Olsen, G.J., Pace, N.R & Stahl, D.A. Campylobacter pylori, a spiral bacterium associated with human gastritis, is not a true Campylobacter sp. J. Bacteriol. 1987, 169, 2137–41.

52 Paster, B.J. & Dewhirst, F.E. Phylogeny of campylobacters, wolinellas, Bacteroides gracilis, and Bacteroides ureolyticus by 16S ribosomal ribonucleic acid sequencing. Int. J. Systematic Bacteriol. 1988, 38, 56–62.

53 Lau, P.P., DeBrunner-Vossbrinck, B., Dunn, B., Miotto, K., MacDonell, M.T., Rollins, D.M., Pilledge, C.J., Hespell, R.B., Colwell, R.R., Segin, M.L. & Fox,

G.E. Phylogenetic diversity and position of the genus *Campylobacter*. *Systematic Appl. Microbiol.* 1987, **9**, 231–8.

54 Thompson, L.M. III, Smibert, R.M., Johnson, J.L. & Krieg, N.R. Phylogenetic study of the genus *Campylobacter*. *Int. J. Systematic Bacteriol.* 1988, **38**, 190–200.

55 Vandamme, P. & DeLey, J. 1988. Phylogenetic relationships in and of the genus *Campylobacter*. In Kaijser, B. & Falsen, E. (eds) *Campylobacter IV*. Goterna, Kungälv, pp. 47–8.

56 Owen, R.J. & Pitcher, D. 1985. Current methods for estimating DNA base composition and levels of DNA–DNA hybridization. In Goodfellow, M. & Minnikin, D.E. (eds) *Chemical Methods in Bacterial Systematics*. Academic Press, London, pp. 67–93.

57 Von Wulffen, H. Low degree of relatedness between *Campylobacter pyloridis* and enteropathogenic *Campylobacter* species as revealed by DNA–DNA blot hybridization and immunoblot studies. *FEMS Microbiol. Lett.* 1987, **42**, 129–33.

58 Fox, J.G., Edwards, P., Taylor, N.S., Paster, B. & Dewhirst, F. 1988. Comparison of the phylogenetic, biochemical, phenotypic, and morphological characteristics of gastric campylobacters from humans and ferrets. In Kaijser, B. & Falsen, E. (eds) *Campylobacter IV*. Goterna, Kungälv, pp. 50–4.

59 Bukholm, G., Nedenskov-Sorensen, P. & Bovre, K. DNA–DNA hybridization incompatibility of *Campylobacter pylori* with other *Campylobacter* and *Wolinella* species. *APMIS* 1989, **97**, 472–4.

60 Pearson, A.D., Bamforth, J., Booth, L., Holdstock, G., Ireland, A., Walker, C., Hawtin, P. & Millward-Sadler, H. Polyacrylamide gel electrophoresis of spiral bacteria from the gastric antrum. *Lancet* 1984, **i**, 1349–50.

61 Mégraud, F., Bonnet, F., Garnier, M. & Lamouliatte, H. Characterisation of 'Campylobacter pyloridis' by culture, enzymatic profile, and protein content. *J. Clin. Microbiol.* 1985, **22**, 1007–10.

62 Costas, M., Owen, R.J. & Jackman, P.J. Classification of *Campylobacter sputorum* and allied campylobacters based on numerical analysis of electrophoretic protein patterns. *Systematic Appl. Microbiol.* 1987, **9**, 125–31.

63 Owen, R.J., Costas, M., Morgan, D.D., On, S.L.W., Hill, L.R., Pearson, A.D. & Morgan, D.R. Strain variation in *Campylobacter pylori* detected by numerical analysis of one-dimensional electrophoretic protein patterns. *Antonie van Leeuwenhoek J. Microbiol.* 1989, **55**, 253–67.

64 Owen, R.J., On, S.L.W. & Costas, M. The effect of cooling rate, freeze-drying suspending fluid and culture age on the preservation of *Campylobacter pylori*. *J. Appl. Bacteriol.* 1989, **66**, 331–7.

65 Tanner, A.C.R. & Socransky, S.S. 1984. Genus *Wolinella*. In Krieg, N.R. & Holt, J.G. (eds) *Bergey's Manual of Systematic Bacteriology*, vol. I. Williams & Wilkins, Baltimore, pp. 646–50.

66 Tanner, A.C.R., Badger, S., Lai, C.-H., Listgarten, M.A., Visconti, R.A. & Socransky, S.S. *Wolinella* gen. nov., *Wolinella succinogenes* (*Vibrio succinogenes* Wolin *et al.*) comb. nov., and descriptions of *Bacteroides gracilis* sp. nov., *Wolinella recta* sp. nov., and *Eikenella corrodens* all from humans with periodontal disease. *Int. J. Systematic Bacteriol.* 1981, **31**, 432–45.

67 Collins, M.D. & Fernendez, F. Menaquinone-6 and thermoplasmaquinone-6 in *Wolinella succinogenes*. *FEMS Microbiol. Lett.* 1984, **22**, 273–6.

68 Owen, R.J. 1989. Taxonomy of *Campylobacter pylori*. In Rathbone, B.J. & Heatley, R.V. (eds) *Campylobacter pylori and Duodenal Disease*. Blackwell Scientific Publications, Oxford, pp. 12–23.

69 Stackebrandt, E., Murray, R.G.E. & Trüper, H.G. Proteobacteria classis nov., a name for the phylogenetic taxon that includes the 'purple bacteria and their relatives'. *Int. J. Systematic Bacteriol.* 1988, **38**, 321–5.

70 Owen, R.J., Bickley, J., Moreno, M., Costas, M. & Morgan, D.R. Biotypic and genotypic variation of *Helicobacter pylori* and association with cytotoxin production. *Rev. Esp. Enf. Dig.* 1990, **78**, Suppl. 1, 19.

71 Owen, R.J. & Desai, M. Preformed enzyme profiling of *Helicobacter pylori* and *Helicobacter mustelae* from human and animal sources. *Lett. Appl. Microbiol.* 1990, **11**, 103–5.

72 Majewski, S.I.H. & Goodwin, C.S. Restriction endonuclease analysis of the genome of *Campylobacter pylori* with a rapid extraction method: evidence for considerable genomic variation. *J. Infect. Dis.* 1988, **157**, 465–71.

73 Langenberg, W., Rauws, E.A.J., Widjojokusomo, A., Tytgat, G.N.J. & Zanen, H.C. Identification of *Campylobacter pyloridis* isolates by restriction endonuclease DNA analysis. *J. Clin. Microbiol.* 1986, **24**, 414–17.

74 Morgan, D.D. & Owen, R.J. Use of restriction endonuclease digest and ribosomal RNA gene probe patterns to fingerprint *Helicobacter pylori* and *Helicobacter mustelae* isolated from human and animal hosts. *Molec. Cell. Probes* 1990, **4**, 321–34.

75 Fox, J.G. & Lee, A. Gastric *Campylobacter*-like organisms: their role in gastric disease of laboratory animals. *Lab. Anim. Sci.* 1989, **39**, 543–53.

76 Lee, A., Eckstein, R.P., Fevre, D.I., Dick, E. & Kellow, J.E. Non *Campylobacter pylori* spiral organisms in the gastric antrum. *Aust. NZ J. Med.* 1989, **19**, 156–8.

77 Jones, D.M. & Eldridge, J. 1988. Gastric *Campylobacter*-like organisms (GCLO) from man ('C. pyloridis') compared with GCLO strains from the pig, baboon and ferret. In Kaijser, B. & Falsen, E. (eds) *Campylobacter IV*. Goterna, Kungälv, pp. 44.

78 Curry, A., Jones, D.M. & Eldridge, J. Sprial organisms in the baboon stomach. *Lancet* 1987, **ii**, 634–5.

79 Morgan, D.D., Owen, R.J. & Costas, M. 1989. Characterization of *Campylobacter pylori* strains from different animal sources by determination of electrophoretic protein pattern similarities and urease isoelectric points. In Mégraud, F. and Lamouliatte, H. (eds) *Gastroduodenal Pathology and Campylobacter pylori. Proceedings of the First Meeting of the European Campylobacter pylori Study Group, Bordeaux, France.* Excerpta Medica, Elsevier Science Publishers BV, Amsterdam, pp. 89–93.

80 Bronsden, M.A. & Schoenknecht, F.D. *Campylobacter pylori* isolated from the stomach of the monkey *Macaca nemestrina. J. Clin. Microbiol.* 1987, **26**, 1725–8.

81 Newell, D.G. & Baskerville, A. 1988. Experimental and natural *Campylobacter pylori* infections in the rhesus monkey. In Kaijser, B. & Falsen, E. (eds) *Campylobacter IV.* Goterna, Kungälv, pp. 436–7.

82 Eaton, K.A., Radin, M.J., Kramer, L., Wack, R., Sherding, R., Krakowka, S. & Morgan, D.R. Epizootic gastritis in captive cheetahs associated with two kinds of gastric spiral bacteria. *Rev. Esp. Enf. Dig.* 1990, **78**, Suppl. 1, 51–2.

83 Fox, J.G., Edrise, B.M., Cabot, E.B., Beaucage, C., Murphy, J.C. & Prostak, K.S. *Campylobacter*-like organisms isolated from gastric mucosa of ferrets. *Am. J. Vet. Res.* 1986, **47**, 236–9.

84 Rathbone, B.J., West, A.P., Wyatt, J.I., Johnson, A.W., Tompkins, D.S. & Heatley, R.V. *Campylobacter pyloridis*, urease, and gastric ulcers. *Lancet* 1986, **ii**, 400.

85 Tompkins, D.S., West, A.P., Goodwin, P.G.R., Wyatt, J.I. & Rathbone, B.J. 1988. Characterization of ferret gastric *Campylobacter*-like organisms. In Kaijser, B. & Falsen, E. (eds) *Campylobacter IV.* Goterna, Kungälv, pp. 46.

86 Fox, J.G., Taylor, N.S., Edmonds, P. & Brenner, D.J. *Campylobacter pylori* subsp. *mustelae* subsp. nov. isolated from the gastric mucosa of ferrets (*Mustela putorius furo*), and an emended description of *Campylobacter pylori. Int. J. Systematic Bacteriol.* 1988, **38**, 367–70.

87 Fox, J.G., Chilvers, T., Goodwin, C.S., Taylor, N.S., Edmonds, P., Sly, L.I. & Brenner, D.J. *Campylobacter mustelae*, a new species resulting from the elevation of *Campylobacter pylori* subsp. *mustelae* to species status *Int. J. Systematic Bacteriol.* 1989, **39**, 301–3.

88 Lee, A., Hazell, S.L., O'Rourke, J. & Kouprach, S. Isolation of a spiral-shaped bacterium from the cat stomach. *Infect. Immun.* 1988, **56**, 2843–50.

89 Paster, B.J., Lee, A., Fox, J.G., Dewhirst, F.E., Tordoff, L.A., Fraser, G.J., O'Rourke, J.L., Taylor, N.S. & Ferrero, R. Phylogeny of *Helicobacter felis* sp. nov., *Helicobacter mustelae*, and related bacteria. *Int. J. Systematic Bacteriol.* 1991, **41**, 31–8.

90 Bronsdon, M.A. *Helicobacter nemestrinae* sp. nov., a spiral bacterium found in the stomach of a pigtailed macaque (*Macaca nemestrina*). *Int. J. Systematic. Bacteriol.* 1991, **41**, 148–53.

91 Vandamme, P., Falsen, E., Rossau, R., Hoste, B., Segers, P., Tytgat, R. & De Ley, J. Revision of *Campylobacter, Helicobacter* and *Wolinella* taxonomy: emendation of generic descriptions and proposal of *Arcobacter* gen. nov. *Int. J. Systematic Bacteriol.* 1991, **41**, 88–103.

92 Vandamme, P., Falsen, E., Pot, B., Kesters, K. & De Ley, J. Identification of *Campylobacter cinaedi* isolated from blood and faeces of children and adult females. *J. Clin. Microbiol.* 1990, **28**, 1016–20.

93 Bryner, J.H. 1988. *Flexispira rappini* gen. nov., sp. nov. A motile, urease producing rod similar to *Campylobacter pyloridis*. In Kaijser, B. & Falsen, E. (eds) *Campylobacter IV.* Goterna, Kungälv, pp. 440–2.

94 Fennell, C.L., Totten, P.A., Quinn, T.C., Patton, D.L., Holmes, K.K. & Stamm, W.E. Characterization of *Campylobacter*-like organisms isolated from homosexual men. *J. Infect. Dis.* 1984, **149**, 58–66.

95 McNulty, C.A.M., Dent, J.C., Curry, A., Uff, J.S., Ford, G.A., Gear, M.W.L. & Wilkinson, S.P. New spiral bacterium in gastric mucosa. *J. Clin. Pathol.* 1989, **42**, 585–91.

96 Queiroz, D.M.M., Cabral, M.M.D.A., Noguera, A.M.M.F., Barbosa, A.J.A., Rocha, G.A. & Mendes, E.N. Mixed gastric infection by *Gastrospirillum hominis* and *Helicobacter pylori. Lancet.* 1990, **ii**, 336–7.

3 Isolation and Characteristics of Helicobacter pylori

D.S.TOMPKINS

The spiral bacteria which had been observed by many pathologists in gastric specimens were first isolated when culture plates were left for a prolonged incubation of 6 days over the Easter holiday period in 1982 [1]. In this original study, gastric antral biopsies were obtained from patients at routine elective gastroscopy. The biopsies were transported to the laboratory in a chilled anaerobic broth transport medium, and cultured within 1 hour of collection. The biopsy specimens were minced and inoculated on to blood agar, 'chocolate agar' and Skirrow's *Campylobacter* medium and incubated microaerobically at 37 °C. After the initial isolation was made on 'chocolate' agar, it was found that colonies of this new organism were usually visible after 3–4 days' incubation. This spiral, microaerophilic organism shared many characteristics with campylobacters, and was named *Campylobacter pyloridis* and then *C. pylori*, but has now been placed in the genus *Helicobacter* along with a similar organism, *H. mustelae*, isolated from ferrets [2, 3].

Since the preliminary report of this original isolation in 1983 [4], many workers, all over the world, have successfully isolated *Helicobacter pylori*. The bacteria are present in a site previously thought to be colonized only by transient oral flora in most human subjects, because gastric acid rapidly destroys the majority of bacteria [5]. They live closely attached to gastric epithelial cells, beneath a protective layer of mucus, in a situation where the pH is virtually neutral [6]. *H. pylori* has also been visualized histologically in association with metastatic gastric-type epithelium in the duodenum [7], oesophagus [8], Meckel's diverticulum [9] and,

in one case, in the rectum [10]. Apart from a single report of the isolation of *H. pylori* from dental plaque [11], there are no reports of culture from sites other than gastric juice and the mucosa of the stomach and the adjacent oesophagus and duodenum, and no reports of invasion and spread to other sites.

Survival in the stomach

Most bacteria are rapidly killed in an acid environment of pH less than 4.0 [5]. Studies of the bacterial flora of the stomach in normal human subjects and those with gastric diseases reveal a varied flora, with few bacteria in the gastric juice of the normal, fasting stomach but large numbers (10^8/ml) of a large variety of species in acid-deficient subjects [5, 12]. Gastric microbial flora studies have, until recently, been carried out on samples of gastric juice and the presence of *H. pylori* has not been sought. *H. pylori* has been detected in juice in the more recent studies [13, 14] and it has been shown that there is a rich and varied mucosal flora, similar to that found in juice of achlorhydric patients [12]. A varied and substantial mucosal flora has also now been demonstrated in biopsies taken from patients with normal gastric acid levels [15]. No relationship was found between the pH of the gastric juice and the numbers of bacteria and yeasts found in the mucosa. It appears that various micro-organisms are protected by the mucus layer from the acidic gastric juice although, when present, *H. pylori* was always found in higher numbers than other micro-organisms [15].

The presence of a human gastric mucosal

urease activity, which varies between subjects and is greater than the activity seen in small bowel or colon [16], had been recognized for many years before the urease activity of *H. pylori* was first reported [17]. Helicobacters are as susceptible to acid as *Campylobacter jejuni*, *Escherichia coli*, and *Proteus mirabilis* [18, 19]. However, in the presence of physiological amounts of urea, *H. pylori* and *H. mustelae* are able to survive at a pH of < 3.0 whereas the other bacteria are killed, including *P. mirabilis*, which produces less urease activity than the helicobacters [18, 19]. The obvious conclusion to be drawn from these studies supports the hypothesis of Goodwin *et al.* [20] that, *in vivo*, *H. pylori* survives in gastric acid surrounded by a cloud of ammonia. However, Lee & Hazell [21] believe that it is unlikely that large amounts of urease would be produced for protective purposes by bacteria normally attached to the gastric mucosa beneath a layer of mucus. They suggest that *H. pylori* utilizes the extracellular ammonia generated as a nitrogen source for protein synthesis, although they concede that protection against the effects of acid could be of secondary advantage.

In vitro work has demonstrated that *H. pylori* is inhibited by 1% bile salts [1] and is less tolerant of bile than *C. jejuni* and other bacteria commonly found in the lower intestinal tract [18]. *H. pylori* is seen less often in patients with 'reflux gastritis' and those who have had gastric surgical procedures resulting in the reflux of bile compared with other patients with chronic gastritis [22]. Intragastric bile acid concentrations are also significantly higher in *H. pylori*-negative patients [22, 23]. Areas of gastric epithelial cell metaplasia of the gall-bladder are not colonized by *H. pylori*, unlike areas of metaplasia seen elsewhere in the gastrointestinal tract [24]. The inhibition of *H. pylori* growth by individual bile acids varies, and this may depend on the polarity and detergent effect of the individual bile acid [23].

Microaerophilism

Oxygen is potentially toxic to all living cells [25]

and tolerance of different bacterial species varies [26]. However, in aerobic metabolism molecular oxygen is used as a terminal electron acceptor and as a substrate in metabolic oxygenase-catalysed reactions, in which oxygen atoms are incorporated into organic compounds [25]. Campylobacters and helicobacters are micro-aerophilic organisms; they are cultured *in vitro* in a 'microaerobic' atmosphere with a reduced oxygen content, and die if exposed for more than a short period to air with 21% oxygen [27]. It is likely that the natural gastric environment of *H. pylori* is microaerobic [21]. Some campylobacters will grow anaerobically when supplied with an alternative respiratory electron acceptor such as fumarate or nitrate [26].

The reasons for the toxicity of oxygen for microaerophilic organisms are not clear. Oxygen may be converted into superoxide anion radical, hydrogen peroxide, hyroxyl radical or singlet molecular oxygen [28, 29]. These toxic products may be produced either by metabolism within the bacterial cells or by auto-oxidation and photochemical oxidation processes in growth media [28–30]. Bacteria produce enzymes such as catalases, superoxide dismutase (SOD) and peroxidases to protect themselves from these toxic products but the relationship of oxygen toxicity to production of these enzymes is not direct [25, 26]. Catalase and SOD activities are present in *C. jejuni* [31] and *H. pylori* [32]. SOD activity has been shown to be related directly to the aerotolerance of certain strains of *C. jejuni* [31].

The growth and aerotolerance of *C. jejuni* is improved by addition of various media components, which may neutralize the effects of toxic radicals produced in the media rather than providing extra nutritional factors [28–30, 33]. Blood contains catalase, peroxidase and SOD; 1% blood or haematin, also probably acting as a detoxifying agent, will support the growth of *C. jejuni* on basal media incubated micro-aerobically [34]. Catalase and SOD have been shown to reduce the deleterious effects produced in media by storage in ultraviolet (UV) light [28, 29, 31]. Ferrous sulphate, sodium pyruvate and sodium metabisulphite have also been used singly and in combination, as FBP supplement, to reduce the effects of oxygen toxicity on the survival and growth of *C. jejuni* [30, 33, 34], as have a number of other scavengers of toxic radicals such as dithionite and histidine [28]. The results of these studies have formed the basis for investigation of the factors affecting the growth of *H. pylori*, described below.

Carbon dioxide is assimilated in many key carboxylation reactions; capneic bacteria, like campylobacters and helicobacters, require an elevated concentration of CO_2 (5–10%) as they have a lower affinity, rather than a special use, for CO_2 [25]. Some campylobacters will grow in air with 8–10% CO_2 on media supplemented with blood or other additives which reduce oxygen toxicity [29, 30], and *H. pylori* will grow in these conditions on subculture [1].

Old cultures of campylobacters, and cultures exposed to atmospheric oxygen, have a tendency to lose their typical spiral morphology and form coccal bodies [27, 31]. Campylobacters may exist for months in the environment in this form, in a viable but non-culturable state [35]. *H. pylori* also forms coccal bodies and survives in a viable state in freshwater microcosms for up to a year [36]. One group [36] have reported that the coccal forms may be converted to spiral rods by increasing substrate concentrations in broth cultures, but this has yet to be confirmed by others. *H. pylori* is recoverable on solid media following suspension in water or saline held unaerated at 7 °C for several days, but dies within 1 day at room temperature [37].

Primary isolation

Ideally, specimens taken for isolation of *H. pylori* should be set up for culture as quickly as possible. Gastric biopsies should be maintained in either broth or saline to prevent the organisms from drying out and also to protect them from the effects of atmospheric oxygen. Nutrient broth contains very little dissolved oxygen [25]. Normal and phosphate-buffered saline [38, 39], nutrient broth [40] and thioglycollate broth [41] have all been used as transport media.

Biopsies have been stored for up to 5 hours at 4 °C without adverse effects on the recovery of *H. pylori* [42]. As stated above, *H. pylori* survives much better at 4–7 °C than at room temperature [37]. A small volume of transport medium should be used, as the biopsy may then be homogenized in this fluid prior to inoculation of solid media and any bacteria detached from the biopsy during transit will be recovered.

A different approach is to use a small amount of hypertonic fluid, e.g. 20% glucose, as the transport medium [42, 43]. This should maintain the structure of the biopsy so that bacteria and the mucus layer will not become detached. A biphasic transport system, comprising an enriched blood agar slant with brucella broth plus 10% horse serum, was used in one study [44]. This medium was then incubated after the biopsy was removed for routine culture and some isolations were made only on the agar slope of the transport medium. If biopsies cannot be processed within a few hours they may be frozen at −70 °C in a cryopreservative fluid such as 1% peptone water with 25% glycerol [45] or brucella broth with 20% glycerol (used by the author); losses should be minimal [45].

The biopsy should be ground in a tissue grinder with a little broth or saline, or finely minced [42]. The homogenate is then inoculated on agar plates and most microbiologists use a medium incorporating 5–10% sheep or horse blood. The plates should not be dried, as *H. pylori* grows best in a moist environment, but may be stored for several days in an airtight container before use without adversely affecting isolation [42]. It is advisable to use selective antibiotics in the medium to inhibit the growth of other contaminating bacteria and fungi [46]. Details of media will be given in the section below.

H. pylori grows best in a microaerobic atmosphere of 5% oxygen with 5–10% CO_2 [42]. A suitable atmosphere can be obtained in 'anaerobe' jars by the use of commerical gas-producing sachets which are activated by adding water. A moist atmosphere is generated using sachets. If the microaerobic atmosphere is produced in the jar by evacuation and replacement of the air by a suitable gas mixture, the humidity can be increased by including some blotting-paper soaked in water. Variable atmosphere incubators have been developed as an alternative to the use of jars. The author has used an incubator manufactured by Don Whitley Scientific Ltd for the successful isolation and subculture of helicobacters and campylobacters. It is possible to grow *H. pylori* on subculture in a humidified CO_2 incubator containing 8–10% CO_2 [1] but this is not recommended for optimal recoveries on primary isolation [42].

The plates are incubated at 37 °C for up to 7 days. *H. pylori* will grow over a temperature range of 33–40 °C [47, 48]. Only a minority of strains grow at 42 °C [3, 38] so the conditions used for the selective isolation of thermophilic campylobacters from faeces are not appropriate. Colonies will usually be visible after 2–3 days but occasionally, particularly after storage by freezing, are not visible until 6–7 days of incubation. The characteristic, small (1–2 mm), translucent colonies produce slight haemolysis on blood agar and are greyish in colour but take up a tan colour appearance on heated blood agar. Triphenyl-tetrazolium chloride (TTC) has been incorporated in media at a concentration of 40 mg/litre to simplify the identification of *H. pylori* colonies, which become a characteristic golden-yellow [41]; no other bacteria give this pigmentation. Colonies are confirmed as *H. pylori* by Gram stain, which shows characteristic curved or spiral Gram-negative rods, and by positive catalase, oxidase and rapid urease tests [45].

H. pylori may be isolated from gastric juice, even from acidic juice, but the isolation rate is lower than that obtained from biopsies [14, 49]. The distribution of *H. pylori* in the stomach may be uneven or patchy [42]. In about 14% of cases one biopsy may be positive when a second, taken at the same time, is negative [43]. However, in some studies culture was as sensitive as histology for the detection of *H. pylori* [43, 45]. Other detection methods include Gram or acridine orange staining of smears made from biopsies [50, 51] (less sensitive than culture) and the biopsy urease test [51]. Nucleic acid hybridization [52, 53] and the polymerase chain reaction [54, 55] may be more sensitive than culture for the detection of *H. pylori* but, at present, culture is required for the study of the epidemiology of the organism and for antibiotic sensitivity testing.

Media

A variety of basal media with agar and added blood (5–10% v/v, sheep or horse) have been used for the successful culture of *H. pylori*. In some studies, serum has been substituted for blood in media used for subculture or sensitivity testing. The basal media used include: blood agar base no. 2 (Oxoid) [39, 40], Columbia agar base [39], brucella agar [38, 50], brain–heart infusion agar [41, 42], tryptic soy agar [38, 51], Mueller–Hinton agar [38], Wilkins–Chalgren agar [38] and Isosensitest agar [56]. 'Chocolate' agar has also been used in several studies [1, 38, 46]. Two different media are known as 'chocolate' agar, because they resemble chocolate; one is heated blood agar and the other comprises GC agar base with yeast extract, haemoglobin or haemin and other growth supplements. Most diagnostic laboratories will want to use their routine blood agar medium with a second, selective medium for the isolation of *H. pylori*. Fresh isolates are more fastidious than laboratory-adapted strains, so the results of some of the studies on growth requirements given below may not be applicable to primary isolation.

Nutrient agar, made with blood agar base no. 2 (Oxoid), will not support the growth of *H. pylori*, although growth stimulation has been reported on this medium around an X-factor (haemin) disc [57]. However, *H. pylori* does not require haem as a source of porphyrin [56]. Poor growth is obtained on GC agar base and Mueller–Hinton agar, which both contain starch [58]. Enhanced growth is achieved on GC agar base supplemented with an extra 1% starch or 0.2% activated charcoal [58] and on Isosensitest agar with added 5% bovine serum albumin plus 0.1% catalase [56]. The role of all of these supplements may be to absorb or inactivate toxic factors [58], such as peroxidation products from long-chain fatty acids [59]. The requirement for catalase in media may be lost on sub-culture and is not dependent on endogenous catalase production by the bacterial cells [59].

In one study [51], 10% extra serum and 1% cholesterol were found to improve the colony size of *H. pylori* grown on a medium containing 10% blood, but this would be an expensive medium for routine use and the observations have not been confirmed by others. A primary isolation medium has been developed containing activated charcoal (2 g/litre), yeast extract (10 g/litre) and 10% horse serum in brain–heart infusion agar with TTC (40 mg/litre) to aid the visualization of colonies and antimicrobial agents to suppress contaminants [60]. This medium was superior to other selective and non-selective blood and 'chocolate' agar media. FBP supplement, commonly added to *Campylobacter* media to facilitate growth and aerotolerance, was reported as inhibitory to some strains of *H. pylori* [42]. Sodium metabisulphite (0.25 g/litre) was found to be the component responsible. brucella agar and broth have both been used in many studies [38, 50, 61, 62] for the successful culture of *H. pylori*; they contain sodium meta-bisulphite at a lower concentration (0.1 g/litre). Isovitalex (BBL), identical in composition to Vitox (Oxoid), is a chemically defined mixture of growth factors and has been used to supplement blood agar media and broth. A heavier growth of *H. pylori* may be obtained in a shorter time on an agar medium containing 7% lysed horse blood and 1% Isovitalex, when compared with growth on other media [42, 45]. No experimental details, however, have been given to support this claim. The individual components that may be of value have not been investigated and in one study Vitox was found to have no effect on growth in broth [61].

For primary isolation, antibacterial and anti-fungal agents are added to media to inhibit contaminants. Skirrow's supplement contains vancomycin, trimethoprim and polymyxin B and is widely used for the isolation of thermo-philic campylobacters from faeces [27]. This supplement, in media with lysed blood, has been used by many workers to isolate *H. pylori* [48, 51, 57], giving improved isolation rates in com-parison with non-selective media [63]. Goodwin *et al.* [42] have used nalidixic acid with vancomycin and amphotericin B as selective agents. However, some strains are sensitive to nalidixic acid and others to polymyxin B or colistin [46]. An alternative agent, which inhibits pseudomonads and other bacterial flora, is cefsulodin. Dent & McNulty [46] described the use of this antibiotic (5 mg/litre) with vancomycin (10 mg/litre), amphotericin B (5 mg/litre) and trimethoprim (5 mg/litre) and this selective supplement is commercially avail-able (Oxoid, SR 147). Occasionally, fungal contaminants can cause problems in gas jars and moist incubators but may be suppressed in culture media by cycloheximide (50 mg/litre).

Culture in broth is dependent on an adequate dispersion of a microaerobic gas mixture throughout the medium and this may be achieved in static culture by using a small volume of broth with a large surface area, e.g. using tissue culture flasks [20, 64], or by agitation of the broth in a microaerobic atmos-phere [61, 65]. Suitable liquid media include brain–heart infusion broth with 10% horse serum and 0.25% yeast extract [64], brucella broth with 1–10% fetal calf serum [61] or 5–10% horse serum [58, 66], nutrient broth with 5% horse serum and 0.25% yeast extract [20] and Isosensitest, Columbia and Mueller–Hinton broths, all with 10% fetal calf serum [65]. As stated above, 1% Vitox supplement did not stimulate extra growth in serum-enriched broth [61] but, in one study [58], 1% soluble starch was a satisfactory replacement for serum in liquid media. Growth of *H. pylori* was improved using a biphasic system, a brucella agar slope with overlying brucella broth containing 2.5% heat-inactivated fetal calf serum, in comparison with static or gyrated broth cultures [62]. Growth apparently occurred at the broth/agar interface. This type of system has also been used for the successful culture of campylobacters in broth [67].

A selective enrichment technique for *H. pylori* has been described in which the gastric biopsy specimen is cultured in a gyrated, gassed broth containing antibiotics, before subculture on to

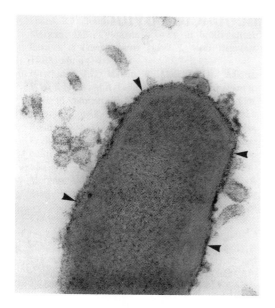

Fig. 4.2 Thin section of *H. pylori* fixed in glutaraldehyde and osmium tetroxide containing ruthenium red. Ruthenium red stabilizes surface polysaccharides, which show up as a thin electron-dense layer covering the surface of the outer envelope (arrowheads). Magnification × 76 800.

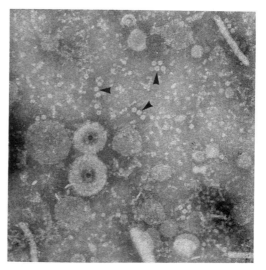

Fig. 4.3 Negatively stained preparation of sarcosinate-treated culture of *H. pylori*. In addition to fragmented flagellar filaments and fragments of membrane, discs perforated by a central hole and surface proteins shaped like doughnuts are present (arrowheads). Magnification × 152 000.

tightly packed structures are seen covering the cell surface. These surface structures are roughly 12 nm in diameter with a central, darkly staining hole 4 nm in diameter. In sarcosinate preparations (Fig. 4.3), which disrupts the plasma membrane and membrane-like wall components covering the body of the organism, these 'doughnut' structures are readily dissociated from the surface. Proteolytic enzymes degrade these 'doughnuts', showing that they are wholly or partially composed of protein. Such protein structures are not readily seen in campylobacters but are not unusual in other bacteria [13]. Those found in *H. pylori* seem to incorporate the urease enzyme [14]. The 'doughnuts' may also have a structural function and, in addition, restrict access of substances through the cell wall.

Internal appearance

Thin sections of *H. pylori* show typical prokaryotic structures. the central region of the organism is filled with the filamentous nucleoid and is surrounded by a dense granular cytoplasm comprising large numbers of bacterial ribosomes. Occasional electron-lucent spherical (up to 150 nm) storage bodies are located in the proteoplasmic matrix. Bode *et al.* [15] have also seen crystal-like inclusions in *H. pylori*, when grown in liquid media. The protoplasmic cylinder is covered by the true plasma membrane, which, in turn, is covered by the membrane-like outer wall component. A small gap 7 nm wide (the periplasmic space) separates the plasma membrane and the outer envelope. In favourable sections, a thin (2 nm) electron-dense layer can be seen in the periplasmic space, which most probably represents the location of the peptidoglycan layer. The terminal region of the flagellated end of the organism shows specializations which are restricted to that region and probably represent terminal strengthening associated with the flagellar insertion (Fig. 4.4). The terminal specializations consist of an electron-lucent region immediately below the terminal region of the plasma membrane. Additional structures are found on the protoplasmic face of the plasma membrane but are

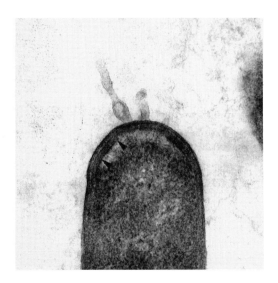

Fig. 4.4 Thin section through flagellated terminal dome of *H. pylori*. Note membrane-like nature of flagellar sheath, electron-lucent zone and terminal plasma membrane decorations on inner (protoplasmic) surface (arrowheads). Magnification × 80 000.

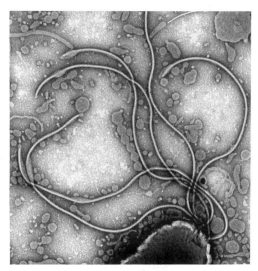

Fig. 4.5 Negatively stained preparation of flagella terminations showing dilated sheath and occasional terminal 'paddles'. Magnification × 28 000.

restricted to a distance of about 400 nm from the tip of the organism although the extreme tip appears to be devoid of these additions. These comprise additional decorations to this membrane: a 6 nm thick electron-dense layer is intimately associated with the membrane, with another electron-dense layer approximately 20 nm thick being found internally. In favourable sections these two layers (separated by 15 nm) appear to have links joining them together. Similar structures are to be seen in many polar-flagellated organisms including true campylobacters [16, 17].

Flagellar structure

The flagellar apparatus consists of the external filaments with associated membrane-like sheaths and basal rotatory structures embedded in the wall of the terminal region. Although in some cultures non-flagellated cells can be found, usually from one to eight filaments are inserted into the terminal dome. Two-day cultures more commonly show cells with five or six filaments; 4-day cultures often possess up to nine flagellar filaments. The average number of filaments

present appears to increase with age of the culture.

Individual sheathed filaments are helical but assume a sinusoidal or curved form when dried down on to electron microscope specimen support films. They are up to 3 μm in length and have an overall diameter (including the sheath) of 30 nm. In favourable preparations the wavelength would appear to be 2–3 μm. The terminal regions or subterminal regions of the sheathed filaments often show a paddle-like or dilated form (Fig. 4.5). These dilatations are expressed in the membrane-like sheaths. Empty terminal sheaths can also be found devoid of their internal filament. Occasionally the internal filament, 15 nm in diameter, is seen to extend through and beyond the termination of the sheath. This form is most probably an artefact produced during preparation for examination under the electron microscope.

Sheathed flagellar filaments are found in several species of bacteria. Those found in *H. pylori* probably reflect an adaptation to living in and moving through mucus, and a protection against stomach acid, which would depolymerize naked filaments [18]. Such degradation of the filament would not allow the organism to

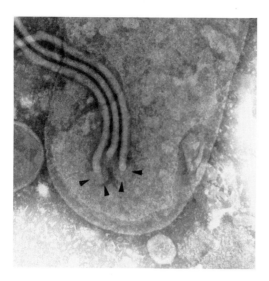

Fig. 4.6 Fortuitous negatively stained preparation showing location of large discs of the flagellar insertions (arrowheads). Magnification × 92 000.

move away from hostile acid conditions [19]. An additional survival factor in *H. pylori* is the presence of the urease enzyme, whose products could locally neutralize stomach acid. Other mucus-inhabiting bacteria have a spiral body form and sheathed flagella, which may be optimal adaptations for living in and moving through mucus [20]. The flagella sheaths are continuous with the outer membrane-like component of the body wall, although there is some evidence to indicate that they are composed almost entirely of protein [21]. The interal flagellar filament, which probably rotates within the flexible sheath [22], penetrates a large disc associated with the outer envelope. These insertion discs can sometimes be seen in favourably stained whole organisms (Fig. 4.6), but are best viewed in sarcosinate preparations, where they separate from the membranous wall components (Fig. 4.3). The discs are about 90 nm in diameter and have a central hole of 19 nm diameter, which is surrounded by a more densely staining zone about 40 nm in diameter. This disc is probably located on the inner surface of the outer membrane, the annular morphology reflecting adherence to this membrane. The function of the disc is not fully understood but

probably acts both as a bearing for the rotational movements of the flagellar filaments and as a strengthening structure, stabilizing the flagellar insertion [17, 23]. Two smaller discs, 22 nm in diameter, can also be found associated with the proximal region of the flagellar apparatus where it originates from the plasma membrane. Such small discs have been identified in other motile bacteria, particularly *Escherichia coli*, *Salmonella typhimurium* and *Bacillus subtilis*, as providing the motive force to drive the rotational movements of the flagellar filament [24]. Such discs are fixed to or rotate about a central rod, which in turn is connected to the flexible hook region at the cell surface and the rigid filament. The structure of this flagellar apparatus is summarized in Fig. 4.7.

Division

Division in *H. pylori* is by transverse fission (Fig. 4.8). The plasma membrane initially invaginates to divide the protoplasmic cylinder into halves. The membrane-like outer wall component then completes separation by invagination between the plasma membranes of the two incipient daughter cells. During this division process, one half of the cell retains the original flagellar apparatus. The daughter cell without the original flagellar apparatus produces these structures sequentially at the opposite pole from the original (Fig. 4.9), but will not have produced a full complement at the time of separation. Thus the division septum region does not produce flagellar filaments.

Spherical and other forms

Atypical forms of *H. pylori* are seen in some cultures of various ages and passages. Such forms have been observed *in vivo* [25]. This phenomenon is also apparent with true campylobacters and other bacteria [26, 27]. Spherical forms can also be seen in campylobacters from aqueous environments. The spherical form would minimize the surface in contact with unfavourable external conditions and may, therefore, be a survival adaptation in both true

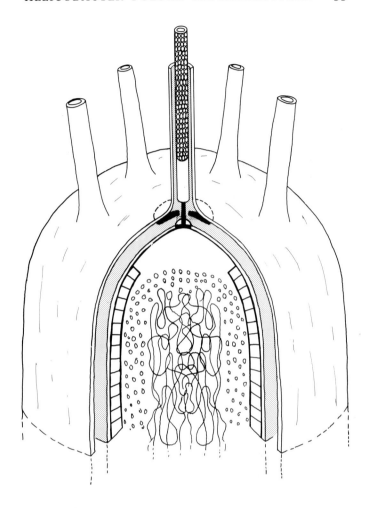

Fig. 4.7 Diagram of terminal region showing flagellar insertions and terminal specializations.

campylobacters and *H. pylori*. Thus 'atypical' forms may be adaptations to marginal or hostile environments or may, in culture, reflect a response to defects in the cultural conditions, nutrients provided, build-up of waste products, prolonged passage or antibiotics. Naturally occurring spherical forms may be a transmission form in both *H. pylori* and true campylobacters [28].

In culture U-shaped, V-shaped and spherical forms of *H. pylori* can be found in negatively stained preparations (Fig. 4.10). The mechanism of genesis of these various forms seems to involve protoplasmic growth within a restricted outer envelope which has failed to expand in synchrony with the outer cell components and has become loosened from the protoplasmic

cylinder. Some of these forms show features of early division septum formation. If the proto-plasmic cylinder bounded by the plasma membrane continues to elongate within a non-expanding or more slowly expanding outer envelope, then bending of the cylinder occurs, producing U-shaped forms. Equally, if the organism divides but the outer envelope fails to induce separation or expand adequately (Fig. 4.11), then growth of the daughter cells would produce the V-shaped forms. Rupture of the plasma membrane would fill the space enclosed by the outer envelope with protoplasm, although this seems to self-heal. Entirely spherical forms then result from the outer envelope losing the last vestiges of its rigidity or cylindrical form, presumably because of defects

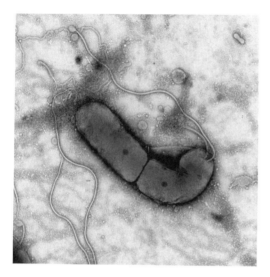

Fig. 4.8 Negatively stained preparation of dividing *H. pylori* in culture. Note loose outer membrane where organism has bent, which indicates that this organism may develop into an atypical form. Magnification × 16 800.

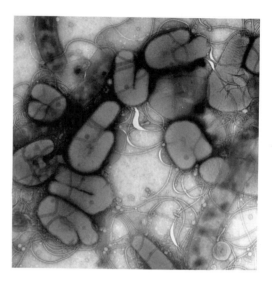

Fig. 4.10 Negatively stained preparation of *H. pylori* culture showing abnormal, mainly U-shaped forms. Magnification × 11 200.

in this wall. Evidence for this mechanism can be found by examination of both negatively stained, and thin-sectioned cultured organisms (Figs 4.8 and 4.11–4.16).

By negative staining, organisms bent double can be found enclosed within a loose outer envelope (Figs 4.12–4.14). A division septum can be found in some of the aberrant forms. Occasionally an organism bent double within an envelope shows flagellation on one side of the

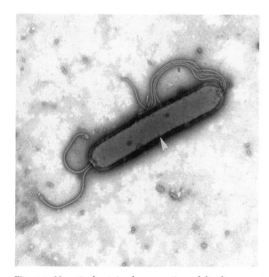

Fig. 4.9 Negatively stained preparation of dividing organism. Note central division septum (arrowhead) and two flagella filaments from previously non-flagellated pole. Magnification × 16 000.

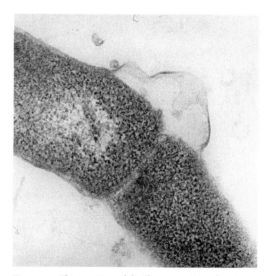

Fig. 4.11 Thin section of dividing organism showing septum and outer membrane-like wall component blebbing away from plasma membrane. Magnification × 90 400.

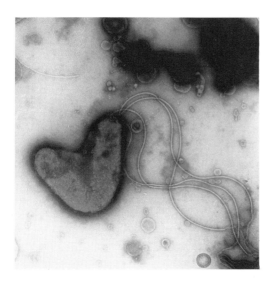

Fig. 4.12 Negatively stained V-shaped organism. Note flagella from one pole only and loose outer wall membrane between arms of V. Magnification × 19 200.

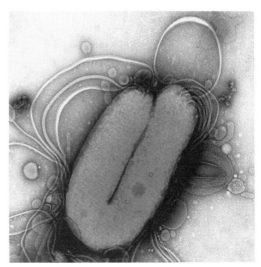

Fig. 4.14 U-shaped form showing flagellar filaments from both poles of both arms. A division septum is faintly visible. Magnification × 31 200.

bend but not the other, indicating that bending had occurred in an organism with previously normal morphology. Thin sections of these organisms show a membrane-like wall enclosing a U-shaped protoplasmic cylinder surrounded by the plasma membrane. The folded or twisted protoplasmic cylinder retains its shape, indicating that this, at least, has retained some rigidity. This rigidity may, perhaps, indicate that the peptidoglycan layer remains firmly attached to the plasma membrane [29]. Some less dense

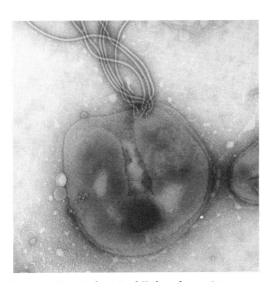

Fig. 4.13 Negatively stained U-shaped organism showing single bunch of filaments and loose outer membrane enclosing both arms of the U form. Magnification × 29 600.

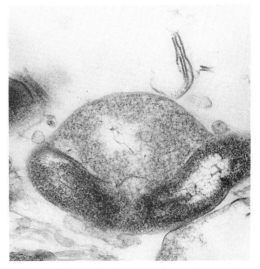

Fig. 4.15 Thin section of abnormal organism showing bend in protoplasmic cylinder with less electron-dense protoplasm filling the space between it and the outer membrane-like wall. Magnification × 51 200.

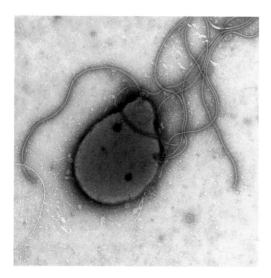

Fig. 4.16 Spherical form of *H. pylori*. Note non-degenerative look of this organism. Magnification × 18 400.

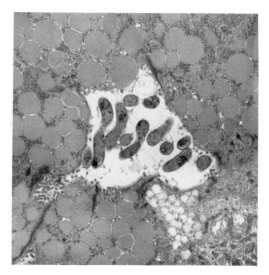

Fig. 4.17 *H. pylori* in crypt of baboon stomach. Magnification × 7360.

protoplasm can be found in the space between the halves of the protoplasmic cylinder, indicative of protoplasmic leakage (Fig. 4.15). The resultant spherical forms have the appearance of viability and do not show degenerative changes (Fig. 4.16), perhaps indicating that they are indeed viable transmissible forms.

Appearance in vivo

In gastric biopsy material, *H. pylori* is predominantly an extracellular, mucus-living organism which is found either in crypts or on the microvillus surface. Its distribution is patchy and the size of the organism is variable, depending upon the region of the stomach sampled [25]. In crypts the organisms do not appear to be attached to the epithelial cells (Fig. 4.17) but on the mucosal surface a proportion of organisms are intimately associated with the cell surface. Here, fine threads or strands are seen linking the bacteria to the epithelial cell surfaces (Figs 4.18 and 4.19). The sheathed flagellar filaments do not show such attachments [25]. The attachment of bacterium and epithelial cell probably involves interaction between surface polysaccharides (glycocalyx), probably mediated by lectin binding. Pedestals and surface pits are

sometimes seen in such associations. Occasionally *H. pylori* can be found directly above the junction between epithelial cells (Fig. 4.20) and there is evidence that this is a preferred location because of the leakage of metabolites at these sites [30, 31]. There are also reports of organisms

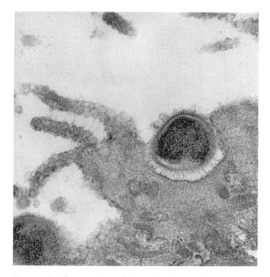

Fig. 4.18 Thin section of *H. pylori* from a human biopsy showing organism partially embedded in an epithelial cell. Note filamentous material surrounding the organism and faint links anchoring it to cell surface. Magnification × 48 000.

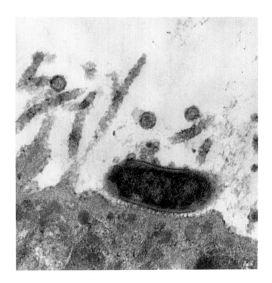

Fig. 4.19 Thin section of *H. pylori* on epithelial cell surface. Magnification × 34 000.

being seen in intercellular [32] and intracellular [32–35] locations. The present authors have not found intracellular *H. pylori* in humans but have seen a different, tightly spiralled organism, resembling *Gastrospirillum hominis* [8], with a predilection for the canaliculi of HCl-secreting oxyntic cells in baboons [10]. Further examination of biopsy material needs to be undertaken

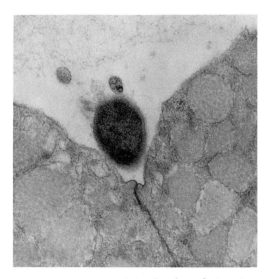

Fig. 4.20 Thin section of *H. pylori* above the junction between two epithelial cells. Magnification × 36 000.

to determine if *H. pylori* can penetrate oxyntic cells or become truly intracellular or whether previous reports have misidentified the organism involved.

Ultrastructure of colonies

Little work has been performed on the ultrastructure of *H. pylori* colonies. Forty-eight-hour cultures show organisms of normal morphology, many of which are orientated into parallel arrays (Fig. 4.21). A few atypical forms are also found (see above). Four-day cultures show many more atypical forms and, in addition, degraded organisms.

Appearance in other animals

Organisms closely resembling *H. pylori* have been found in various animal species in addition to man [36]. Primates, pigs and ferrets have been shown to harbour these bacteria (Figs 4.22–4.24). From baboons, monkeys and pigs, organisms that are structurally, biochemically and serologically identical to *H. pylori* have been isolated. The ferret organism has a number of differences including some important morphological features. It tends to be shorter and less sinusoidal than *H. pylori*. In addition, the sheathed flagellar filaments originate from lateral or subterminal locations and not just a single pole. The surface 'doughnuts' in the ferret organism have a slightly different appearance and are also smaller in diameter (10 nm, with a 5 nm central hole). All these differences have dictated that the ferret organism is allocated to a different species within the same genus *Helicobacter*. Thus *H. mustelae* is the second species of the genus [12].

All these helicobacters are easily distinguishable on morphological grounds from campylobacters and the tightly spiralled organisms described in baboons [9, 10], dogs [31], cats [37] and humans [7, 8]. The human organism has been provisionally named *Gastrospirillum hominis* [8].

A tightly spiralled organism has been isolated from the cat stomach and tentatively described

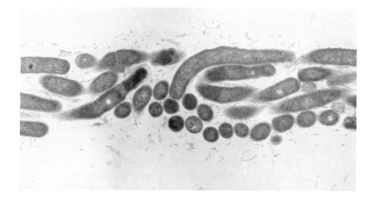

Fig. 4.21 Thin section through 2-day-old colony of *H. pylori*. Note that some degree of alignment is apparent. Magnification × 9200.

as *Helicobacter felis* [38]. This feline organism shows little morphological resemblance to *H. pylori*, but has features in common with *Gastrospirillum*. However, this cat organism has periplasmic fibres that run helically the length of the cell, which have not been seen in either the genus *Gastrospirillum* or the genus *Helicobacter*. It may be that this feline tightly spiralled organism represents yet another genus of spiral organisms from the animal stomach.

Comparison with other spiral organisms

Until recently, *H. pylori* was conveniently, if erroneously, classified as belonging to the genus *Campylobacter*, despite significant morphological differences being apparent between these two genera. True campylobacters, such as *C. jejuni*, have a single, unsheathed flagellum at each end of the organism which originates in a shallow terminal pit (Figs 4.25 and 4.26). In addition, the ends of the organism are truncated cones rather than the hemispherical form of *H. pylori*. The flagellar discs associated with the flagellar apparatus are different, those of *C. jejuni* and *C. fetus* having radial spokes [17] (Fig. 4.27), whereas those of *H. pylori* show an annular differentiation. Thus, there was little morphological commonality between true campylobacters and *H. pylori*. A true campylobacter has been isolated from human gastric epithelium

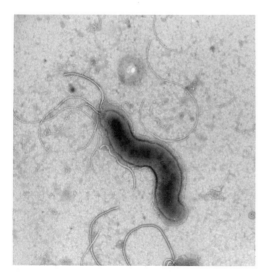

Fig. 4.22 *H. pylori* isolated from a baboon stomach. Magnification × 16 800.

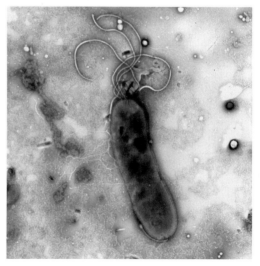

Fig. 4.23 *H. pylori* isolated from a pig stomach. Magnification × 16 000.

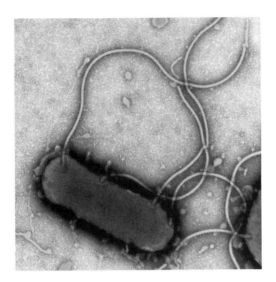

Fig. 4.24 Organism isolated from the ferret stomach. Note lateral insertions of flagellar filaments. Magnification × 41 600.

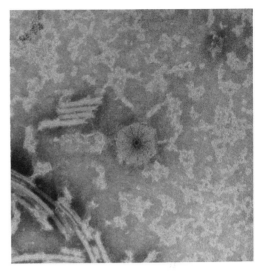

Fig. 4.26 Flagellar disc isolated from a sarcosinate-treated *C. jejuni* preparation. Note radial spokes originating from the central darkly staining hole. Magnification × 131 200.

[39, 40] and this is now designated *C. jejuni* subsp. *doylei* and is more normally found in the lower gut.

Gastrospirillum hominis, which has recently been described from the human stomach, is distinct from both *H. pylori* and the true campylobacters [7, 8]. A very similar tightly

spiralled organism has been described from baboon stomachs [9, 10]. Both these newly described organisms show similar overall morphology, possessing multiple sheathed flagella at

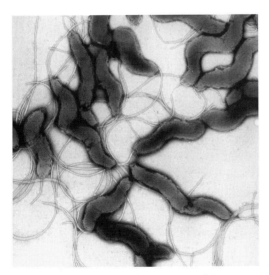

Fig. 4.25 Negatively stained preparation of *C. jejuni*. Note different form of this organism compared with *H. pylori*. Magnification × 18 400.

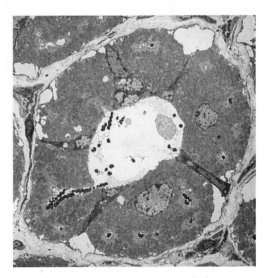

Fig. 4.27 Thin section of baboon stomach showing tightly spiralled organisms in a crypt. Note that this organism lives in the crypt lumen but is also commonly found in the canaliculi of the oxyntic cells. Magnification × 1840.

each end. The human organism, *Gastrospirillum hominis*, may be associated with gastritis [8], whereas the baboon organism was not [10]. Neither organism has been cultured so their true affinities remain to be elucidated. However, the presently unclassified baboon organism will probably be allocated to the genus *Gastrospirillum*. The baboon organism has been commonly found in the canaliculi of the HCl-secreting oxyntic cells (Fig. 4.27) as well as in the mucus of the mucosal surface and crypts. Ultrastructurally it appears to be able to bend and contract within the extensive canalicular system of the oxyntic cells. Internally a complex tubular system is present which may mediate these movements, thus enabling this organism to exploit this niche [10]. It may be unique, but many animal species remain to be examined. From our present knowledge several different types of spiral bacteria exist in stomachs of various mammals including man. Workers in this field should be careful to evaluate the morphological differences between these bacteria.

References

1 Freedberg, A.S. & Barron, L.E. The presence of spirochaetes in human gastric mucosa. *Am. J. Dig. Dis.* 1940, **7**, 443–5.

2 Palmer, E.D. Investigation of the gastric mucosa spirochaetes of the human. *Gastroenterology* 1954, **27**, 218–20.

3 Kasia, K. & Kobayashi, R. The stomach spirochete occurring in mammals. *J. Parasitol.* 1919, **6**, 1–10.

4 Doenges, J.L. Spirochetes in the gastric glands of *Macacus rhesus* and of man without related disease. *Arch. Pathol.* 1939, **27**, 469–77.

5 Lim, R.K.S. A parasitic spiral organism in the stomach of the cat. *Parasitology* 1920, **12**, 108–12.

6 Tompkins, D.S., Foulkes, S.J., Godwin, P.G.R. & West, A.P. Isolation and characterisation of intestinal spirochaetes. *J. Clin. Pathol.* 1986, **39**, 535–41.

7 Dent, J.C., McNulty, C.A.M., Uff, J.C., Wilkinson, S.P. & Gear, M.W.L. Spiral organisms in the gastric antrum. *Lancet* 1987, **ii**, 96.

8 McNulty, C.A.M., Dent, J.C., Curry, A., Uff, J.S., Ford, G.A., Gear, M.W.L. & Wilkinson, S.P. New spiral bacterium in the gastric mucosa. *J. Clin. Pathol.* 1989, **42**, 585–91.

9 Curry, A., Jones, D.M. & Eldridge, J. Spiral organisms in the baboon stomach. *Lancet* 1987, **ii**, 634–5.

10 Curry, A., Jones, D.M. & Skelton-Stroud, P. Novel ultrastructural findings in a helical bacterium found in the baboon (*Papio anubis*) stomach. *J. Gen. Microbiol.* 1989, **135**, 2223–31.

11 Thomsen, L.L., Gavin, J.B. & Tasman-Jones, C. Relation of *Helicobacter pylori* to the human gastric mucosa in chronic gastritis of the antrum. *Gut* 1990, **31**, 1230–6.

12 Goodwin, C.S. & Armstrong, J.A. Microbiological aspects of *Helicobacter pylori* (*Campylobacter pylori*) *Eur. J. Clin. Microbiol. Infect. Dis.* 1990, **9**, 1–13.

13 Dickson, M.R., Downing, K.H., Wu, W.H. & Glaeser, R.M. Three-dimensional structure of the surface layer protein of *Aquaspirillum serpens* VHA determined by electron crystallography. *J. Bacteriol.* 1986, **167**, 1025–34.

14 Hawtin, P.R., Stacey, A.R. & Newell, D.G. Investigation of the structure and localization of the urease of *Helicobacter pylori* using monoclonal antibodies. *J. Gen. Microbiol.* 1990, **136**, 1995–2000.

15 Bode, G., Malfertheiner, P., Lehnardt, G. & Ditschuneit, H. 1990. Virulence factors of *Helicobacter pylori* – ultrastructural features. In Malfertheiner, P. & Ditschuneit, H. (eds) *Helicobacter pylori, Gastritis and Peptic Ulcer*. Springer-Verlag, Berlin, Heidelberg, pp. 63–73.

16 Rowles, C.R., Parton, R. & Jeynes, M.H. 1976. Some aspects of the cell walls of *Vibrio* spp. In Fuller, R. & Lovelock, D.W. (eds) *Midrobial Ultrastructure: the Use of the Electron Microscope*. Academic Press, London, pp. 109–15.

17 Curry, A., Fox, A.J. & Jones, D.M. A new bacterial flagellar structure found in campylobacters. *J. Gen. Microbiol.* 1984, **130**, 1307–10.

18 Ibrahim, G.F., Fleet, G.H., Lyons, M.J. & Walker, R.A. Method for the isolation of the highly purified *Salmonella* flagellins. *J. Clin. Microbiol.* 1985, **22**, 1040–4.

19 Hazell, S.L. & Lee, A. 1985. The adaptation of motile strains of *Campylobacter pyloridis* to gastric mucus and their association with gastric epithelial intercellular spaces. In Pearson, A.D., Skirrow, M.B., Lior, H. & Rowe, B. (eds) *Campylobacter III: Proceedings of the Third International Workshop on Campylobacter Infections, Ottawa, 7–15 July 1985*. Public Health Laboratory Service, London, pp. 189–91.

20 Ferrero, R.L. & Lee, A. Motility of *Campylobacter jejuni* in a viscous environment: comparison with conventional rod-shaped bacteria. *J. Gen. Microbiol.* 1988, **134**, 53–9.

21 Hranitzky, K.W., Mulholland, A., Larson, A.D., Eubanks, E.R. & Hart, L.T. Characterization of a flagellar sheath protein of *Vibrio cholerae*. *Infect. Immun.* 1980, **27**, 597–603.

22 Thomashow, L.S. & Rittenberg, S.C. Isolation and composition of sheathed flagella from *Bdellovibrio bacteriovirus* 109 J. *J. Bacteriol.* 1985, **163**, 1047–54.

23 Jones, D.M., Curry, A. & Fox, A.J. An ultrastructural

study of the gastric campylobacter-like organism 'Campylobacter pyloridis'. *J. Gen. Microbiol.* 1985, **131**, 2335–41.

24 De Pamphilis, M.L. & Alder, J. Fine structure and isolation of the hook–basal body complex of flagella from *Escherichia coli* and *Bacillus subtilis*. *J. Bacteriol.* 1971, **105**, 384–95.

25 Steer, H.W. 1989. Ultrastructure of *Campylobacter pylori in vivo*. In Rathbone, B.J. & Heatley, R.V. (eds) *Campylobacter pylori and Gastroduodenal Disease*. Blackwell Scientific Publications, Oxford, pp. 146–54.

26 Buck, G.E., Parshall, K.A. & Davis, C.P. Electron microscopy of the coccoid form of *Campylobacter jejuni*. *J. Clin Microbiol.* 1983, **18**, 420–1.

27 Jai-King, N.G., Sherburne, R., Taylor, D.E. & Stiles, M.E. Morphological forms and viability of *Campylobacter* species studied by electron microscopy. *J. Bacteriol.* 1985, **164**, 338–43.

28 Rollins, D.M. & Colwell, R.R. Viable but non culturable stage of *Campylobacter jejuni* and its role in survival in the natural aquatic environment. *Appl. Environ. Microbiol.* 1986, **52**, 531–8.

29 Jones, D.M. & Curry, A. 1990 The genesis of coccal forms of *Helicobacter pylori*. In Malfertheiner, P. & Ditschuneit, H. (eds) *Helicobacter pylori, Gastritis and Peptic Ulcer*. Springer-Verlag, Berlin, Heidelberg, pp. 29–37.

30 Hazell, S.L., Lee, A., Brady, L. & Hennessy, W. *Campylobacter pyloridis* and gastritis: association with intercellular spaces and adaptation to an environment of mucus as important factors in colonization of the gastric epithelium. *J. Infect. Dis.* 1986, **153**, 658–63.

31 Lee, A. & Hazell, S.L. *Campylobacter pylori* in health and disease: an ecological perspective. *Microb. Ecol. Health Dis.* 1988, **1**, 1–16.

32 Kazi, J.L., Sinniah, R., Zaman, V., Ng, M.L., Jafarey, N.A., Alam, S.M., Zuberi, S.J. & Kazi, A.M. Ultrastructural study of *Helicobacter pylori*-associated gastritis. *J. Pathol.* 1990, **161**, 65–70.

33 Rollason, T.P., Stone, J. & Rhodes, J.M. Spiral organisms in endoscopic biopsies of the human stomach. *J. Clin. Pathol.* 1984, **37**, 23–6.

34 Chen, X.G., Correa, P., Offerhaus, J., Rodriguez, E., Janney, F., Hoffmann, E., Fox, J., Hunter, F. & Diavolitis, S. Ultrastructure of the gastric mucosa harboring campylobacter-like organisms. *Am. J. Clin. Pathol.* 1986, **86**, 575–82.

35 Marshall, B.J. *Campylobacter pyloridis* and gastritis. *J. Infect. Dis.* 1986, **153**, 650–7.

36 Curry, A., Jones, D.M., Eldridge, J. & Fox, A.J. 1985. Ultrastructure of *Campylobacter pyloridis* – not a *Campylobacter*? In Pearson, A.D., Skirrow, M.B., Lior, H. & Rowe, B. (eds) *Campylobacter III: Proceedings of the Third International Workshop on Campylobacter Infection, Ottawa, 7–10 July 1985*. Public Health Laboratory Service, London, abstr. no. 117.

37 Lee, A., Hazell, S.L., O'Rourke, J. & Kouprack, S. Isolation of a spiral-shaped bacterium from the cat stomach. *Infect. Immun.* 1988, **56**, 2843–50.

38 Lee, A., Fox, J.G., Otto, G. & Murphy, J. A small animal model of human *Helicobacter pylori* active chronic gastritis. *Gastroenterology* 1990, **99**, 1315–23.

39 Kasper, G. & Dickgiesser, N. Isolation from gastric epithelium of *Campylobacter*-like bacteria that are distinct from '*Campylobacter pyloridis*'. *Lancet* 1985, **i**, 111–12.

40 Goodwin, S., Blincow, E., Armstrong, J., McCulloch, R. & Collins, D. *Campylobacter pyloridis* is unique: GCLO-2 is an ordinary *Campylobacter*. *Lancet* 1985, **ii**, 38–9.

5 Ultrastructure of Helicobacter pylori in vivo

H.W.STEER

The microenvironment of the bacterium *Helicobacter pylori* is unique, displaying a number of unusual features necessitating the conclusion that only a highly specialized bacterium could survive at such a site. Electron microscopy has helped to define this microenvironment aiding in determining the characteristics of the bacterium and its role in any pathological process. To examine the ultrastructural features of this microenvironment, the *in vivo* appearance of *H. pylori* will be considered prior to its relationship with its surroundings.

In vivo appearance of H. pylori

The shape of *H. pylori in vivo* can vary from spiral to kidney-shaped to a coccal form. Spiral and kidney-shaped forms have been observed with both the transmission and scanning electron microscopes [1, 2], confirming previous observations made with the light microscope. It had not been possible to define the coccal shape with transmission electron microscopy because of possible cross-cutting of the bacteria, but this form of bacterium has been observed with the scanning electron microscope [3]. Evidence is lacking without any possible pattern of distribution of the various forms of *H. pylori* or any relationship between the different forms. The coccal form is seen in older bacteriological cultures and has been considered degenerate, although this concept may have to be reconsidered in the light of recent evidence that the coccal form is capable of regrowth.

The size of *H. pylori* has been reported to vary in patients with chronic duodenal ulceration, depending upon the site at which the bacterium is located. Thus, *H. pylori* are larger in antral biopsies compared with those biopsies taken from the edge of the duodenal ulcer [3].

Helicobacter pylori have four to six unipolar sheathed flagella, which have terminal bulbs [4]. The flagella are attached to the bacterial body by a spherical body or basal granule. The terminal bulbs are infrequently observed *in vivo* because of their diameter but occasional terminal bulbs, flagella and basal granules are seen (Figs 5.1 and 5.2). There are two types of terminal bulbs seen. The larger terminal bulbs (Fig. 5.1) have a diameter of 0.28 µm with a sheathed flagellum, which has an overall diameter of only 67 nm and a basal granule diameter of only 50 nm. The substructure of the larger terminal bulb includes an organized array of microtubules (seen in cross-section in Fig. 5.1) with a diameter of 17 nm. The precise arrangement of these microtubular structures cannot be determined from the *in vivo* studies but in cross-section they are separated by a space of 20–25 nm. It appears that some of these microtubules open on to the surface of the terminal bulb. This profile of the terminal bulb is larger than that described by Goodwin *et al.* [4]. The substructure of this smaller terminal bulb (Fig. 5.2) differs from that already described and this type of terminal bulb has a diameter of only 58 nm. The flagella attached to these smaller terminal bulbs have a diameter of 25 nm. These differences in the flagella and terminal bulbs may represent a dimorphism as far as the bacteria are concerned and may reflect different dynamic states of the bacteria.

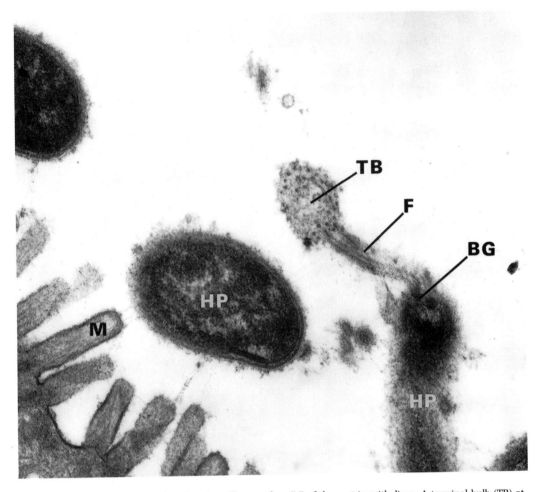

Fig. 5.1 *H. pylori* (HP) are related to the microvillous surface (M) of the gastric epithelium. A terminal bulb (TB) at the end of the flagellum (F) is seen together with two basal granules (BG). Transmission electron micrograph, ×45 600.

Helicobacter pylori and its environment

The localization of *H. pylori* is limited to cells derived from the gastric-type mucosa [1–5]. They are never related to intestinal-type mucosal cells. The bacteria are most frequently found deep to the layer of mucus overlying the epithelial cells and are therefore not apparent unless this layer of mucus is removed [1]. Some *H. pylori* are present in the overlying gastric mucus and at this site tend to be aggregated in 'cave-like' structures [3]. Some of these bacteria have been identified in the gastric juice of patients when the appropriate bacteriological analyses have been performed.

The distribution of the epithelium-related bacteria is 'patchy' with frequent clusters of bacteria apparent [6]. *Helicobacter pylori* are most frequently found near the neck of gastric mucosa although bacteria have been seen in the depths of gastric glands and even in the canaliculi of parietal cells [7]. The *H. pylori* in the duodenum are always related to areas of gastric metaplasia. The reasons for this specificity of mucosal relationship include the differences in the physicochemical properties of the mucus at the sites of intestinal metaplasia where the globlet cells produce an acidic mucus [8]. Differences in the antigenic recognition and

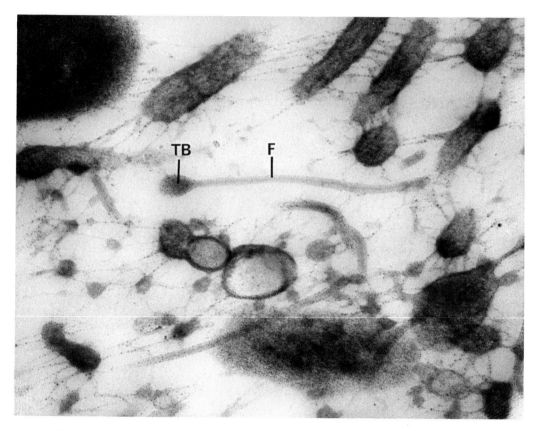

Fig. 5.2 The flagellum (F) and an attached terminal bulb (TB) from an *H. pylori*. Transmission electron micrograph, × 73 000.

expression of the two types of cell surface could influence bacterial adhesion but if this is a criterion for their absence at areas of intestinal metaplasia it would be reasonable to expect to find non-adherent *H. pylori* at these sites. However, even non-adherent *H. pylori* are not found at the areas of intestinal metaplasia, making this possibility untenable. *Helicobacter pylori* can be related to any part of the lumenal surface of gastric mucus-secreting cells but are most frequently sited in the 'grooves' at the junction of individual epithelial cells (Figs 5.3 and 5.4). The epithelial cells related to bacteria have a decreased number of surface microvilli [1, 3, 4]. In addition, the length of the microvilli is significantly decreased but their diameter is unchanged [9]. The siting of the bacteria in the 'grooves' between the neighbouring epithelial cells results in their close proximity to the inter-

cellular junctions [1, 3, 4, 10]. The localization of the bacteria at these sites, seen most clearly with the scanning electron microscope, is unlikely to be artefactual resulting from the removal of the overlying mucus, because such a localization has been confirmed with the transmission electron microscope. This siting must confer benefits for individual bacteria and may enable the bacteria to avoid the principal flow of mucus from the cell surface. Mucus is secreted from the gastric mucus-secreting cells by a process of merocrine secretion, with the mucus passing from the apex of individual cells into the overlying mucus layer. Bacteria located at the apex of actively secreting mucus cells would be continually forced into the mucus layer in transit to other hostile parts of the gastro-intestinal tract. This may account for the aggregates of bacteria present in the overlying

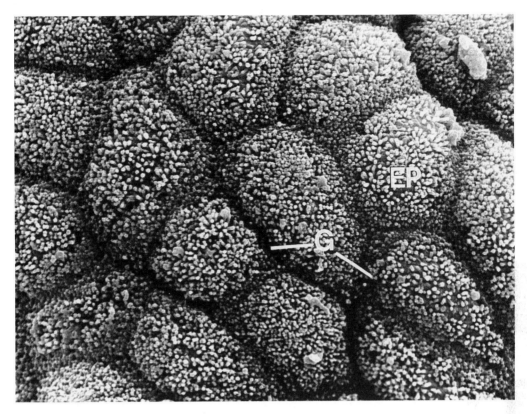

Fig. 5.3 The gastric epithelial surface in a normal stomach showing individual epithelial cells (EP) covered with microvilli. The 'grooves' (G) between the surface of individual cells is clearly seen. Scanning electron micrograph, × 5936.

mucus [3] and those *H. pylori* isolated from the gastric juice. It is possible that large numbers of bacteria are lost in this way, so that those bacteria observed in the 'grooves' at the epithelial surface would be more appropriately termed the 'resident' bacterial population.

The three-dimensional net-like structure of the gastric mucus helps stabilize the unstirred layer of the gastric mucus and physically assists in the pH gradient. This net-like structure is disrupted in the presence of *H. pylori* infection [9] and rapidly restored on successful treatment of the infection. The disruption would, of necessity, reduce the gastric mucosa/mucus defensive barrier.

Most *H. pylori* are found between the epithelial cell surface and the overlying mucus barrier. The reason for this localization may be related to the pH gradient across the gastric mucus barrier

[11]. At the epithelial cell surface many *H. pylori* are adherent to the epithelial surface. This adherence is a characteristic of bacterial pathogenicity and can be so intimate that they are only separated by a distance of 10 nm. Adhesion may take one of three forms. Most frequently the bacterial surface and the epithelial cell surface are separated by part of the glycocalyx [6]. Such initial adhesion may involve non-specific interactions before a more specific process occurs. The accompanying adhesive mechanisms result in a thickening of the cell membrane [3, 4], forming an adhesive pedestal. Adhesion is usually between the bacterial bodies rather than the flagellae or terminal bulbs. Whether the different forms of adhesion have any pathogenic significance has not been investigated.

The zona occludens, zona adherens and macula adherens are specialized intercellular

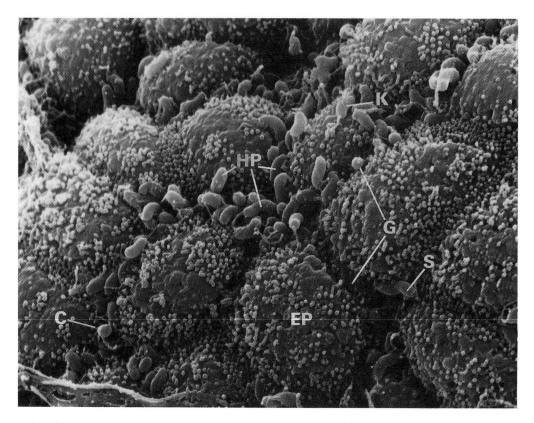

Fig. 5.4 The epithelial surface of gastric mucus-secreting cells from the prepyloric area of a patient with chronic duodenal ulceration. The number of surface microvilli is decreased. The *H. pylori* (HP) are numerous and present in the 'grooves' (G) between individual epithelial cells (EP). Coccal (C), kidney-shaped (K) and spiral (S) forms of *H. pylori* are seen. Scanning electron micrograph, × 3907.

junctions vital to the integrity of the epithelial cell surface. The continuity of this layer remains in spite of the different and often highly specialized cells of the gastrointestinal tract. Disruption of this epithelial cell continuity either by premature cell death or disintegration of the intercellular junction will result in a sequence of events leading to epithelial ulceration. The location of *H. pylori* near the zona occludens (Fig. 5.5) enables these bacteria to be ideally sited to disrupt these junctions (Fig. 5.6) and participate in the processes of ulceration. There is ultrastructural evidence for the disruption of these intercellular junctions near *H. pylori* and the siting of *H. pylori* in the intercellular spaces [3, 7, 10]. Whether this disruption of the intercellular junction results from the presence of

bacteria and what the mechanisms for this disruption are yet to be elucidated.

Ultrastructural evidence has also been produced for the intracellular invasion of *H. pylori*. These bacteria have been described in mucus granules, in lysosomes and closely related to such structures [3, 12, 13]. The frequency of such *H. pylori* invasion has been reported to be 10% in patients with active duodenal ulceration [3]. Whether such invasion is a characteristic of *H. pylori*, an alteration to *H. pylori* when subjected to appropriate conditions, or the crosscutting of ultra-thin sections is debatable. *In vitro*, *H. pylori* are characteristically non-invasive [14] and contrast with *Campylobacter jejuni*.

Helicobacter pylori are found in areas of acute and chronic gastritis. They are most numerous

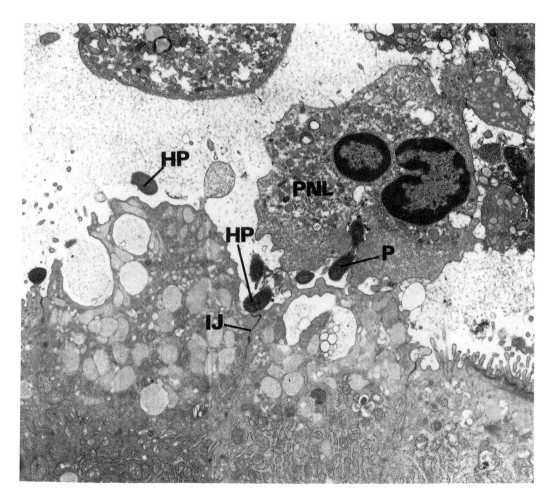

Fig. 5.5 *H. pylori* (HP) and a polymorphonuclear leucocyte (PNL) are closely related to gastric mucus-secreting cells. A bacterium is being phagocytosed (P) by the polymorphonuclear leucocyte. The close relationship between the *H. pylori* and the intercellular junctions (IJ) is apparent. Transmission electron micrograph, × 6350.

in those areas of active chronic gastritis [5, 6] when bacteria are frequently associated with migrating polymorphonuclear leucocytes (Fig. 5.7). At such sites there is positive correlation between the number of intraepithelial polymorphonuclear leucocytes and the number of bacteria [8]. This correlation is not absolute [6] and depends upon the site from which the biopsy has been taken. Thus, at the edge of a benign ulcer, there is a disproportionate number of intraepithelial polymorphonuclear leucocytes. At the edge of the ulcer, the protective mucus barrier is incomplete. This enables the gastric/duodenal fluid to reach the epithelial surface,

resulting in a hostile environment for *H. pylori* survival but acting as a potent stimulator of polymorphonuclear leucocyte migration. The nature of the chemotactic factors responsible for the migration of polymorphonuclear leucocytes at the sites of active chronic gastritis has not been fully elucidated. After migrating from the subepithelial layer through the overlying epithelium, phagocytosis of *H. pylori* by polymorphonuclear leucocytes does, however, occur [3–6, 15]. A bacterium in the process of being phagocytosed by an intraluminal polymorphonuclear leucocyte is seen in Fig. 5.5. This phagocytosis is less frequent than might be

teristics of the patient population tested and how *H. pylori* positivity is defined.

Urea concentration

2% Tests. All the modified 2% urea broth tests produce more rapid results than the originally described Christensen's broth, with a sensitivity of between 65% and 75% at 1 hour [6–9]. The increased sensitivity with the modified broths is either due to the smaller volume of broth used, the temperature of incubation or the increased concentration of phenol red, which makes the colour change easier to detect. Specimens yielding false negatives with these tests probably contain insufficient organisms to produce the pH change required. McNulty *et al.* [8] found that 70% (9 of 13) of specimens yielding a false negative modified urease test grew less than 10 colonies on culture. With all the 2% urea broth tests so far described there is a correlation between the degree of infection with *H. pylori* and the speed of the test. This difference in speed is not seen with the *Campylobacter*-like organisms (CLO) test [10], the 4-hour rapid urease test (RUT) of Vaira *et al.* [11] or the rapid tests. If in the future it became evident that the severity of infection was important, it might be useful to have a test which would differentiate scanty from profuse colonization.

6 and 10% Tests. The concentration of the urea has been increased in the tests described by Vaira *et al.* [11] and Arvind *et al.* [12] to 6% and 10% urea, respectively, to increase the speed of the results and attain a diagnosis before the patient leaves the endoscopy department. The ideal concentration of substrate in an enzyme reaction is usually 50–100 times the K_m value of the enzyme (a measure of affinity of an enzyme for its substrate), so that the substrate is in a large excess and the reaction rate is dependent only on the enzyme activity. *H. pylori* urease has a K_m value of 0.32 g/litre (8 mM [13]); the ideal concentration of urea would therefore be about 16–32 g/litre (1.6–3.2%). In theory too much substrate may result in inhibition of an enzyme;

however, in practice the 6% and 10% solutions do increase the sensitivity of the test and are very promising. Vaira *et al.* [9, 11] have described in short communications several rapid tests, including the 6% RUT. The constituents and methods described in their reports are not complete and have been modified with each communication. Their latest test contains 6% urea with no buffer, plus another ingredient that increases the stability and shelf-life of the test so that it can be made in advance and stored [11]. The test has similar specificity to and higher sensitivity than all the other tests at 1 hour but can be read at 20 min post-incubation – although many tests are positive immediately.

Arvind *et al.* [12] have described a 1-min test which must be freshly prepared in the endoscopy unit to avoid false positive results. It contains 1 ml of 10% urea in deionized distilled water with two drops of 1% phenol red solution added. The rapid results produced with this test may outweigh the disadvantages of the extra nursing time required to prepare the test. As the 1-min test has only been assessed in 40 patients thus far, further studies are required to confirm its high predictive value.

pH and pH indicator

The concentration of the pH indicator has been increased in some of the tests [8], which may decrease the time taken for the colour change by making it easier to detect. So far the pH of the urea broths has not been changed. Changing the pH of the broth so that it is closer to the ideal pH for urease activity (pH 8.2 [13]) might increase the sensitivity and speed of the test. This change will necessitate the use of an indicator with a higher pH range, for example *m*-cresol purple (pH range 7.4–9.0) or thymol blue (pH range 8.0–9.6), and a buffer with a higher pH range.

Liquid or agar?

Agar tests are easier to transport and inoculate and several workers have investigated their use. In the CLO test developed by Marshall *et al.* [10]

the urea is incorporated in a small bleb of agar, into which the biopsy specimen is placed. This eases transport of the test and due to the small volume of agar sensitivity remains high – 75% at 20 min. Simor *et al.* [14] inoculated biopsy specimens on to 2% agar slants. Despite incubation at 37 °C, these tests had only a 62% sensitivity at 4 hours. Diffusion of urease through the large volume of agar is probably poor and therefore this method would not be recommended.

Volume

The volume of broth or agar used in the tests varies between 50 μl and 1 ml. This will lead to great differences in urease concentrations attained by the same biopsy specimen. A small-volume test should produce more rapid and sensitive results. Hazell *et al.* [7] use a microtitre tray for the test. Biopsy specimens are dropped into only 50 μl of urea broth, which, because of the small volume, improves the sensitivity and speed of the test. The wells of the microtitre tray in this method must be sealed or the ammonia produced may diffuse to neighbouring wells and cause false positive results. Most of the other tests used between 0.2 ml and 0.5 ml of broth. Abdalla *et al.* [15] used 1 ml of 10% urea broth. When left at room temperature this test gave a sensitivity at 1 hour of only 62% – it is likely that superior results would have been obtained with a smaller volume. Sweeney *et al.* [16] drop a urea Minitek disc (BBL Microbiology Systems, Cockeysville, Md) into 0.2 ml of bacteriostatic saline. This simple test has a sensitivity of 75% at 1 hour. To obtain the best results workers should use the smallest volume they can handle and inoculate with ease – in practice this is probably 0.2 ml.

Temperature

The optimum temperature for urease is 45 °C [13]. Fewer organisms may be needed to produce a positive result if a test is incubated at or near this temperature. The sensitivity of all tests improves if incubated above room tem-

perature. Incubated at 30 °C the CLO test of Marshall *et al.* [10] has at least a 75% sensitivity [10, 17]. The original Christensen's urea broth is more sensitive when incubated at 37 °C (sensitivity 61% at room temerature, 67% at 37 °C [18]). When read at 1 hour the sensitivity of the 10% 1 ml urea test described by Abdalla *et al.* [15] improves from 62% when incubated at room temperature to 93% at 55 °C (Table 7.1).

Time of inoculation

The method and timing of inoculation are also important. Deltenre *et al.* [6] have found that immediate inoculation in the endoscopy unit, crushing the specimen and avoiding the use of transport media increase sensitivity.

False positives

Although false positives are a potential problem with these tests the specificity is near 100% even in the nutrient containing Christensen's broth. There are several reasons for this high specificity: contaminating bacteria are usually present in low numbers compared with *H. pylori*; no other organism produces urease with such high affinity or rate of activity [13]; the specimens are left at room temperature or read at 1 hour, or a bacteriostatic agent has been incorporated which prevents the rapid growth of other organisms.

Buffer

Buffer maintains the stability of the test during storage. Vaira *et al.* [9, 11] and Arvind *et al.* [12] have omitted the buffer from their tests and this produces very rapid results at room temperature. False positives may occur if read after the designated time. If a buffer is not used, it is better to prepare the tests just before inoculation.

Cost

Cost may be an important factor in the choise of biopsy urease test. The CLO test and Minitek urea disc are both commercial products and will therefore be more expensive, but they may be performed with ease without the use of a microbiology department. In contrast the 'home-made' urea broth tests can be made by the majority of microbiology departments for use in endoscopy and cost less than 5 p/test.

Advantages and disadvantages of the biopsy urease tests

The major advantage of the biopsy urease tests for the diagnosis of *H. pylori* infection is that they can be performed very simply and, with modification, results are obtainable before the patient leaves the endoscopy department. All the tests are extremely cheap when compared with the cost of culture or microscopy of histology sections.

There are several disadvantages. Despite the high sensitivity of the biopsy urease test, some positives will be missed. In a study of 1445 patients attending endoscopy *H. pylori* was detected in 628 patients. The Gram stain was positive in 582 patients, culture in 583, histology in 575 and the biopsy urease test in 553 [8]. The small lack of concordance is probably due to sampling variation; *H. pylori* infection can be patchy and organisms may be present in one specimen and not another. The test is not as sensitive when performed with specimens from patients who have received antimicrobial or bismuth treatment and Deltenre *et al.* [6] would not recommend their use in these circumstances.

If biopsy specimens are not sent for culture and histology, strains of *H. pylori* will not be available for serotyping or sensitivity testing and histology sections will not be available for histological assessment of the gastric mucosa – a major disadvantage during treatment trials. I consider the gold-standard diagnostic method required for research studies should still include detection by culture and histology, with the addition of the biopsy urease test if a rapid diagnosis is required.

Conclusion

In summary, all the biopsy urease tests have a specificity of near 100% and sensitivity of at least 70% at 1 hour and 90% at 24 hours. Several very rapid tests have now been described that give almost immediate results. All the tests so far described can be made quite easily in most microbiology departments for use by endoscopy units; alternatively several tests are now available commercially. The most sensitive and rapid test would contain a small volume (0.2 ml) of 4% urea solution with a high concentration of pH indicator, and would be incubated at or near to 45 °C. The tests can replace, at negligible expense, the diagnosis by culture or histology; if sensitivities and serotyping or histology of the gastric mucosa is required the other diagnostic methods should still be used. Although non-invasive diagnostic tests are now available, clinicians will probably continue to perform endoscopy and biopsy for the investigation of upper gastrointestinal disease and the biopsy urease test will continue to be a very useful rapid diagnostic test for *H. pylori* infection for many years to come.

References

1 Luck, J.M. & Seth, T.N. Gastric urease. *Biochem. J.* 1924, **18**, 1227–31.
2 Fitzgerald, O. & Murphy, P. Studies on the physiological chemistry and clinical significance of urease and urea with special reference to the stomach. *Ir. J. Med. Sci.* 1950, **292**, 97–159.
3 Kornberg, H.L., Davies, R.E. & Wood, D.R. The activity and function of gastric urease in the cat. *Biochem. J.* 1954, **56**, 363–72.
4 Langenberg, M.L., Tytgat, G.N., Schipper, M.E.I., Rietra, P.J.G.M. & Zanen, H.C. *Campylobacter*-like organisms in the stomach of patients and healthy individuals. *Lancet* 1984, **i**, 1348.
5 McNulty, C.A.M. & Wise, R. Rapid diagnosis of *Campylobacter*-associated gastritis. *Lancet* 1985, **i**, 1443–4.
6 Deltenre, M., Burette, A., Glupczynski, Y., Dekoster, E., De Prez, C. & Jonas, C. 1988. Rapid identification of *Campylobacter pylori* in gastric biopsies. In Menge, H., Gregor, M., Tytgat, G.N.J. & Marshall, B.J. (eds) *Campylobacter pylori*. Springer-Verlag, Berlin, pp. 135–44.
7 Hazell, S.L., Borody, T.J., Gal, A. & Lee, A. *Campylobacter pyloridis*. Gastritis I: detection of urease as a marker of bacterial colonization and gastritis. *Am. J. Gastroenterol.* 1987, **82**, 292–6.
8 McNulty, C.A.M., Dent, J.C., Uff, J.C., Gear, M.W.L. &

Wilkinson, S.P. Detection of *Campylobacter pylori* by the biopsy urease test: an assessment in 1445 patients. *Gut* 1989, **30**, 1058–62.

9 Vaira, D., Holton, J., Cairns, S., Falzon, M. & Salmon, P. Four hour rapid urease test (RUT) for detecting *Campylobacter pylori*: is it reliable to start treatment? *J. Clin. Pathol.* 1988, **41**, 355–6.

10 Marshall, B.J., Warren, J.R., Francis, G.J., Langton, S.R., Goodwin, C.S. & Blincow, E.D. Rapid urease test in the management of *Campylobacter pyloridis*-associated gastritis. *Am. J. Gastroenterol.* 1987, **82**, 200–10.

11 Vaira, D., Holton, J., Cairns, S., Polydorou, A., Falzon, M., Dowsett, J. & Salmon, P.R. Urease tests for *Campylobacter pylori*: care in interpretation. *J. Clin. Pathol.* 1988, **41**, 812–13.

12 Arvind, A.S., Cook, R.S., Tabaqchali, S. & Farthing, M.J.G. One-minute endoscopy room test for *Campylobacter pylori*. *Lancet* 1988, **i**, 704.

13 Mobley, H.L.T., Cortesia, M.J., Rosenthal, L.E. & Jones, B.D. Characterization of urease from *Campylo-bacter pylori*. *J. Clin. Microbiol.* 1988, **26**, 831–6.

14 Simor, A.E., Cooter, N.B. & Low, D.E. Comparison of four stains and a urease test for rapid detection of *Helicobacter pylori* in gastric biopsies. *Eur. J. Clin. Microbiol. Infect. Dis.* 1990, **9**, 350–2.

15 Abdalla, S., Marco, F., Perez, R.M. *et al.* Rapid detection of gastric *Campylobacter pylori* colonization by a simple biochemical test. *J. Clin. Microbiol.* 1989, **27**, 2604–5.

16 Sweeney, L., Garcia, L.P., Talbert, M., Silverman, M. & Needham, C.A. Minitek urea disk test, a sensitive and cost-effective method to screen for *Campylobacter pylori* in gastric biopsies. *J. Clin. Microbiol.* 1989, **27**, 2684–6.

17 Morris, A., McIntyre, D., Rose, T. & Nicholson, G. Rapid diagnosis of *Campylobacter pyloridis* infection. *Lancet* 1986, **i**, 149.

18 Westblom, T.U., Madan, E., Kemp, J. & Subik, M.A. Evaluation of a rapid urease test to detect *Campylobacter pylori* infection. *J. Clin. Microbiol.* 1988, **26**, 1393–4.

8 The Serology of Helicobacter pylori Infections

D.G.NEWELL AND A.R.STACEY

Introduction

It is now widely accepted that there is an association between *Helicobacter pylori* colonization of the gastric antrum and non-autoimmune (type B) gastritis and peptic ulceration. Histologically definable gastritis is, undoubtedly, a consequence of the local immune response of the host to this infection and involves the infiltration of lymphocytes, plasma cells, histiocytes and, frequently, polymorphonuclear cells into the lamina propria.

The role of antibodies in H. pylori-associated gastritis

A large proportion of the lymphoid cells infiltrating the gastric mucosa are immunoglobulin-secreting B cells [1]. These mature B cells in the gastric mucosa produce a local antibody response, which is primarily of the immunoglobulin A (IgA) and IgG classes [2].

The role of these local antibodies in the disease process is debatable. The extent of the response does not correlate with either the degree of inflammation or the presence of ulceration [3–6]. Although organisms attached to the gastric epithelium are coated with human immunoglobulin [7], the antibodies neither eliminate the colonization of the gastric mucosa nor prevent the re-establishment of the infection after clearance [8]. As *H. pylori* is sensitive *in vitro* to both antibody-dependent and antibody-independent, complement-mediated, bactericidal mechanisms [9, 10], this suggests that the organisms have a means of protecting themselves from the host response. Moreover, the localized immune response is so extensive that the possibility of a pathological role for host antibody in the disease process cannot be ignored.

The host circulating antibody response during infection

Most patients colonized with *H. pylori* elicit a measurable systemic antibody response, which may reflect the specificity of those antibodies produced at the gastric mucosa [11].

The immunoglobulin classes and subclasses of these circulating anti-*H. pylori* antibodies are consistent with a prolonged chronic mucosal infection, with IgG and IgA predominating and IgM antibodies rarely seen [2, 5], even in children with acute infections [12]. Serum levels of the IgG-1 and IgG-4 antibodies are significantly raised, and so is specific IgG-2, but not in all cases. IgG-3 antibodies, which generally indicate acute infection, are not detected [5]. In the singe well-documented volunteer study, where ingestion of *H. pylori* eventually led to chronic gastritis, IgG seroconversion occurred between 22 and 33 days post-infection [13]. Subsequent studies showed that there was also an initial, short-lived IgM response and a seroconversion of specific IgA [14].

The antigenic specificity of anti-H. pylori antibodies

The response of the host to those bacterial antigens to which it is exposed during infection, and thereby the antibodies produced, is directed by a variety of both host and bacterial factors. Little is known of the immune response to infection at the gastric mucosal surface or of how that response spills over into the circulation. However, epithelial damage, the massive infiltration of immunocompetent cells, the efficiency of the antigen-presenting cells and the chronic nature of the infection will all affect the molecular basis of the host response. There are two main methods for analysing antibody specificity at the molecular level. The first is the radio-immuno-precipitation assay (RIPA), which involves the separation and identification, by sodium dodecyl sulphate polyacrylamide gel electrophoresis (SDS-PAGE), of ^{125}I-labelled bacterial surface antigens bound to the antibodies and immuno-precipitated on to agarose beads. The second, and easier, method is western blotting, which involves the electrophoretic transfer on to nitrocellulose of bacterial antigens separated by PAGE. Antibodies bound to these immobilized antigens are detected by an enzyme-linked antibody system. A sophisticated alternative to western blotting is the electroelution of separated polypeptides from the PAGE gel and the analysis of their antigenicity by enzyme-linked immunosorbent assay (ELISA) [15]. Because of conformational changes potentially induced in the antigen by PAGE or the limitations of the radio-labelling techniques, these techniques may not provide identical results but should be considered as complementary. An alternative, with limited resolution, is the use of purified, or partly purified, antigens bound to a plastic support in an ELISA system [16].

Significant differences in the molecular weights of the major protein antigens have been reported. Such variations are largely due to the PAGE systems used. However, it seems that most *H. pylori*-positive patients produce antibodies that react against 61 and 28 kD polypeptides, which are specific for *H. pylori* and which are probably urease components [17, 18]. Other, apparently specific, antigens frequently detected by positive sera include a 110–120 kD protein [6, 19, 20], a 56 kD polypeptide associated with urease [18], and several series of high (87–86, 63–57 kD) and low (20–22, 14–16 kD) molecular weight proteins [4, 6]. Almost all sera react with polypeptides of 54 kD, which is flagellin, and 56 kD, which appears to comprise

flagella-associated proteins. Some of these polypeptides are not specific for *H. pylori* [21, 22]. At present no single protein antigen has been detected which consistently reacts with all the positive sera investigated. Most reports, therefore, agree that the antibody response to *H. pylori* is both complex and highly variable. The observation that individual sera will detect the same major antigens in heterologous strains as in the homologous strain [21] supports the contention that this variation in antibody specificity is host-mediated rather than a reflection of antigenic differences between infecting strains.

Nevertheless, serological tests to detect circulating anti-*H. pylori* antibodies could be useful, not only for epidemiological and research investigations but also as tools for the pre-endoscopic screening of dyspeptic patients and the monitoring of treatment.

Techniques for serodiagnosis

Serum anti-*H. pylori* antibodies can be detected by a variety of serological assays. Such tests include the complement fixation test (CFT), haemagglutination, bacterial agglutination, immunofluorescence and ELISA [20, 23, 24]. ELISA is currently the technique of choice in most laboratories, because of its speed, low cost, simplicity and reproducibility. However, both western blotting and RIPA may be ultrasensitive tools in serodiagnosis. Although the variation in human antibody specificity at the molecular level is great, sufficiently specific antigens are present to allow accurate diagnosis.

The ELISA technique involves the absorption of antigen on to a plastic support, usually the well of a 96-well microtitre plate. Excess antigen is removed by washing and diluted serum is incubated with the immobilized antigen. After washing, human immunoglobulin bound to the antigen is detected using an anti-human immunoglobulin coupled to an enzyme, such as peroxidase. The peroxidase indirectly bound to the antigen can then be visualized using a chromogenic enzyme substrate. The assay is quantitative, with the optical density of the coloured product being directly proportional to the

Table 8.1 Criteria for the selection of suitable ELISA antigens.

Contains a high proportion of immunogenic
 components
Immunogens should be common to all *H. pylori* strains
Absence of antigenic cross-reactions with other
 organisms
Absence of non-specific immunoglobulin binding
Easily prepared and purified
Bind effectively to the plastic support
Stable on storage

amount of antibody bound. The antibody concentration in the serum can be measured by reference to standard curves or antibody titres obtained by serial dilution of the serum.

Antigens for ELISA serodiagnosis

The sensitivity and specificity of the ELISA is largely dependent on the nature of the antigenic material bound to the solid plastic support. The criteria essential for the selection of a suitable antigenic material for ELISA are given in Table 8.1.

Several antigens have now been investigated for ELISA serodiagnosis. Originally crude antigens, such as whole-cell sonicates, were used but these tended to give high backgrounds, a high proportion of false positive sera and a poor sensitivity. It is now widely considered that these crude antigens are generally unsatisfactory for the accurate diagnosis of *H. pylori*-related gastritis. However, some serodiagnostic tests based on such a crude antigen provide acceptable sensitivities and specificities [25].

Partly purified antigens have now been developed. The most common of these antigens in use at present is an acid-extractable material eluted from the surface of whole organisms in 0.2 M glycine buffer, pH 2.2. Both this antigen and an ultracentrifuged whole-cell sonicate antigen comprise a number of polypeptides as determined by SDS-PAGE (Fig. 8.1). ELISAs with these complex antigens generally detect approximately 95% of patients with *H. pylori* infection with a specificity of over 90% [25–27].

More recently several highly purified anti-

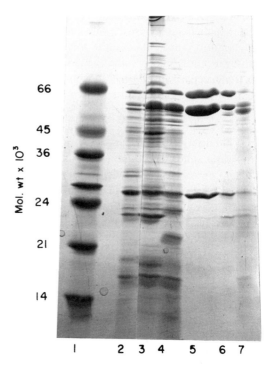

Fig. 8.1 Total protein profile of antigens used in serodiagnosis determined by SDS-PAGE using 10–25% gradient gel. Track 1 – standards; track 2 – acid extract; tract 3 – whole-cell sonicate; track 4 – French Press urease preparation; tracks 5 and 6 – fast protein liquid chromatography (FPLC)-purified urease; track 7 ultracentrifuged cell sonicate (prepared by B.J. Rathbone) (from Newell & Rathbone 1989 [26]).

gens, including urease and the 120 kD polypeptide, have been described, which are discussed in detail below.

Without doubt the ability of the serodiagnostic test to accurately detect *H. pylori*-associated disease would be further improved with the development of even better antigens. Several major problems, discussed below, inherent in the antigenic material have now been identified which influence the specificity and sensitivity of the ELISA test.

Antigenic variation between H. pylori strains

A proportion of sera from patients with proved *H. pylori* infection do not appear to have a detectable antibody response. As most antigen preparations are the product of a limited number of *H. pylori* strains (one to five strains), the presence of antigenic variation within the species could prevent the detection of antibody responses in those patients infected with the less common variants. There is some evidence for the presence of serotype-specific antigens on *H. pylori*, detectable by hyperimmune rabbit sera in agglutination systems [28] and by western blotting [29], and that this serotype specificity is geographically distributed [29]. However, it is unlikely that antibody specificity observed with hyperimmune rabbit antisera will reflect the specificity of the human antibody responses induced by infection. In agglutination systems the serotype differences probably result from the diversity in *H. pylori* lipopolysaccharides [30]. Lipopolysaccharides bind indifferently to micro-ELISA plate plastics and may only marginally influence ELISA results. However, the inclusion of more strains in the antigen preparation only marginally increases the sensitivity of the sero-diagnostic test, if at all [31]. Moreover, antigen derived from only one strain provided excellent results in sera from a geographically remote country [25]. The serotypic differences observable in agglutination techniques, therefore, are probably not relevant when using the ELISA technique.

Non-specific immunoglobulin binding

H. pylori can non-specifically bind human immunoglobulin. Such processes could be advantageous to the host, enhancing opsinophagocytosis [9], but may also, by virtue of Fc receptor-like properties, form the basis of the organism's protection from host antibody responses. Nevertheless, this non-specific immunoglobulin binding can also cause unacceptable high backgrounds in the ELISA technique. The use of Fab$_2$ fragments conjugated to the enzyme reduces some of this non-specific binding (A.R. Stacey, unpublished data). However, the major components mediating this non-specificity appear to be confined to a high-molecular-weight fraction of sonicated *H. pylori*, which can be largely eliminated from the whole-cell sonicate [16].

Antigenic cross-reactivity with other bacteria

Some of the surface antigens of *H. pylori*, in particular the flagella-associated proteins, have epitopes in common with *Campylobacter* species [23, 32–34]. Unfortunately these flagella-associated proteins are extremely immunogenic. The presence of such proteins in the antigen preparation would prevent the exclusion of those seropositive patients with, for example, a recent *C. jejuni* infection [21]. Some authors advise the screening of sera for anti-*C. jejuni* as well as anti-*H. pylori* antibodies [4]. In general flagellins would be difficult to selectively exclude from a crude antigen without significantly reducing sensitivity.

Although it is generally considered that the urease antigens are specific for *H. pylori*, in fact, antigenic cross-reactivity exists with the ureases of other gastric-colonizing organisms, including *Gastrospirillum hominis* [35]. Evidence suggests that such antigenic cross-reactivity may be a complicating factor in serodiagnosis. However, infection with *G. hominis* is a relatively rare event, except in non-human primates.

In view of these problems, second-generation serodiagnostic tests incorporating the development of purified ELISA antigens has become necessary.

The choice and isolation of purified antigens for ELISA

Both the sensitivity and specificity of the serodiagnostic test may be significantly improved using species-specific antigens. Preferably these should be proteins or glycoproteins, which bind most effectively to ELISA plates and are readily purified.

A major problem in the production of purified antigens is the large-scale growth of *H. pylori*. Recently chemostat culture techniques have been developed which can produce up to 1 g bacterial mass per day under defined growth conditions. The antigenic composition of this material is directly comparable to plate-grown cells (M.Hudson & K.Lee, unpublished data).

As mentioned previously, few proteins, if any, are detected by all *H. pylori*-positive sera using techniques like western blotting or RIPA. One such antigen is a 120 kD protein [21]. This antigen, which is probably equivalent to the antigen 9 described by Hirschl *et al.* [15], can be isolated by electroelution after preparative SDS-PAGE [15] with retention of antigenicity. However, there is evidence to suggest that this protein is not expressed by all strains of *H. pylori* [21]. Therefore, although this material is unsuitable as a univalent antigen, the selective enrichment of complex antigens, such as the acid extract, by the 120 kD polypeptide results in a significantly improved sensitivity and specificity [36]. Nevertheless, electroelution is not an easy technique for large-scale production, and other preparative techniques should be considered.

Another protein that is generally specific to *H. pylori*, although also found in *G. hominis*, is the urease. Several methods of urease production and purification have been described. The supernatant retained following ultracentrifugation of antigens disrupted by French Press [37] or by sonication [16] has a high urease activity. As an ELISA antigen this crude urease preparation has a very good sensitivity [16]. However, the specificity of antigens prepared by these methods is similar to that of the whole-cell sonicate [31], which they closely resemble as seen by SDS-PAGE analysis (Fig. 8.1).

A high-molecular-weight protein of 400–700 kD is also reported to have urease activity [38]. This antigen is eluted from the surface of the organism in 1% *n*-octyl-glucose and is then purified by size-exclusion gel filtration on an agarose A-5m column. The effect of the detergent treatment on urease conformation appears to be minimal as enzyme activity is retained. In an ELISA system this antigen appears to have an excellent sensitivity (98.3%) and specificity (100%) in comparison with the ^{13}C breath test and/or culture and biopsy observation.

A significantly purified urease preparation can also be obtained from disrupted cells by means of size-exclusion gel filtration by fast protein liquid chromatography (FPLC) [16]. The material obtained by this method comprises a single protein with urease activity, by PAGE, under non-denaturing conditions and has a molecular weight of approximately 500 kD. By SDS-PAGE analysis, under reduced conditions, this material comprises three major polypeptide bands with molecular weights of 61, 56 and 28 kD. Although only two of these polypeptides are essential components of the urease, all three have been shown to be antigenic during human infections by western blotting techniques (A.R. Stacey, unpublished data). In an ELISA this purified urease antigen has, once again, an excellent specificity but appears to have a slightly reduced sensitivity when compared with the acid-extract antigen [16]. All investigations to date suggest that partly purified urease is highly immunogenic during infection. This has been confirmed using urease affinity purified by monoclonal antibodies directed against the 28 kD polypeptide [16]. Although the majority of *H. pylori*-infected patients produced anti-urease antibodies, some patients, known to have anti-*H. pylori* antibodies by the acid-extract ELISA and to be ^{14}C breath test-positive, did not have circulating anti-urease antibodies detectable either by ELISA or by western blotting (A.R. Stacey, unpublished data).

The results obtained so far with purified material confirm that the antibody response to *H. pylori* is, in general, unique to every patient, with individuals responding to different immunogenic proteins on the surface of the organism. Consequently, antigen preparations comprising single proteins, like the urease, cannot provide the sensitivity necessary for an ideal ELISA antigen. However, antigens with enhanced proportions of urease, purified by chromatographic fractionation procedures, now form the basis of second-generation serodiagnostic tests [39]. To this end, the expression of the genes of immunodominant antigens in *Escherichia coli* [40] and the use of monoclonal anti-urease antibodies for affinity purification [18] will allow the large-scale production of this pure antigenic material. Chromatographic fractionation can also be used to selectively remove unwanted components like the cross-reactive flagellin or non-specific binding material [16, 39].

The value of immunoglobulin class analysis in serodiagnosis

The detection of IgA as well as IgG antibodies can significantly increase sensitivity [41], although in some cases IgG antibodies are present in the absence of raised specific IgA [5]. It is possible that an assay which detects both classes may be the best method of enhancing the sensitivity. The value of IgG subclass detection has yet to be investigated; however, preliminary evidence suggests that specific circulating IgG-4 is an excellent indicator of infection.

The role of serology in epidemiological investigations

Serology is a non-invasive method of diagnosing H. pylori infection with a reasonable accuracy. Moreover, it is a relatively inexpensive and simple technique, now readily available from commercial sources. Seroepidemiology, therefore, is a significant tool in the investigation of the prevalence of H. pylori infection, its sources and its modes of transmission.

In studies of normal healthy blood donors the overall prevalence of anti-H. pylori antibodies appears to be about 20–30% [4, 42, 43]. However, this prevalence is both age- and geographically dependent. In Great Britain the frequency of anti-H. pylori antibodies in asymptomatic children under the age of 15 years is about 5%, rising gradually to 50–75% in the general population over the age of 50 years [4]. The prevalence then generally plateaus, or falls, in the elderly. This trend is similar in populations throughout the developed world [44–47]. Preliminary studies indicate that the fall in seropositivity in the elderly is probably not a true fall in infection but is, more probably, a reflection of age-associated immune incompetence. Age is, therefore, an important consideration in seroepidemiological studies.

The geographical location of the population under investigation is also important. Not only the country, but also the province, is relevant, as the prevalence of infection may vary significantly from region to region [48]. Raised antibodies are common in children from Third World areas

[49, 50]. Moreover, the proportion of seropositive adults tends to be higher in underdeveloped countries. It should also be remembered that a high prevalence of asymptomatic carriage of C. jejuni occurs in underdeveloped countries, which could influence the serological data.

Finally, ethnic origin should be considered in seroepidemiological studies. For example, higher proportions of asymptomatic individuals of Chinese and Indian origin living in Texas [50] and Asians living in Birmingham, UK [51], are H. pylori-positive than their age-matched Caucasian controls.

The role of serology in diagnosing histological gastritis and peptic ulceration

Potentially the major clinical role for serodiagnosis is the screening of dyspeptic patients for H. pylori infection. Dyspepsia is a considerable clinical problem in general practice [52, 53]. Traditionally these patients are investigated by endoscopy or radiology, both expensive and time-consuming techniques.

Although up to 75% of patients attending gastroenterology clinics with upper abdominal pain are diagnosed as having non-ulcer dyspepsia [54], a significant proportion of these patients will have H. pylori-associated gastritis. Serological tests currently available diagnose chronic gastritis with acceptable accuracy. The prevalence of anti-H. pylori antibodies in patients with histologically defined gastritis is 80–90% (specificity >90%, sensitivity >80% and positive predictive value 80–95%) [26]. As these figures depend on the pathologist's definition of chronic gastritis and its distinction from normal histology, the real correlation is probably even greater. However, the value of serodiagnosis in these patients is debatable, particularly as the role of H. pylori infection in non-ulcer dyspepsia is questionable [55]. Nevertheless, should eradication of the infection be shown to alleviate dyspeptic symptoms, then a serodiagnostic test would have significant therapeutic implications. Similarly, the identification of H. pylori infection in those patients with peptic ulcers will not necessarily influence patient management, although the choice of those anti-ulcer drugs with antimicrobial activity may affect the ulcer relapse rate [26].

Serology is potentially very useful in diagnosing *H. pylori*-related gastroduodenal disease in children. However, it seems likely that the criteria for seropositivity may need to be adjusted from those already established for adults in order to allow accurate detection of the low antibody levels expected in childhood acute infections.

It is generally considered that up to 50% of all dyspeptic patients are histologically, and thereby endoscopically, normal. The prior selection of only those patients who would benefit from further investigation could, therefore, reduce endoscopic workloads, releasing substantial National Health Service resources [26, 53]. In this case a non-invasive technique to diagnose gastritis could become an essential pre-endoscopic procedure. Such a test may be used either to exclude seronegative patients from further investigation by endoscopy or to treat seropositive patients. As seropositive individuals would also include the majority of high-risk patients, especially those with peptic ulcer and gastric cancer, it would seem that the first option is preferable in order to avoid missing those patients with treatable gastric cancer [53]. To this end, it is additionally recommended that an age limit (40–45 years of age) is imposed on those patients screened in order to avoid missing those at higher risk from gastric cancer. The incorporation of such a screening procedure into the routine management of the patient will, of course, require evaluation in controlled trials. However, an initial retrospective study, using a strategy which was designed to detect patients with gastric cancer or peptic ulcer disease, indicates that a significant proportion (about 22%) of younger (under 40 years) *H. pylori*-negative patients could be excluded from endoscopy [56]. Such a strategy failed to detect only 3.1% of all peptic ulcers.

The role of serology in monitoring treatment

The specific serum IgG response remains con-

stant throughout the infection [47, 57]. However, several studies now suggest that both IgG and IgA levels decrease after treatment and concomitant clearance of the organism [6, 8, 58, 59]. Nevertheless, the fall is generally slow, with patients attaining normal levels only after 6 months or so [59]. Reinfection is accompanied by a rapid rise in titre [57]. It is therefore considered that serology is a reliable, albeit slow, indicator of effective treatment. Certain improvements in technology may allow more accurate prediction of eradication in the future. For example, it seems likely that some antibodies, particularly those directed against certain surface antigens and those of the short-lived subclasses of IgG, such as IgG-2, fall more rapidly following treatment and are therefore more suitable for monitoring treatment.

Conclusion

The majority of people colonized with *H. pylori* elicit a specific antibody response. Immunochemical techniques have shown that the host response to *H. pylori* is not only complex but extremely variable. This, coupled with the fact that up to 20% of the normal population are infected with *H. pylori* while remaining asymptomatic, indicates that the ability of the host to respond to the organism may be an important factor in the aetiology of *H. pylori*-associated gastritis. It seems likely, therefore, that research focusing on these areas of investigation should be profitable.

Serological tests have become an important tool in the detection of *H. pylori*-associated gastritis. In comparative studies, the sensitivities and specificities of both ELISA and western blotting correlate well with the invasive methods of detection, biopsy bacterial culture and histology. However, western blotting is costly and time-consuming and requires considerable expertise, so the ELISA system would be preferred since the technique is already in use in many routine laboratories. Recently, several commercial serodiagnostic kits, generally based on ELISA, have become available which compare favourably with current laboratory-based tests.

The antigens currently employed routinely in the serodiagnosis of *H. pylori* have been improved in terms of their sensitivity, specificity and reliability. Nevertheless, the development of better antigens is still necessary. Second-generation antigens are now being identified. Nevertheless, the unicomponent antigens, such as the purified urease, whilst having good specificity are still insufficiently sensitive. This is probably due to the variation in the patient antibody response. Future research should concentrate on the identification and isolation of multiple specific antigens from the organism and the establishment of techniques to prepare these antigens in reasonable quantities.

References

1 Kirchner, T., Melber, A., Fischbach, W., Heilmann, K.L. & Hermelink, H.K. 1990. Immunohistological patterns of the local immune response in *Helicobacter* gastritis. In Malfertheiner, P. & Ditschuneit, H. (eds) *Helicobacter pylori, Gastritis and Peptic Ulcer*. Springer-Verlag, Berlin, pp. 213–22.

2 Rathbone, B.J., Wyatt, J.I., Worsley, B.W., Shires, S.E., Trejdosiewicz, L.K., Heatley, R.V. & Losowsky, M.S. Systemic and local antibody responses to gastric *Campylobacter pyloridis* in non-ulcer dyspepsia. *Gut* 1986, **27**, 642–7.

3 Booth, L., Holdstock, G., MacBride, H., Hawtin, P., Gibson, J.R., Ireland, A., Bamforth, J., DuBoulay, C.E., Lloyd, R.S. & Pearson, A.D. Clinical importance of *Campylobacter pyloridis* and associated serum IgG and IgA antibody responses in patients undergoing upper gastrointestinal endoscopy. *J. Clin. Pathol.* 1986, **39**, 215–19.

4 Jones, D.M., Eldridge, J., Fox, A.J., Sethi, P. & Whorwell, P.J. Antibody to the gastric campylobacter-like organism ('*Campylobacter pyloridis*') – clinical correlations and distribution in the normal population. *J. Med. Microbiol.* 1986, **22**, 57–62.

5 Steer, H.W., Hawtin, P.R. & Newell, D.G. An ELISA technique for the serodiagnosis of *Campylobacter pyloridis* infection in patients with gastritis and benign duodenal ulceration. *Serodiagnosis Immunother.* 1987, **1**, 253–9.

6 Von Wulffen, H., Grote, H.J., Gaterman, S., Loning, T., Berger, B. & Buhl, C. Immunoblot analysis of immune response to *Campylobacter pylori* and its clinical associations. *J. Clin. Pathol.* 1988, **41**, 653–9.

7 Wyatt, J.I., Rathbone, B.J. & Heatley, R.V. Local immune response to gastric *Campylobacter* in non-ulcer dyspepsia. *J. Clin. Microbiol.* 1986, **39**, 863–70.

8 Langenberg, W., Rauws, E.A.J., Widjojokusumo, A., Tytgat, G.N.J. & Zanen, H.C. Identification of *Campylobacter pyloridis* isolates by restriction endonuclease DNA analysis. *J. Clin. Microbiol.* 1986, **24**, 414–17.

9 Das, S.S., Karin, Q.N. & Easmon, C.S.F. Opsonophagocytosis of *Campylobacter pylori*. *J. Med. Microbiol.* 1988, **27**, 125–30.

10 Pruul, H., Lee, P.C., Goodwin, C.S. & McDonald, P.J. Interaction of *Campylobacter pyloridis* within human immune defence mechanisms. *J. Med. Microbiol.* 1987, **23**, 233–8.

11 Stacey, A.R., Hawtin, P.R. & Newell, D.G. 1990. Local immune responses to *Helicobacter pylori*. In Malfertheiner, P. & Ditschuneit, H. (eds) *Helicobacter pylori, Gastritis and Peptic Ulcer*. Springer Verlag, Berlin, pp. 162–6.

12 Mitchell, H.M., Bohane, T.D., Berkowicz, J., Hazell, S.L. & Lee, A. Antibody to *Campylobacter pylori* in families of index children with gastrointestinal illness due to *Campylobacter pylori*. *Lancet* 1987, **ii**, 681–2.

13 Morris, A. & Nicholson, G. Ingestion of *Campylobacter pyloridis* causes gastritis and raised fasting pH. *Am. J. Gastroenterol.* 1987, **82**, 192–9.

14 Morris, A. & Nicholson, G. 1989. *Campylobacter pylori*: human ingestion studies. In Rathbone, B.J. & Heatley, R.V. (eds) *Campylobacter pylori and Gastroduodenal Disease*. Blackwell Scientific Publications, Oxford, pp. 185–9.

15 Hirschl, A.M., Pletschette, M., Hirschl, M.H., Berger, J., Stanek, G. & Rotter, M.L. Comparison of different antigen preparations in an evaluation of the immune response to *Campylobacter pylori*. *Eur. J. Clin. Microbiol. Infect. Dis.* 1988, **7**, 570–5.

16 Stacey, A.R., Hawtin, P.R. & Newell, D.G. Antigenicity of fractions of *Helicobacter pylori* prepared by fast protein liquid chromatography and urease captured by monoclonal antibodies. *Eur. J. Clin. Microbiol. Infect. Dis.* 1990, **9**, 732–7.

17 Hu, L.T. & Mobley, H.L.T. Purification and N-terminal analysis of urease from *Helicobacter pylori*. *Infect. Immun.* 1990, **58**, 992–8.

18 Hawtin, P.R., Stacey, A.R. & Newell, D.G. Investigation of the structure and localization of the urease of *Helicobacter pylori* using monoclonal antibodies. *J. Gen. Microbiol.* 1990, **136**, 1995–2000.

19 Apel, I., Jacobs, E., Kist, M. & Bredt, W. Antibody response of patients against a 120 kDa surface protein of *Campylobacter pylori*. *Zentralbl. Bakteriol. Mikrobiol. Hyp.* 1988, **268**, 271–6.

20 Kaldor, J., Tee, W., Nicolacopolous, C., Demirtzoglou, K., Noonan, D. & Dywer, B. Immunoblot confirmation of immune response to *Campylobacter pyloridis* in patients with duodenal ulcers. *Med. J. Aust.* 1986, **145**, 133–5.

21 Newell, D.G. Human antibody responses to the surface protein antigens of *Campylobacter pyloridis*. *Serodiagnosis Immunother.* 1987, **1**, 209–17.

22 Newell, D.G. Identification of the outer membrane proteins of *Campylobacter pyloridis* and antigenic

9 Detection of Helicobacter pylori by the ^{14}C-urea Breath Test

G.D.BELL AND J.WEIL

Helicobacter pylori has extremely high urease activity: it has been shown to be between 20 and 70 times that of, for instance, *Proteus* [1]. This important observation has become the basis of the various 'rapid urease tests' now available. Endoscopy is required to obtain gastric biopsies for the detection of *H. pylori* organisms, whether this is by culture, the rapid urease test or examination of histological specimens by one of the various stains currently in use. The serological detection of *H. pylori* is of considerable value for epidemiological studies as to whether particular groups of patients and healthy volunteers are infected with *H. pylori*. However, the demonstrated falls in titres of antibody to the organism which have been reported following bismuth/antibiotic therapy are unlikely to be sufficiently sensitive to accurately predict in which patient the organism has been successfully eradicated from the stomach, rather than, as so frequently happens, merely temporarily suppressed [2]. Many groups have now reported their experience of serological follow-up after eradication of *H. pylori*. Although the mean antibody levels fall progressively with time after successful eradication, our experience suggests that some patients' immunoglobulin G (IgG) antibody levels may take several years to return to the 'normal' range. Figure 9.1 shows the total IgG response of five *H. pylori*-positive patients who were successfully treated with various bismuth/antibiotic combinations. Figure 9.2 shows the ^{14}C-urea breath test performed on the same five patients. It can be seen that the 1 month post-treatment ^{14}C-urea breath test was unequivocally negative and remained so throughout the period of 1 year's observation, while in contrast, in Fig. 9.1, the serum IgG levels dropped much more slowly. Some of the patients' total IgG levels took many months to show any response.

It is our belief that the ^{14}C-urea breath test is a reasonably sensitive, inexpensive, non-invasive and reproducible test for *H. pylori* detection and may have a particular role to play in serially monitoring the efficacy (or otherwise) of different forms of treatment designed to eradicate the organism. The ^{13}C-urea test has the advantage of using a stable non-radioactive isotope [3]. It has, however, the major disadvantage that the $^{13}CO_2$ expired in the patient's breath requires the use of a mass spectrometer, which costs over 10 times as much as a simple scintillation beta counter and is thus unlikely to be widely available outside teaching hospitals/university centres.

In this chapter, we shall concentrate on discussing the technique involved in the ^{14}C-urea breath test, giving examples of its use before discussing the points for and against its use as a diagnostic test. We have relied heavily on our own experience at the Ipswich Hospital [2, 4–14]. The results from other groups, such as Marshall & Surveyor in Australia [15], Rauws, Tytgat and co-workers in Amsterdam [16], Hunt's group in Ontario (Veldhuyzen van Zanten *et al.* [17]), Phillips' group from the Mayo Clinic (Ormand *et al.* [18]), Husebye *et al.* from Oslo [19], Conti-Nibali *et al.* from Messina, Italy [20], and Glupczynski *et al.* from Brussels [21], are compared and contrasted with our own experience. Many other groups are using the ^{14}C-urea breath test to monitor the efficacy of various treatment regimens designed to suppress/eradicate *H. pylori*, as well as the effect of

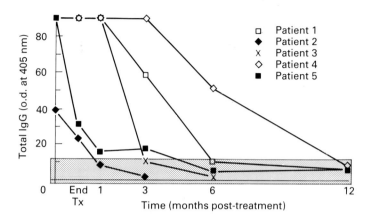

Fig. 9.1 Total IgG levels in five patients taken on the same day as attendance for ^{14}C-urea breath test. The authors are grateful to Dr Diane Newell who analysed the serum samples. A figure of > 10 μg per ml is used as a 'cut-off' between positive and negative individuals. Tx = treatment.

inhibition of *H. pylori* urease activity with aceto-hydroxamic acid [22] or the suppression of gastric urease activity by antacids [23]. Finally, a ^{14}C-urea breath test has been developed to study ferrets colonized with *Helicobacter mustelae*, looking particularly at the effects of urease inhibitors, bismuth and antibiotics [24].

The ^{14}C-urea breath test – standard 2-hour test

Technique

Our patients are fasted overnight. At 9 a.m. each patient is given 350 ml of a liquid meal, followed immediately by 0.4 MBq ^{14}C-urea (Amersham International) in 20 ml of water. The patients are asked to lie on their right side for a few seconds and then on the left for a few more seconds in an attempt to get the labelled urea evenly distributed over the lining of the stomach. Breath samples are collected at 10, 20,

30, 40, 60, 80, 100 and 120 min after ingestion of the ^{14}C-urea. The patients exhale through a tube of anhydrous calcium chloride into a vial containing 2 mmol of hyamine (a trapping agent for CO_2) in 2 ml of ethanol, with phenolphthalein as indicator; decolorization of this solution indicates the collection of 2 mmol of exhaled CO_2. Then 10 ml of toluene-based scintillate is added, and the ^{14}C activity measured by liquid scintillation counting. A 1% standard is also counted and the activity expressed as the percentage of the administered dose per millimole of expired CO_2. This is multiplied by body-weight (kg) to allow for endogenous CO_2 production. The area under the curve (AUC) is then computed, using the trapezoid rule for each individual 2-hour breath test. The single figure derived is then used as an expression of the cumulative excretion of [14]CO_2.

The principle of the test is illustrated in Fig. 9.3, and an example of the breath test on a

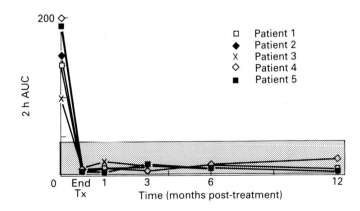

Fig. 9.2 ^{14}C-urea breath test (UBT) results for the same five patients as in Fig. 9.1 before, at the end of and following treatment (Tx) resulting in *H. pylori* eradication. Shaded area represents negative UBT.

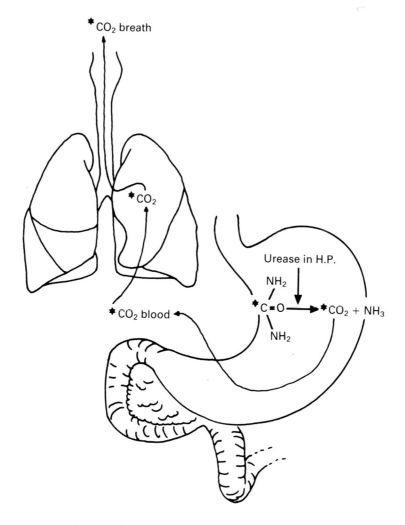

Fig. 9.3 Schematic drawing of the principle of the ^{14}C-urea breath test. When ^{14}C-labelled urea is administered orally, urea-derived labelled CO_2 appears in the breath of *H. pylori*-infected individuals.

patient who was *H. pylori*-positive (by culture and histological criteria) before and again at the end of a 1-month course of bismuth subcitrate (De-Nol Brocades) is shown in Fig. 9.4. It can be seen that ^{14}C-labelled CO_2 rapidly appears in the breath of the patient. (The peak, in our experience, may be anywhere between 20 min and 60 min, with a mean of 40 min.)

The patient may need to exhale into the hyamine for between 1 and 3 min to achieve decolorization of the solution (thus indicating the collection of 2 mmol of exhaled CO_2). Marshall & Surveyor [15] employ only 1 mmol of hyamine,

which halves the time the patient needs to blow into the solution, since only 1 mmol of CO_2 is trapped. Since the radioactive counts obtained are high and there is reasonably clear separation between *H. pylori*-positive and *H. pylori*-negative groups, this appears to us to be a perfectly reasonable 'short cut'.

The dose of ^{14}C-urea used by both Marshall & Surveyor [15] and ourselves [4–14] is much higher than is necessary. We now use 0.2 MBq (5 μCi). The Amsterdam group [16] use 110 kBq (3 μCi) of ^{14}C-labelled urea. Hunt's group [17] use 5 μCi while others use 2.5 μCi [19]. Interes-

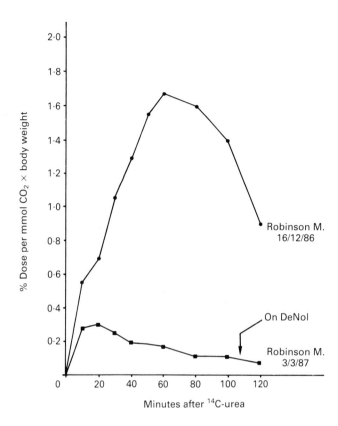

Fig. 9.4 Typical ^{14}C-urea breath test result in an *H. pylori* positive individual before and again while taking the bismuth preparation, De-Nol.

tingly, Conti-Nibali and colleagues [20] are now using a patient dose of only 37 kBq (1 μCi) of ^{14}C-urea. They have used the test on children, as well as their parents, and achieved good separation between *Helicobacter*-positive and negative patients.

Our own discussions with Amersham International led us to suspect that it probably was not necessary to give ^{14}C-urea mixed with 'cold' ^{12}C-urea. We have never included any ^{12}C-urea in our protocol, although we are aware that others are doing so [16, 17].

We do not agree with the Australian workers [15] that it is necessary to avoid giving H$_2$ blockers for 48 hours prior to the ^{14}C-urea breath test, or to wash out the mouth of the patient prior to examination because of the theoretical risk of urease-splitting mouth organisms affecting the test. It is perfectly true that high counts are obtained in the first 2–3 min after ingesting the ^{14}C-urea. However, most groups now (see below) consider that taking samples between

20 min and 2 hours and avoiding taking samples in the first few minutes dispose of this problem.

We have always given the ^{14}C-urea with a test meal in the hope that this might delay gastric emptying, and thus increase the time for which the radioactive urea is in contact with the organism. We have no personal evidence to suggest that the test would not work equally well without giving a test meal. The Amsterdam group [16] have looked at the effects of the test meal on the recovery of ^{14}CO$_2$ in nine patients by repeating the test within 24 hours without the test meal. The test meal had no effect on the ability of the test to identify *H. pylori*-positive individuals. When the breath test was carried out with a test meal, however, the resolution of the curves increased substantially. In *H. pylori*-negative subjects, no significant effect was recorded. In *H. pylori*-positive subjects, the values obtained with a test meal exceeded those obtained without. The authors [16] concluded that the addition of a test meal increased the resolution of the curves, probably by increasing the retention time of the ^{14}C-urea in the stomach. They felt that, because of the increased resolution of the curves when using a test meal, lower doses of ^{14}C-urea could be used to reliably detect *H. pylori*.

As stated above, it had previously always been our custom in Ipswich to collect a number of samples over a 2-hour period and compute an AUC. We had argued that this was likely to give a more accurate reflection of total bacterial urease activity in the stomach as compared with taking one sample at 20–40 min after ingestion of the radioactive urea. We readily accept, however, that, in a busy district general hospital, it would be much simpler to take a single sample somewhere between 10 min and 1 hour after receiving the isotope. Rauws *et al.* [16] calculated the mean values of the ^{14}C activity for each time period between 10 min and 90 min after ingestion of the ^{14}C-urea. A receiver operator characteristic (ROC) analysis was then performed by increasing step-wise the cut-off value of the test separating the *H. pylori*-positive from the *H. pylori*-negative subjects. Likelihood analysis revealed a most favourable cut-off level at 40 min [16]. At a time when our own group had performed well in excess of 500 tests [11], we reanalysed our own data and correlated the 2-hour AUC with the single 40-min sample technique on 146 patients of known *H. pylori* status before they received any drug therapy – for example, antibiotics or bismuth-containing substances that might affect the result of the test. The correlation between the 2-hour AUC and the much simpler 40-min test was 0.956 ($P < 0.01$, slope 0.011). Our group now simply takes a 20-min, 40-min and 60-min sample, using the 40-min sample to compute the 2-hour AUC.

Different groups appear to be getting very good sensitivity and specificity results, using different single time points varying between 10 min and 1 hour. Presumably, anyone wishing to set up the ^{14}C-urea breath test in their own hospital would initially study their own culture-positive and negative subjects to define their own normal range and upper limit of normal. The Amsterdam group [16] reported that an arbitrary cut-off level of 0.07% of the dose of ^{14}C-urea/mmol CO_2 × body-weight (kg) at 40 min conveniently separated culture-positive and culture-negative subjects. In their series, sensitivity of the test was 95% and specificity 98%.

In this chapter, as previously [2], we have deliberately presented our data as distrbution tables, rather than taking single 'cut-off points' and giving sensitivity and specificity figures for that arbitrary value. For instance, one group setting up the test might wish to use the test of an epidemiological study. Another might wish to use it to monitor the success (or failure) of bismuth/antibiotic treatment to eradicate the organism from the stomach of a series of patients already known to be *H. pylori*-positive on endoscopic biopsy. The first group might, thus, opt for a higher 'cut-off point', as it would be important not to get too many false positives, while in the second case a much lower arbitrary cut-off figure would be more appropriate.

Two groups [17, and see below] challenged the necessity of expressing the ^{14}C-urea breath test results in terms of breath radioactivity multiplied by body-weight to correct for the influence of endogenous CO_2 production on the breath-specific activity of ^{14}C. With the latter method, the results are expressed as percentage of the administered dose/mmol CO_2 × weight (kg). Both groups [17, and see below] have instead expressed their results simply in terms of counts per minute (CPM) (× 1000). As discussed by Hunt and his colleagues [17]:

> . . .the impact of any possible variants in endogenous CO_2 production due to differences in body weight on the result of breath tests in resting patients, to our knowledge, has never been studied in detail. We repeated the calculations in a random sample of eighteen patients, applying the formula used by Marshall and Surveyor [15] which accounts for differences in endogenous CO_2 production due to body weight. This resulted in a less clear distinction between *H. pylori*

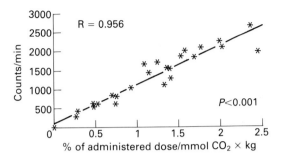

Fig. 9.5 ^{14}C-urea breath test result at 30 min, showing the correlation between CPM and percentage of administered dose per mmol of CO$_2$ × body-weight. The authors are grateful to Dr Shao Kai Lin and Dr John Lambert for kindly allowing us to publish this figure from their data.

positive and negative patients. It is important to realise that the breath test does not measure between patient but rather within patient differences where the patient serves as his own control. Furthermore, the counts per minute in all patients who were *H. pylori* negative are so close to background radiation levels that a correction for body weight does not seem necessary.

The results of Dr J.R. Lambert's group from Melbourne, Australia, are illustrated in Fig. 9.5. It can be seen that there was a statistically significant correlation between the results expressed as percentage of administered dose – mmol CO$_2$ × body-weight (kg) – and CPM, using logistic regression analysis. Their feeling was that endogenous CO$_2$ production was not influenced by body-weight and that in the clinical setting the ^{14}C-urea breath test results using CPM alone is adequate to define positive and negative subjects.

Results and examples of usage

Table 9.1 shows the Ipswich results for a series of 27 *H. pylori*-negative patients, expressed both as percentage of administered dose per mmol of CO$_2$ × body-weight (kg) for 10–40 min and also the AUC over 2 hours. It will be seen that we have divided the *H. pylori*-negative patients arbitrarily into two groups: one in which our

pathologist felt the mucosa was entirely normal and a second group of 13 in which minor histological abnormalities were seen (not active chronic gastritis – which is believed by many to be a histological 'hallmark' of *H. pylori* colonization). It will be seen that in both groups relatively low counts were obtained but, interestingly, those with the normal mucosa were significantly lower. We did not perform serological tests on the *H. pylori*-negative controls with abnormal histology. It may be that some of these patients had organisms present in small numbers which we failed to detect by simply taking two biopsies from the antrum (one for histology and the other for bacterial culture). Had we taken biopsies from the body of the stomach as well as the antrum, some of these *H. pylori*-'negative' controls might well have been positive.

Table 9.2 shows the results we obtained in 75 patients who were known to be *H. pylori*-positive (on culture of antral biopsies). It can be seen that in this group ^{14}CO$_2$ appears in the breath in much higher quantities than in the controls (see Table 9.1). The differences in the cumulative excretion expressed as AUC in 2 hours was not significantly different in the patients with duodenal ulcers or gastric ulcers and those with active chronic gastritis in whom no active ulcer was demonstrated.

The distribution and mean of estimated AUC of breath ^{14}CO$_2$ excretion of ^{14}C-labelled urea by both endoscopic diagnosis and the presence of *H. pylori* on culture is shown in Table 9.3, and a similar exercise, taking the 40-min ^{14}CO$_2$ excretion data, is shown in Table 9.4. In order to assess the reproducibility of the ^{14}C-urea breath test, we studied 16 individuals, on two occasions within 1 month of each other, while the subjects were on no treatment likely to affect the *H. pylori* status. As can be seen from Fig. 9.6, the test was fairly reproducible. The mean AUC on the first occasion of 147.3 ± 80.2 was not significantly different from that on the second occasion of 145.2 ± 87.2 (mean ± SD).

We have also studied the ^{14}C-urea breath test in *H. pylori*-positive individuals both before and after being put on cimetidine at a dose of 400 mg

Table 9.1 ^{14}C-urea breath test in *H. pylori*-negative patients (mean $\pm$ SD) expressed as a percentage of administered dose per millimole CO_2 $\times$ body-weight (kg) for times 10–40 min and also as AUC over 2 hours.

Group	n	Time (min)				AUC in 2 hours
		10	20	30	40	
H. pylori-negative controls with normal histology	14	0.21[a] (0.13)	0.16[a] (0.11)	0.16[a] (0.11)	0.18[a] (0.16)	18.4[a] (14.7)
H. pylori-negative controls with abnormal histology	13	0.47 (0.40)	0.46 (0.44)	0.50 (0.47)	0.52 (0.50)	54.6 (46.5)

[a] Significantly different from the *H. pylori*-negative controls with abnormal histology ($P < 0.05$).

b.d. There was the theoretical possibility that the suppression of acid secretion with an H_2 antagonist would alter the environment of the *H. pylori* organism and either increase or decrease the number/enzyme activity. In our experience (see Table. 9.5), this was not the case, with AUC on the first occasion of 184 ± 100 being similar to that after treatment of 167 ± 65.6 (mean $\pm$ SD).

In contrast (see Fig. 9.7), the 2-hour AUC result of *H. pylori*-positive patients was significantly reduced by 20–40 mg of Omeprazole daily for 1 month. As can be seen from Fig. 9.7, several of the patients' tests moved into the 'negative' range at the end of treatment. One month later all but one of these subjects had again developed a positive ^{14}C-urea breath test. The single individual who was still negative was again positive when tested 3 months later, suggesting that in every case Omeprazole had simply suppressed rather than eradicated the organism [13].

We had previously elected to take an AUC of 70 as our arbitrary cut-off point between *H. pylori*-positive and negative individuals [2]. In those with intact stomachs and who were *H. pylori*-positive (on either histological and/or bacterial criteria), 76/81 (93.8%) had AUCs of > 70. No *H. pylori*-negative patient with normal histology had an AUC of >61.9 but 5/13 of those who were *H. pylori*-negative with abnormal histology were above this arbitrary figure.

We recently [11] looked at the results of our breath tests in *H. pylori*-positive patients: (i) while on active treatment ($n = 110$); and (ii) 1, 3, 6, 12 and 24 months post-treatment in 151, 60, 40, 11 and 8 patients, respectively. As we previously reported [11], the breath test results while on active treatment were of limited value, as the 'success rate' of 84.5% fell to 46.4% when

Table 9.2 ^{14}C-urea breath test in *H. pylori*-positive patients (on culture of antral biopsies) expressed as a percentage of administered dose per millimole CO_2 $\times$ body-weight (kg) for times 10–40 min and also as AUC over 2 hours (mean $\pm$ SD).

Group	n	Time (min)				AUC in 2 hours
		10	20	30	40	
Active chronic gastritis	24	1.58 (1.07)	1.69 (1.10)	1.88 (1.02)	1.90 (0.98)	178.4 (76.1)
Duodenal ulcer	43	1.56 (0.85)	1.72 (0.76)	1.84 (0.77)	1.88 (0.71)	174.9 (66.0)
Gastric ulcer	8	1.74 (0.89)	2.21 (1.31)	2.35 (1.53)	2.35 (1.5)	209.2 (118.0)
Total	75	1.58 (0.92)	1.77 (0.94)	1.91 (0.95)	1.95 (0.90)	179.7 (75.5)

Table 9.3 Distribution and mean of estimated areas under curve (AUC) of breath $^{14}CO_2$ excretion of ^{14}C-labelled urea by endoscopic diagnosis and presence of *Helicobacter pylori* (HP) on culture.

AUC	Normal controls all HP −ve (n = 19)	Abnormal controls all HP −ve (n = 13)	Gastritis only HP −ve (n = 4)	Gastritis only HP +ve (n = 24)	Duodenal ulcer HP −ve (n = 3)	Duodenal ulcer HP +ve (n = 43)	Gastric ulcer HP −ve (n = 1)	Gastric ulcer HP +ve (n = 8)	Total HP −ve (n = 40)	Total HP +ve (n = 75)
0–24	16	6	1[a]	1	1	1			24	2
25–49	2	1			1			1	4	1
50–74	1	3						1	4	1
75–99			1[a]						1[a]	1
100–124	1	1		2		1			1	11
125–149	2	2	1[a]	5	1[a]	9			4	11
150–174			1[a]	3		10		1	1[a]	14
175–199				6		2		1		9
> 200				7		14	1[a]	4	1[a]	25
Mean AUC	18.4	54.6	99.8	178.4	54.0	174.9	325.7	209.2	48.6	179.7
SD	14.7	46.5	68.6	76.1	67.7	66.0	–	118.0	63.7	75.5

[a] These subjects had *H. pylori* found in gastric biopsies on histology only.

Table 9.4 Distribution and mean breath $^{14}CO_2$ excretion at 40 min after ingestion of ^{14}C-labelled urea by endoscopic diagnosis and presence of *Helicobacter pylori* (HP) on culture.

Excretion of $^{14}CO_2$ at 40 min	Normal controls all HP − ve (n = 19)	Abnormal controls all HP − ve (n = 13)	Gastritis only		Duodenal ulcer		Gastric ulcer		Total	
			HP − ve (n = 4)	HP − ve (n = 24)	HP − ve (n = 3)	HP − ve (n = 43)	HP − ve (n = 1)	HP − ve (n = 8)	HP − ve (n = 40)	HP − ve (n = 75)
0	18	8	1[a]	1	2	1		1	29	3
0.5	1	3	1[a]	3	–	1		1	5	5
1.0		1	1[a]	5	–	13		1	2	19
1.5		1	–	6	1[a]	11		–	2	17
2.0			1[a]	2		8		1	1[a]	11
2.5				4		6		1	–	11
3.0				2		2		1	–	5
3.5				–		1		1	–	2
4.0				–			1[a]	1	1[a]	1
4.5				1				1	1	1
> 5										
Mean excretion	0.18	0.52	0.99	1.90	0.71	1.88	4.24	2.35	0.51	1.94
SD	0.16	0.50	0.86	0.98	0.88	0.71	–	1.50	0.79	0.90

[a] These subjects had *H. pylori* found in gastric biopsies on histology only.

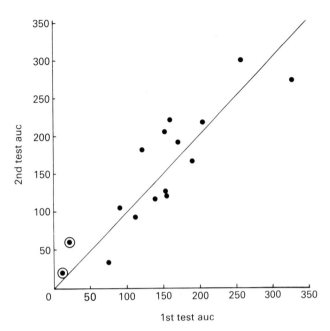

Fig. 9.6 Reproducibility results of ^{14}C-urea breath test of 16 individuals having tests repeated within 1 month of no treatment for *H. pylori*. The two ringed dots are biopsy-proved *H. pylori*-negative patients while the remainder are all *H. pylori*-positive.

assessed 1 month post-treatment. The vast majority of those who were *H. pylori*-negative at the 1 month post-treatment stage remained so. Carefully reviewing the breath test follow-up data of those who were *H. pylori*-negative by breath test criteria at the 1 month post-treatment stage, we now believe that in this situation one should probably adopt a much lower 'cut-off' value than, for instance, when screening

groups of patients simply to divide them into *H. pylori*-positive and negative groups where one is keen to avoid false positives. Using the much stricter 'cut-off' values of either a 2-hour AUC of <40 or a 40-min breath test value of <0.45, we found few patients whose breath tests were

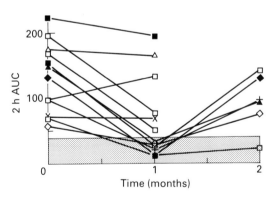

Table 9.5 ^{14}C-urea breath test in 10 *H. pylori*-positive individuals repeated after 1 month's treatment with cimetidine (400 mg b.d.) (mean ± SD).

Subject no.	Age	Sex	AUC$_1$	AUC$_2$
1	65	M	119.2	253.10
2	61	F	143.40	175.60
3	53	M	194.40	122.80
4	49	M	259.30	229.60
5	54	M	116.10	155.50
6	53	F	146.40	171.40
7	50	F	422.60	251.70
8	59	M	88.60	46.50
9	72	F	233.60	135.20
10	46	M	122.50	130.90
Mean ± SD	56.2 ± 8.0		184.6 ± 100.0	167.2 ± 64.6

Fig. 9.7 ^{14}C-urea breath test results in a series of *H. pylori* patients before and again at the end of 1 month's treatment with Omeprazole in doses ranging from 20 to 40 mg daily. In those patients whose breath tests become negative (arbitrarily defined as a 2-hour AUC of <40), all but one of the individuals' tests become positive again when tested 1 month later. The solitary patient whose test was still negative 1 month post-treatment subsequently relapsed when tested 3 months later.

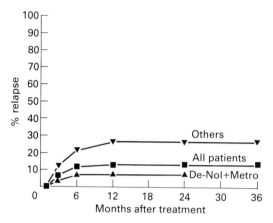

Fig. 9.8 Results in 153 *H. pylori*-positive patients who had apparently had their organism successfully eradicated (eradication defined as a 1 month post-treatment breath test of <40). The relapse rate of the patients treated with De-Nol and metronidazole was significantly lower than those patients treated with other combinations of antibiotics and bismuth salts. This suggests that the vast majority of the relapses are due to a recrudescence of a suppressed organism and not true reinfection.

negative by these criteria at 1 month post-treatment who subsequently relapsed. Our figures for cumulative relapse after apparently successful eradication of the organism, using the criteria of a 1 month post-treatment AUC of <40, were 6.7% at 3 months and 11.8% at 6 months. At 1 year the cumulative relapse had only risen very slightly, to 13.2%. At 2 years and 3 years the cumulative relapse remains at 13.2%. Figure 9.8 shows the cumulative relapse rate of: (i) all 153 patients; (ii) the 105 patients treated with De-Nol and metronidazole; and (iii) the 48 patients treated with either De-Nol alone or other antibiotic combinations. The cumulative relapse rate at 1 year was significantly higher in group (iii) than Group (ii) ($P < 0.05$). The marked difference between the relapse rate at 1 year post-treatment between our patients treated with De-Nol and metronidazole, compared with those treated withn De-Nol either alone or in combination with other antibiotic regimes, probably indicates that: (i) the De-Nol/metronidazole combination is more effective [12]; and (ii) most relapses following apparently

successful eradication of the organisms are due to recrudescence of a suppressed organism and not true reinfection.

As can be seen from Table 9.6, the urea breath test was extremely disappointing in patients who were *H. pylori*-positive and had undergone previous gastric surgery. Only 3/8 (37.8%) of these post-operative stomach patients had an AUC > 70. One must thus conclude that the ^{14}C-urea breath test is unreliable following gastric surgery. It could, however, be regarded as being a predictable outcome if retention of the ^{14}C-urea in the stomach is a critical factor. We feel that the ^{14}C-urea breath test is of particular value in monitoring the effect of various treatments designed to suppress or, hopefully, eradicate the organism from the stomach. The fact that the ^{14}C-urea breath test is negative when restudied while the patient is on a bismuth preparation, either alone or in combination with an antibiotic, does not, of course, mean that the organism has been totally eradicated. In many cases, the number of organisms has simply been reduced to a level that is no longer detectable and, once active treatment is withdrawn, there is a recrudescence of the same organism [25]. It is now generally agreed [6] that it is necessary to wait at least 1 month after discontinuing active treatment before either rebiopsying the patient or doing a repeat urea breath test, in order to obtain a realistic idea of true eradication rates. When tested 1 month after conventional 1–2-month courses of De-Nol, eradication rates of only about 10–20% are achieved. In our experience a combination of De-Nol and Amoxil increases this figure to appproximately 40%. In patients with *H. pylori* organisms which are sensitive to metronidazole, we find a greater than 85% eradication rate using De-Nol in combination with metronidazole [12]. The value of the ^{14}C-urea breath test in serially monitoring patients has already been illustrated in Figs 9.2 and 9.7. As stated above, it is our experience, using the ^{14}C-urea breath test to monitor patients serially – and also the experience of Rauws *et al.* [26], using serial endoscopic biopsy criteria – that the majority of patients whose test is negative at 1 month remain so.

Table 9.6 Individual details of eight *H. pylori*-positive patients who had undergone previous gastric surgery.

| Subject no. | Age | Sex | Operation | H. pylori status | | ^{14}C-urea breath test AUC |
				Bacterial culture	Histology	
I	43	M	Polya	+	+	32.0
2	80	F	Billroth I	+	+	109.6
3	77	M	Gastrojejunostomy	+	+	197.7
4	54	M	Polya	+	+	53.4
5	72	F	Polya	+	+	22.1
6	57	M	Polya	+	+	36.4
7	57	M	V & P	+	+	63.8
8	68	M	V & P	+	+	86.8
Mean ± SD	63.4					72.3
	± 12.9					± 57.5

Use as a diagnostic tool – points for and against

Clearly, if a patient is undergoing endoscopy, the easiest way to confirm or refute the presence of *H. pylori* in the stomach would be to take a series of biopsies. Depending on local interest and expertise, either the biopsies can be looked at by the histopathologist using an appropriate stain (in Ipswich we find the half Gram stain simple and inexpensive [10]), or the nearest co-operative microbiologist can carry out the appropriate culture. For a very rapid answer, one of the many forms of rapid urease tests may be used. Additionally, if the local histopathologist or microbiologist cannot be persuaded to show an interest, one can rely almost entirely on the rapid urease test in most cases. Since most regimens for attempted eradication of *H. pylori* now contain metronidazole [12], if the organism is being cultured it seems sensible to perform metronidazole sensitivity testing. Using combinations of De-Nol and metronidazole, we have had a success rate of 43/50 (86%) if the organism was metronidazole-sensitive, compared with only 1/7 (14.3%) in the case of the metronidazole-resistant group (chi-square with Yates' correction = 14.095, $P < 0.01$) [12].

If one is endoscoping a patient, then only if there is some contra-indication to biopsy (e.g. a clotting disorder or the fact that the patient has been on an oral anticoagulant) would one need the ^{14}C breath test at this stage. For instance, in a patient with a gastric ulcer one would probably wish to do a further endoscopy 1–2 months after starting active anti-ulcer treatment to confirm healing of this ulcer and make quite sure that a malignant process has not been missed. Again, in this case, since one would be repeating the endoscopy, it would be reasonable to see whether the particular form of treatment had eradicated the bacteria, using biopsy criteria. In the case of duodenal ulcers, which are, to all intents and purposes, never malignant, it is not normally necessary (outside clinical trials) to repeat the endoscopy to confirm healing. In this group and also in patients who have *H. pylori*-positive non-ulcer dyspepsia (proved by endoscopy/biopsy), it might be more appropriate (and certainly much less invasive) to monitor the success or failure of a bismuth/antibiotic combination using the ^{14}C-urea breath test, rather than subjecting the patient to an unnecessary second endoscopy.

The main disadvantage of the ^{14}C-urea test appears to be the fact that in the post-operative situation it is unreliable, with a high percentage of false negatives in *H. pylori* patients. Since the test involves ^{14}C-urea, it might be considered unsuitable for certain groups, such as children and premenopausal women. It should, however, be stated that the amount of radioactivity to which the patient is exposed is small. It has been calculated that a patient receiving 10 μCi of ^{14}C-urea receives about one-tenth of the radiation dose of a patient having a single plain abdominal

X-ray. As discussed above, it is almost certainly not necessary to use more than $5 \mu Ci$ and many groups are now using as little as 2.5 or even $1 \mu Ci$ [20]. Although the ^{14}C-urea breath test has been used in children [20], the authors feel that the ^{13}C-urea breath test is more appropriate in this age-group. Until recently, at least in the United Kingdom, only groups who had access to a mass spectrometer were able to use the ^{13}C-urea breath test. However, a number of commercial companies are now offering a testing service for samples transported by mail. Our own results would suggest that the original dose of 250 mg of ^{13}C-urea is unnecessary and we have had good results with as little as 75 mg of ^{13}C-urea [14].

Conclusion

The ^{14}C-urea breath test is a non-invasive, accurate and inexpensive screening test which has a particular use for long-term follow-up studies, particularly when evaluating the therapeutic efficacy of different drug treatments designed to eradicate the organism. It is unreliable in the post-operative stomach. A single breath sample taken between 20 min and 60 min after ingestion of the ^{14}C-urea is adequate to distinguish H. pylori-positive and negative groups, but the 2-hour single AUC figure arguably gives a better assessment of total bacterial count in the patient's stomach. Using these criteria, an AUC of <40 at 1 month post-treatment is a very good predictor of true eradication and few patients subsequently replase. Combining the test with a test meal to delay gastric emptying probably helps but is not essential.

Although most groups are still expressing their results in terms of percentage of the ^{14}C-urea excreted per mmol of CO_2 multiplied by the body-weight, it is probably just as accurate not to allow for either body-weight or endogenous CO_2 production and simply to express the results in CPM. Any group of workers setting up the test are encouraged to define their own normal range. The arbitrary line dividing H. pylori-positive and negative patients should be much lower when the test is used to monitor the success of

eradication treatment than when screening populations. In our experience, the sensitivity and specificity of the ^{14}C-urea breath test and the ^{13}C-urea breath test are virtually identical [14].

Acknowledgements

The authors are grateful to the Ipswich Hospital Medical Library staff for searching out and checking references.

References

1 Ferrero, R.L., Hazell, S.L. & Lee, A. The urease enzymes of Campylobacter pylori and a related bacterium. J. Med. Microbiol. 1988, 27, 33–40.
2 Weil, J. & Bell, G.D. 1989. The ^{14}C breath test. In Heatley, R.V. & Rathbone, B. (eds) Campylobacter pylori in Gastro-duodenal Disease. Blackwell Scientific Publications, Oxford, pp. 83–93.
3 Graham, D.Y., Evans, D.J., Alpert, L.C. et al. Campylobacter pylori detected non-invasively by the ^{14}C-urea breath test. Lancet 1987, i, 1174–7.
4 Bell, G.D., Weil, J., Harrison, G. et al. ^{14}C-urea breath analysis, a non-invasive test for Campylobacter pylori in the stomach (letter). Lancet 1987, i, 1367–8.
5 Weil, J., Bell, G.D., Harrison, G. et al. Campylobacter pylori survives high dose bismuth subcitrate (De-Nol) therapy (abstract). Gut 1988, 29, A1437.
6 Weil, J., Bell, G.D., Jones, P.H. et al. 'Eradication' of Campylobacter pylori: are we being misled? (letter). Lancet 1988, ii, 1245.
7 Weil, J., Bell, G.D., Gant, P. et al. High success rate for eradication of Campylobacter pylori infection using a colloidal bismuth subcitrate (CBS)/metronidazole combination (abstract). Gut 1989, 30, A733.
8 Newell, D.G., Bell, G.D., Weil, J. et al. The effects of treatment on circulating anti-Campylobacter pylori antibodies – a two year follow-up study. European Campylobacter pylori Study Group. Klin. Wochenschr. 1989, 67, 48.
9 Weil, J., Bell, G.D., Harrison, G. et al. Use of the ^{14}C-urea breath test to monitor treatment response in C. pylori positive patients – two year follow-up figures. European Campylobacter pylori Study Group. Klin. Wochenschr. 1989, 67, 70.
10 Trowell, J.E., Yoong, A.K.H., Saul, K.J. et al. A simple half-Gram stain for demonstrating Campylobacter pyloridis in sections. J. Clin. Pathol. 1987, 40, 702.
11 Weil, J., Bell, G.D. & Harrison, G. ^{14}C-urea breath test for C. pylori. Gut 1989, 30, 1656–7.
12 Weil, J., Bell, G.D., Powell, K. et al. Helicobacter pylori infection treated with a tripotassium dicitratobismuthate and metronidazole combination. Aliment. Pharmacol. Ther. 1990, 4, 651–7.
13 Weil, J., Bell, G.D., Powell, K. et al. Omeprazole and

Helicobacter pylori: temporary suppression rather than true eradication. *Aliment. Pharmacol. Ther.* 1991, **5**, 309–13.

14 Brookes, S.T., Prosser, S.J., Harrison, G. *et al.* Rapid analysis of [13]CO$_2$ for ^{13}C-urea breath tests. European *Helicobacter pylori* Study Group. *Rev. Esp. Enf. Dig.* 1990, **78**, suppl. 1, p. 30.

15 Marshall, B.J. & Surveyor, I. Carbon-14 urea breath test for the diagnosis of *Campylobacter pylori* associated gastritis. *J. Nucl. Med.* 1988, **29**, 11–16.

16 Rauws, E.A.J., Royen, E.A.V., Langenberg, W. *et al.* ^{14}C-urea breath test in *C. pylori* gastritis. *Gut,* 1989, **30**, 798–803.

17 Veldhuyzen van Zanten, S.J.O., Tytgat, K.M.A.J., Hollingsworth, J. *et al.* ^{14}C-urea breath test for the detection of *Helicobacter pylori*. *Am. J. Gastroenterol,* 1990, **85**, 399–403.

18 Ormand, J.E., Talley, N.J., Carpenter, H.A. *et al.* ^{14}C-urea breath test for diagnosis of *Helicobacter pylori*. *Dig. Dis. Sci.* 1990, **35**, 879–84.

19 Husebye, E., O'Leary, D., Skar, V. *et al.* How reliable are the ^{14}C-urea breath test and specific serology for the detection of gastric *Campylobacter? Scand. J. Gastroenterol.* 1990, **25**, 725–30.

20 Conti-Nibali, S., Baldari, S., Vitulo, F. *et al.* The [14]CO$_2$ urea breath test for *Helicobacter pylori* infection (letter). *J. Pediatr. Gastroenterol. Nutr.* 1990, **11**, 284–5.

21 Glupczynski, Y., Van Den Borre, C., Goossens, H. *et al.* Study of the epidemiology of *Helicobacter pylori* in a developing country: comparison of serodiagnosis and a ^{14}C-urea breath test. European *Helicobacter pylori* Study Group. *Rev. Esp. Enf. Dig.* 1990, **78**, suppl. 1, p. 92.

22 El Nujumi, A.M., Dorian, C.A. & McColl, K.E.L. Effect of inhibition of *H. pylori* urease activity with acetohydroxamic acid on plasma gastrin in DU subjects. European *Helicobacter pylori* Study Group. *Rev. Esp. Enf. Dig.* 1990, **78**, suppl. 1, p. 111.

23 Berstad, K., Weberg, R. & Berstad, A. Suppression of gastric urease activity by antacids. *Scand. J. Gastroenterol.* 1990, **25**, 496–500.

24 McColm, A.A., Bagshaw, J. & O'Malley, C. Development of a ^{14}C-urea breath test in ferrets colonised with *Helicobacter mustelae*: effects of treatment with urease inhibitors, bismuth and antibiotics. European *Helicobacter pylori* Study Group. *Rev. Esp. Enf. Dig.* 1990, **78**, suppl. 1, p. 97.

25 Langenberg, W., Rauws, E.A.J., Widjojokusomo, A., Tytgat, G.N.J. & Zanen, H.C. Identification of *Campylobacter pyloridis* isolates by restriction endonuclease DNA analysis. *J. Clin. Microbiol.* 1986, **24**, 414–17.

26 Rauws, E.A.J., Langenberg, W., Houthoff, H.J., Zanen, H.C. & Tytgat, G.N.J. *Campylobacter pyloridis*-associated chronic active antral gastritis. *Gastroenterology* 1988, **94**, 33–40.

10 Detection of Helicobacter pylori by the ^{13}C-urea Breath Test

R.P.H.LOGAN

Introduction

Helicobacter pylori is the most common cause of non-immune gastritis and is an important factor in the aetiology of recurrent duodenal ulceration. Initially, detection of *H. pylori* needed endoscopy and biopsy, but in 1987 Graham *et al.* [1] described the ^{13}C-urea breath test (^{13}C-UBT) for non-invasive detection of *H. pylori*. Since then, the ^{13}C-UBT has been developed, is no longer confined to the research laboratory and can be used routinely by clinicians [2–5]. It is the ideal method for serial screening and follow-up of patients after treatment of *H. pylori* [6].

Historical perspective

Although breath tests may appear to be a recent invention, they were first described in 1948 by Leifer and colleagues [7], who were studying gastric urease activity in mice. Using intravenous ^{14}C-urea, they observed that hydrolysis of the urea released ^{14}CO$_2$, which, having been collected in a respiration chamber, could be measured by scintillography. Further, the administration of antibiotics before the ^{14}C-urea abolished this response and so demonstrated a bacterial origin for the urease. Indeed, a bacterial origin for gastric urease activity had been proposed previously [8], but unfortunately most of this early work on gastric bacteria was dismissed as post-mortem artefact, after Palmer [9] failed to detect gastric bacteria *in vivo* on suction biopsy specimens. This was probably because these biopsies were taken from the body rather than the antrum of the stomach.

Principles of ^{13}C-UBT

The principle behind all non-invasive isotopic breath tests is the enzymatic catabolism of a molecule. This produces an isotopically labelled fragment, which is eliminated in exhaled breath and collected for analysis. The enzyme may be endolytic (of endogenous origin), for example lipase or decarboxylase, or may be xenolytic (exogenous, usually bacterial), for example urease or bacterial peptidase [10]. In urease tests, the carbon moiety of urea can be labelled with ^{14}C or ^{13}C and the labelled CO$_2$ collected for analysis in the exhaled breath. Alternatively, the nitrogen moiety can be labelled with ^{15}N. The ^{15}NH$_3$ (from the hydrolysis of ^{15}N-urea) is absorbed and then excreted as ^{15}N-urea (having been re-synthesized), which can be measured in the urine [11].

The ^{13}C- and ^{14}C-UBTs are based on the same principle and use similar methods. The carbon-labelled urea is rapidly hydrolysed in the presence of *H. pylori* urease to $^{13/14}$CO$_2$ and ammonia. The $^{13/14}$CO$_2$ is then absorbed to be excreted (and collected) in the exhaled breath (Fig. 10.1). If *H. pylori* is not present, hydrolysis does not occur and labelled CO$_2$ is not produced. Serial sample collection and analysis permit the construction of excretion curves (Figs 10.2A, B – see pages 90 and 91). In patients with *H. pylori*, ^{13}CO$_2$ can be detected in exhaled breath within 5 min of swallowing ^{13}C-urea. However, there are many different patterns of ^{13}CO$_2$ excretion, the variation including a wide range of ^{13}CO$_2$ concentrations, differing time intervals to peak excretion and different steady states of ^{13}CO$_2$ excretion.

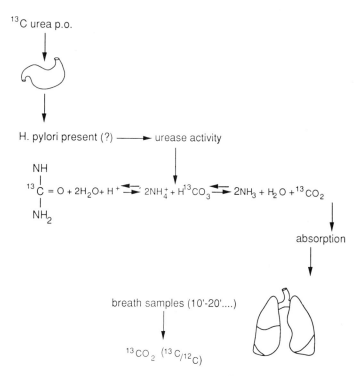

Fig. 10.1 Principle of the ^{13}C-urea breath test (^{13}C-UBT).

Factors affecting the pattern of $^{13}CO_2$ excretion

There are three phases to $^{13}CO_2$ excretion: the initial exponential phase, peak excretion, and steady state before $^{13}CO_2$ excretion returns to baseline levels (Fig. 10.3). The overall shape of the excretion curve depends on conditions adopted for the test, such as the test meal, dose of the isotope, load of *H. pylori* and the host response (Table 10.1).

Table 10.1 Factors affecting $^{13}CO_2$ excretion.

Host factors
Rate of gastric emptying
Intragastric pH
Extent of colonization

H. pylori
Urease activity
Virulence factors
Location within the mucosa

^{13}C-UBT
Test meal
Quantity of isotope
Timing and frequency of sample collection

The test meal

The purpose of the test meal is to slow down gastric emptying, thus prolonging the time the ^{13}C-urea remains within the stomach.

If a test meal is not used, the ^{13}C-urea behaves like an aqueous solution (isotonic glucose) with a gastric residence time ($T_{1/2}$) of less than 10–15 min, remaining in the stomach for less than 6 min before being emptied into the duodenum (Fig. 10.4). This is not long enough for ^{13}C-urea to be evenly distributed in the stomach and may reduce the sensitivity of the ^{13}C-UBT by inadequate coating of ^{13}C-urea over the gastric mucosa.

Rauws *et al.* [12] were the first to show increased discrimination of the ^{13}C-UBT using a test meal of liquid Ensure®. The ideal test meal should effectively inhibit gastric emptying for a known time interval and be equally effective in patients with and without *H. pylori*. Many factors may influence gastric emptying (Table 10.2), especially the total nutrient content, lipid fraction, fibre content and particle size (solid/semisolid/liquid). A liquid test meal containing

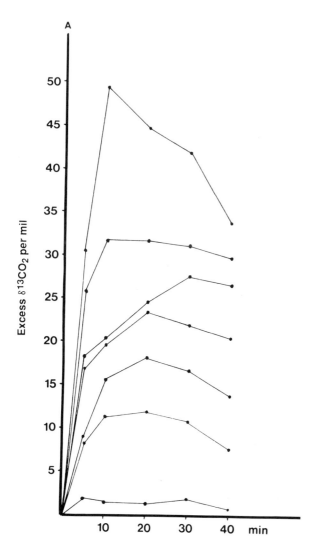

Fig. 10.2 Excretion curves using the European standard ^{13}C-UBT. A series of excretion curves for patients with and one patient without *H. pylori* (bottom curve, (A)). Vertical axis represents excess $\delta^{13}CO_2$ excretion per mil (difference between before and after swallowing ^{13}C-urea 100 mg).

Table 10.2 Factors affecting the rate of gastric emptying.

Promoting
Low nutrient load
Low osmotic load
Liquids – non-particulate
Anticholinergics

Inhibiting
High nutrient load
High lipid content
Solid – particle size
Fibre
Cholinomimetics

60% lipid and 30% carbohydrate has been shown to inhibit gastric emptying for up to 60 min, whilst a liquid meal composed entirely of lipid will inhibit half emptying time for even longer (up to 90 min (Fig. 10.4)). Both of these test meals allow plenty of time for the hydrolysis of ^{13}C-urea. Other studies have used different meals including citric acid [3], simple carbohydrate solution (Maxijul®) and, in children, two scoops of ice-cream [13]. All these meals alter the shape of the excretion curve (increasing the discrimination by shifting the curve to the left and increasing the peak $^{13}CO_2$ excretion (Fig. 10.3)), but their effect on gastric emptying is untested.

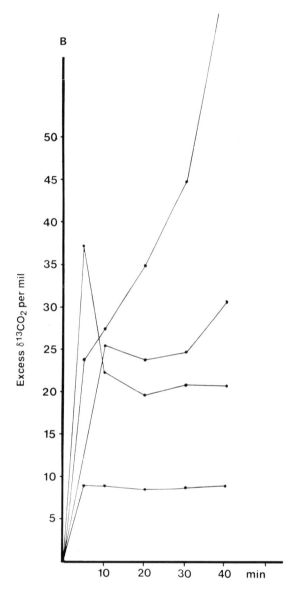

Fig. 10.2 (Continued) The extent and time to reach peak $\delta^{13}CO_2$ excretion varies between patients with *H. pylori*.

The test meal must not contribute to $^{13}CO_2$ excretion by its own catabolism – for example, with carbohydrate-based meals. It must be palatable for the patient, easy to manufacture and distribute and have a long shelf-life. High-fat meals appear to have all of the desirable qualities and can easily be manufactured in the form of a palatable liquid or a solid chocolate bar.

The amount of isotope

At present the quantity of isotope for the ^{13}C-UBT is less than half that used in the original description by Graham *et al.* [1] of the ^{13}C-UBT. Smaller quantities of isotope have since been used in several studies without detrimental effect on the sensitivity, or specificity of the test [3–5]. The overall excretions of $^{13}CO_2$ over the range 75–350 mg of ^{13}C-urea are similar (Fig. 10.5).

Although the trend to use smaller quantities of isotope is welcome, theoretically the intra-gastric concentration of the isotope should be

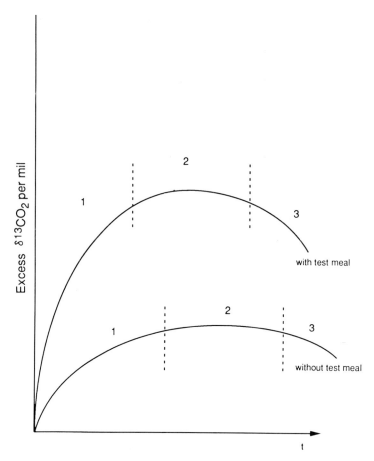

Fig. 10.3 The three phases to $\delta^{13}CO_2$ excretion. Addition of a test meal shifts the curve to the right and increases the peak excretion, thus maximizing the discrimination of the test in patients with and without *H. pylori*.

slightly greater than the K_{max} for the urease of *H. pylori*. At present this value is not accurately known, because the extent of interspecies variation of specific urease activity or the K_{max} of *H. pylori* urease is not known.

Sampling frequency

The shape of the $^{13}CO_2$ excretion curve is influenced by the frequency at which expired breath samples are taken.

Initially, sample collection did not start until 10 min after swallowing the isotope, because of the potential confounding of ^{13}C-urea hydrolysis by oropharyngeal bacterial urease, which could produce an early release of $^{13}CO_2$. The extent to which oropharyngeal contamination may influ-

ence the ^{13}C-UBT has now been more extensively assessed and is not now thought to interfere significantly with the excretion of $^{13}CO_2$; In addition , it is now recognized that the hydrolysis of $^{13/14}$C-urea and the absorption and subsequent exhalation of $^{13/14}CO_2$ in the expired breath can occur within 5 min of the isotope being taken (Fig. 10.6) [14]. In future, therefore, it is likely that sampling will start earlier.

The detailed exhalation pharmacokinetics of $^{13}CO_2$ has been studied in humans by Eggers and colleagues using ^{13}C-sodium bicarbonate [3]. These studies have shown that the exhalation kinetics of $^{13}CO_2$ from ^{13}C-urea and ^{13}C-bicarbonate are similar, with a mean residence time of about 90 min (Fig. 10.6).

The frequency of sampling will also affect the

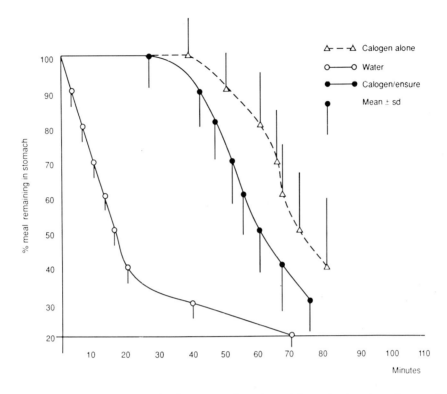

Fig. 10.4 The gastric emptying of test meals. The pattern of gastric emptying, using impedance tomography, with three different test meals. $T_{1/2}$ (half emptying time) is inhibited for up to 90 min using high-fat liquid meal (Calogen® 200 ml), which when flavoured with vanilla Ensure® is still 70 min.

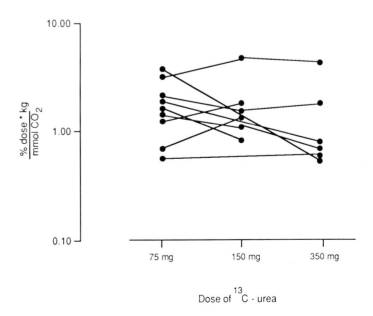

Fig. 10.5 Comparison of different doses of ^{13}C-urea on the ^{13}C-UBT (results expressed as % dose/mmol CO_2/kg). Courtesy Prof. F.E. Bauer.

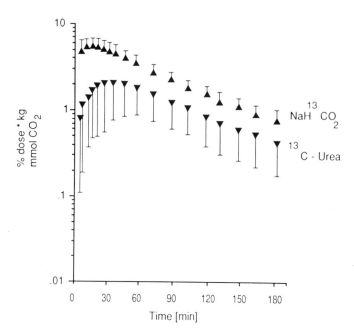

Fig. 10.6 Comparison of the exhalation kinetics of $^{13}CO_2$ after NaH$^{13}CO_3$ ($n = 14$) or ^{13}C-urea ($n = 10$, mean $\pm$ SD). Courtesy Prof. F.E. Bauer.

shape of the excretion curve, being less representative when fewer samples are taken. Single-point samples have been advocated by some groups, and these are considered in detail below.

H. pylori

In contrast to endoscopic biopsy-based methods for detecting *H. pylori*, which may be prone to sampling error, the ^{13}C-UBT assesses a much greater surface area of the stomach for *H. pylori* and theoretically is a quantitative measure of the extent of *H. pylori* infection. This is reflected by the wide range of results obtained with the European Standard ^{13}C-UBT (from 5 to 85 parts per thousand (per mil) excess $\delta^{13}CO_2$ excretion (Fig. 10.7)). Although Rauws *et al.* [12] succeeded in correlating bacterial load with the ^{14}C-UBT, similar attempts at demonstrating the ^{13}C-UBT to be a quantitative measure of *H. pylori* infection have not been so successful, not least because there is no accurate measure of bacterial load. Thus the optimal *in vitro* environment provided by culture may promote greater colony growth than *in vivo*. Histology could more accurately reflect the bacterial load of *H. pylori in vivo* since the severity of gastritis is related to the density of overlying *H. pylori*.

However, histology is a micro- rather than a macroscopic assessment of the load of *H. pylori*, based on sections taken from biopsies which may not necessarily reflect the overall severity of gastritis or extent of *H. pylori* in the rest of the stomach. Moreover, all endoscopy-based methods are liable to sampling error, so that, although *H. pylori* is most frequently found in the antrum, unfavourable factors, such as bile reflux or intestinal metaplasia, may make antral biopsy assessments of the extent of *H. pylori* unreliable. In addition, detailed re-examination of biopsies from patients with apparently false positive ^{13}C-UBT (i.e. false negative antral histology) showed *H. pylori* in only the body or fundus of the stomach [5]. These discrepancies often occur immediately after treatment, with antral endoscopic biopsies being negative on histology and culture, while the ^{13}C-UBT values, although decreased significantly from pretreatment values, remain positive [15]. Within a few days of stopping treatment, the ^{13}C-UBT returns to pretreatment levels, with repeat histology and culture becoming positive for *H. pylori*.

The ^{13}C-UBT result can be stratified and compared with the sensitivity of biopsy-based methods (Table 10.3). At low levels of excess $\delta^{13}CO_2$ excretion the biopsy-based methods have lower

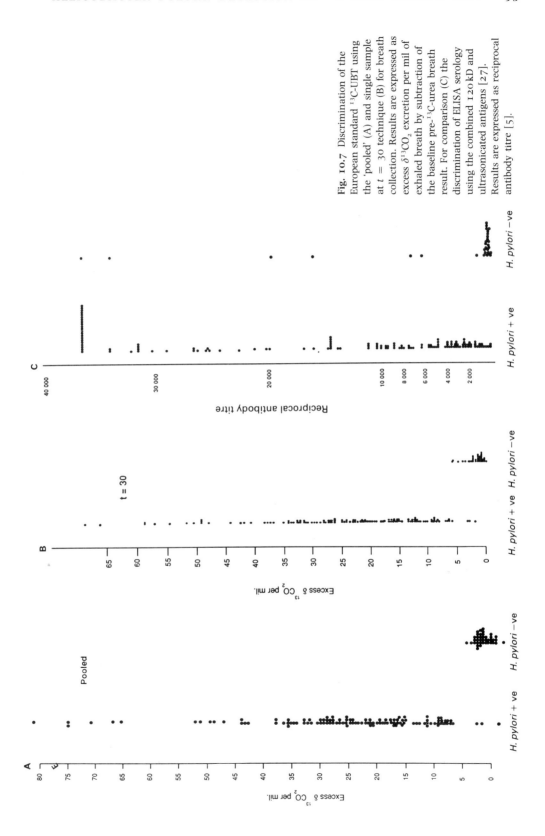

Fig. 10.7 Discrimination of the European standard ^{13}C-UBT using the 'pooled' (A) and single sample at $t = 30$ technique (B) for breath collection. Results are expressed as excess $\delta^{13}CO_2$ excretion per mil of exhaled breath by subtraction of the baseline pre-^{13}C-urea breath result. For comparison (C) the discrimination of ELISA serology using the combined 120 kD and ultrasonicated antigens [27]. Results are expressed as reciprocal antibody titre [5].

Table 10.3 Comparison of the relative sensitivity (Sen.) and specificity (Spec.) of histology, culture and CLO-test, with stratified ^{13}C-UBT.

Excess $\delta^{13}CO_2$ per mil	Histology		Culture		CLO-test	
	Sen.	Spec.	Sen.	Spec.	Sen.	Spec.
5–10	78	100	68	100	92	100
11–20	88	100	67	100	94	100
21–30	95	100	88	100	100	100
31–40	100	100	79	100	100	100
41–60	93	100	62	100	100	100

sensitivities than often recognized, supporting the patchy nature of *H. pylori* infection within the stomach. The ^{13}C-UBT is more sensitive because it reflects the proportion of the gastric mucosa infected by *H. pylori*. Histologically, a more accurate measure of the bacterial load of *H. pylori* could be made by examining biopsies taken from throughout the stomach rather than just the antrum.

We have performed several studies that indirectly support the quantitative nature of the ^{13}C-UBT: the urease activity of *H. pylori* when measured *in vitro* has been shown to be related to the quantity of bacteria present (Fig. 10.8) [16]. If this relationship holds true *in vivo*, the ^{13}C-UBT could be a quantitative measure of *H. pylori*. However, if there is variation in the specific urease activity of different strains of *H. pylori*, then the ^{13}C-UBT may not only be an indicator of bacterial load, but also a measure of overall urease activity within the stomach. Indeed, if urease is an important factor in *H. pyl-*

ori's ability to survive the acidic milieu of the stomach, then it could be expected that any changes in intragastric pH itself would affect the ^{13}C-UBT, not only directly by affecting the pK_a of urease, but also indirectly by altering the pattern of colonization by *H. pylori* within the stomach. Thus, in patients with *H. pylori*, treatment with omeprazole decreases the ^{13}C-UBT (Fig. 10.9), not only by changes in urease activity due to raised intragastric pH but also by changes in the pattern of colonization within the gastric mucosa [17].

Host response

The range of host response to *H. pylori*, including the type and pattern of gastritis and changes in gastric function (secretion and motility), could all potentially affect the shape of the excretion curve. The effect of changes in intragastric pH and rate of gastric emptying on the ^{13}C-UBT has already been discussed. However,

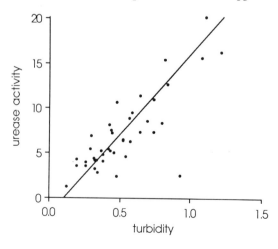

Fig. 10.8 Quantifying the extent of *H. pylori*. The *in vitro* relationship between urease activity (Berthelot method) and number of *H. pylori* (turbidity; absorbance at 750 nm) in pure bacterial suspensions ($n = 40$, $r^2 = 0.77$, $P < 0.01$) [16].

Unusual excretion curves are occasionally seen, with no obvious cause. As we discover more about *H. pylori*, its urease activity, and its favoured microenvironment in different regions of the stomach and mucosa, a better understanding and interpretation of the nuances of these more unusual excretion curves will be achieved.

Measurement of $^{13}CO_2$ and expression of results

The major difference between the ^{13}C-UBT and the ^{14}C-UBT is in the carbon isotope used to label the urea. ^{13}C is a natural non-radioactive isotope that can be measured relative to ^{12}C by isotope ratio mass spectrometry.

Because ^{13}C is always measured as a ratio to ^{12}C, the volume of expired CO_2 for any single analysis is not critical; the analysis can be done on < 0.1 ml of exhaled CO_2. The $^{13}C/^{12}C$ ratio is usually expressed as parts per thousand (per mil) relative to an international primary standard, PDB calcium carbonate (PDB = *Belemnitella americana* extracted from the Pe Dee formation of South Carolina, USA) [18]. This standard has a ^{13}C to ^{12}C ratio close to the natural abundance of ^{13}C and ^{12}C, and is therefore expressed as having a carbon isotope ratio of o per mil. Usually baseline samples are depleted in ^{13}C relative to PDB and therefore have negative per mil values. However, with the amount of ^{13}C-urea used in the breath test, the ratio of $^{13}C/^{12}C$ relative to PDB is often exceeded in patients with *H. pylori*, thereby giving a positive value. By expressing the results as excess $^{13}CO_2$ excretion per mil (difference between before and after ^{13}C-urea), this possible source of confusion and any variation between mass spectrometers in their standardization with PBD are avoided.

The ^{13}C-UBT was previously an expensive technique, not only because mass spectrometers (and the technical expertise required to look after them) are costly, but also because multipoint excretion curves increased the number of samples required for analysis. Fortunately, recent developments in the measurement of stable isotopes have produced smaller and inexpensive

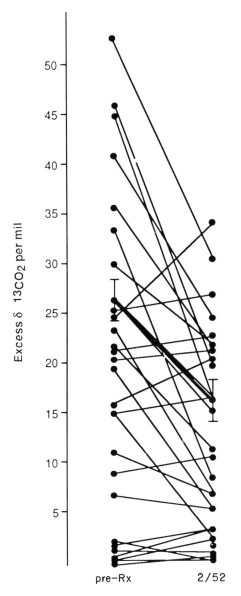

Fig. 10.9 The effect of omeprazole on *H. pylori*. The ^{13}C-UBT in patients with ($n = 20$) and without ($n = 6$) *H. pylori* before and 2 weeks after omeprazole 40 mg *mane*. In no patient previously negative for *H. pylori* did the ^{13}C-UBT become positive [17]. $P < 0.05$.

the extent to which *H. pylori* may cause any pathologically significant changes in gastric secretion or motility is not yet known, so their influence on the ^{13}C-UBT cannot be accurately evaluated.

machines [19], whilst simpler and cheaper methods, based on single-sample analyses, for the ^{13}C-UBT have also been successfully evaluated.

Collection and analysis of breath samples

The construction of excretion curves for each patient, often involving the analysis of up to 10 samples, previously limited the use of the ^{13}C-UBT for the detection of *H. pylori*; this is no longer necessary. Two simpler and cheaper methods of breath collection are now recommended.

Pooled collection

By pooling 2-litre expired breath samples into a large reservoir, and taking one sample from the reservoir bag at the end of the test (Fig. 10.10A, B), a quantitative pooled collection of breath is obtained which averages the excretion of exhaled ^{13}CO$_2$ over the collection period and which approximates to the area under the curve (AUC) (Table 10.4) [4].

Single sample

For a single breath analysis blowing through a straw, the tip is placed in the distal end of a test-tube, or opened vacutainer, until a blush of condensation appears on the container walls around the end of the straw. The straw is then removed and the test-tube promptly sealed (Fig. 10.11A, B).

Using this method, a single diagnostic sample taken 30 min after the isotope has been shown to have a high sensitivity and specificity, and to correlate closely with the AUC and results from the pooled collection (Table 10.4, Fig. 10.7B, Fig. 10.12). Indeed, single samples taken at $t = 10, 20, 40$ and 60 min after the isotope are equally accurate. However, the reproducibility of the single sample is not as good as that of the pooled technique (see below) and should therefore not be used in studies which require serial assessments of *H. pylori* status. The single-sample technique is ideal for routine clinical use

when only pre- and post-treatment assessments of *H. pylori* status are needed.

^{13}C-urea is a stable isotope and does not decay, so special storage conditions are not needed and samples can be analysed at any time.

European standard method

In collaboration with European colleagues, a European standard method for the ^{13}C-UBT has been evaluated and a standard protocol now exists for the ^{13}C-UBT [5]. This allows for direct comparison between studies from different centres and reduces the chance for confusion or disagreement between separate studies, where a full evaluation of individual protocols may not have been made. A brief outline of the European standard protocol is given in Table 10.5. The test meal is known to inhibit gastric emptying for the duration of breath collection, whilst the amount of ^{13}C-urea (100 mg) is considerably less than the 250 mg originally used by Graham *et al.* [1].

Validation

The standardized European protocol for the ^{13}C-UBT has been extensively validated by the participating centres (see Appendix 10.1), with a cumulative experience of over 1000 tests.

Comparisons have been made with enzyme-linked immunosorbent assay (ELISA) serology, histology, culture and biopsy urease tests (*Campylobacter*-like organism test (CLO-test®) and Christensen broth). For comparison of any of these methods, the definition of a 'gold standard' has to be clear [20]. Culture is a theoretical, but impractical, 'gold standard' because of the vagaries and fastidious technique required for successful culture. Histology is an alternative that allows repeated assessments of borderline cases, provides a permanent reference and is easier to process. Urease tests on biopsies are the quickest and simplest invasive method, but provide no information about gastritis or *in vitro* antibiotic sensitivity. In addition, all biopsy-based methods are inherently liable to sampling

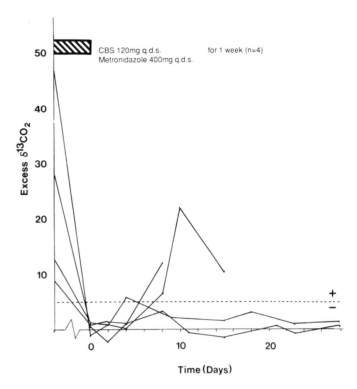

Fig. 10.13 The ^{13}C-UBT after treatment of *H. pylori*. The ^{13}C-UBT pre- and post-treatment with colloidal bismuth subcitrate (CBS) and metronidazole for 1 week. All patients clear *H. pylori*, but within 10 days the ^{13}C-UBT has become positive in two of them, whilst in the remaining patients the test is still negative 28 days after finishing treatment.

Applications

The ^{13}C-UBT can be used in three major areas.

Screening before endoscopy

Dyspepsia is a poor guide to diagnosis and cannot reliably differentiate gastro-oesophageal reflux from peptic ulcer or non-ulcer dyspepsia. However, preliminary results from studies using ELISA serology have suggested that screening patients non-invasively for *H. pylori* before endoscopy may decrease the endoscopic workload. Using the ^{13}C-UBT in a similar context would have the additional important advantage of identifying only patients with active *H. pylori* infection. In patients under 40 years endoscopy could be deferred until *H. pylori* had been successfully eradicated, whilst in those without *H. pylori* alternative diagnosis and management may be more appropriate. However, with the increasing problem of antibiotic resistance, routine pretreatment endoscopy and antral culture of *H. pylori* may still be necessary.

Epidemiological research

A very important advantage of the ^{13}C-UBT over serological methods is that ^{13}C-UBT detects active infection rather than previous exposure [21]. Moreover, it increasingly appears that, in elderly populations, serology may be unreliable, making studies based on these methods difficult to interpret [22]. The choice of antigens used in any ELISA preparations and the extent to which these antigens, and therefore the performance of the ELISA, vary between populations add to the unreliability of serological methods.

Finally, in children the ^{13}C-UBT offers a non-invasive alternative with the additional bonus of ice-cream being used as the test meal.

Follow-up after treatment

The ^{13}C-UBT offers the ideal method of following patients in whom eradication of *H. pylori* is being attempted. The test can clearly identify those patients in which *H. pylori* has been successfully eradicated and can detect those patients not successfully treated more easily and at

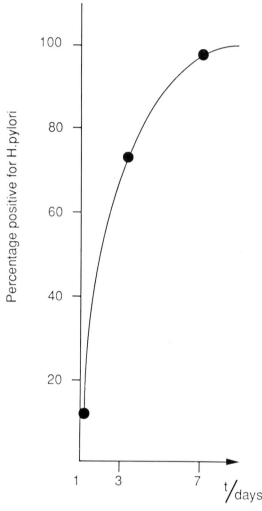

Fig. 10.14 Recurrence of *H. pylorri* after CBS. The ^{13}C-UBT allows frequent assessments of *H. pylori* status to be made and to determine rate of recurrence of *H. pylori* after 1 month colloidal bismuth subcitrate (CBS) (within days of finishing treatment) [26].

an earlier stage than endoscopic biopsy-based methods (Fig. 10.13). Because eradication of *H. pylori* is associated with resolution of histological gastritis and prevention of relapse of duodenal ulcer [23, 24], the ^{13}C-UBT could be used as the sole method of follow-up for patients in whom *H. pylori* is being treated.

The term 'eradication' should be confined to patients without *H. pylori* at least 1 month after the end of treatment [24]. Assessments of *H.*

pylori status between finishing treatment and 1 month provide additional information, such as demonstrating *H. pylori* to have been 'cleared', whilst subsequent assessments will reveal if treatment has failed, enabling appropriate measures to be taken as soon as possible. Unlike the ^{14}C-UBT, the ^{13}C-UBT is ideally suited for such repeat serial assessments of *H. pylori* status, thus measuring the rate of recurrence after different treatment regimens. It is only by making such measurements that the optimal regimen for eradication of *H. pylori* will be established.

Long before the rediscovery of *H. pylori*, bismuth salts had been used for healing duodenal ulcers. Because of possible risks associated with prolonged treatment, it was important to ascertain if long-term therapy was needed for *H. pylori* and to determine the rate of *H. pylori* recurrence after treatment with bismuth. Recent work has now shown that *H. pylori* recurs rapidly, regardless of the length of treatment with bismuth (Fig. 10.14) [26].

Conclusions

The ^{13}C-UBT is now a practical and readily available alternative to endoscopy- and serology-based methods for the detection of *H. pylori*. It can detect very low levels of *H. pylori* colonization within the stomach and, by assessing the entire mucosa, avoids the risks of sampling error. It represents the best practical non-invasive method for the detection of *H. pylori* and as such provides a gold standard, against which other methods can be compared.

Acknowledgements

The author would like to thank Dr David Evans and members of the Parkside Helicobacter Study Group and the European ^{13}C-Urea Breath Test Group for their help and advice.

Appendix 10.1

United Kingdom

BSIA Ltd, 15 Brook Lane Business Centre, Brook Lane North, Brentford, Middlesex TW8 0PP (Fax 081-847-5053, Tel. 081-847 3955)

Dr R. Logan, Parkside *Helicobacter* Study Group, Central Middlesex Hospital, Acton Lane, Park Royal, London. NW10 7NS (Tel. 081-965 5733)

Switzerland

Dr C. Beglinger, Department of Gastroenterology, Kantonsspital, Basle.

Germany

Prof. F.E. Bauer, Department of Clinical Pharmacology, George-August University, D-3400, Göttingen
Dr M.P. Cooreman, Universitätskliniken, D-7900, Ulm

Appendix 10.2: Laboratories offering analysis of ^{13}C:

BSIA Ltd, 15 Brook Lane Business Centre, Brook Lane North, Brentford, Middlesex TW8 0PP (Fax 081-847 5053, Tel. 081-847 3955)

References

1 Graham, D.Y., Klein, P.D., Evans, D.J. *et al. Campylobacter pylori* detected non-invasively by the ^{13}C-urea breath test. *Lancet* 1987, **ii**, 1174–7.

2 Dill, S., Payne-James, J.J., Misiewicz, J.J. *et al.* Evaluation of the ^{13}C-urea breath test in the detection of *Helicobacter pylori* and in monitoring the effect of tripotassium dicitratobismuthate in non-ulcer dyspepsia. *Gut* 1990, **31**, 1237–41.

3 Eggers, R.H., Kulp, A., Tegelet, R. *et al.* A methodological analysis of the ^{13}C-urea breath test for detection of *Helicobacter pylori* infections: high sensitivity and specificity within 30 min using 75 mg of ^{13}C-urea. *Eur. J. Gastroenterol.* 1990, **2**, 437–44.

4 Logan, R.P.H., Polson, R.J., Misiewicz, J.J. *et al.* A simplified single sample ^{13}C-urea breath test for *Helicobacter pylori*: comparison with histology, culture and ELISA serology. *Gut* 1991, **32**, 1461–4.

5 Logan, R.P.H., Dill, S., Bauer, F.E. *et al.* The European ^{13}C-urea breath test for the detection of *H. pylori. Gut* 1991, **3**, 915–21.

6 Logan, R.P.H., Gummett, P.A., Polson, R.J. *et al.* What length of treatment within tripotassium dicitrato-bismuthate (TDB) for *Helicobacter pylori? Gut* 1990, **31**, A1178.

7 Leifer, E., Roth, L.J. & Hempelmann, L.H. *Science* 1948, **108**, 748.

8 Kornberg, H.L., Davies, R.E. & Wood, D.R. The activity and function of gastric urease in the cat. *Biochem. J.* 1954, **56**, 363–72.

9 Palmer, E.D. Investigation of the gastric mucosa spirochetes of the human. *Gastroenterology* 1954, **27**, 218–20.

10 Klein, P.D. & Klein, E.R. Applications of stable isotopes to paediatric nutrition and gastroenterology: measurement of nutrient absorption and digestion using ^{13}C. *J. Pediatr. Gastroenterol. Nutr.* 1985, **4**, 9–19.

11 Guolong, L., Jizong, W., Zhenhua, Z. & Yanglong, M. Detection of *Helicobacter pylori* infection using the ^{13}N method. Proceedings of the III Workship of the European *Helicobacter pylori* Study Group. *Rev. Esp. Enf. Dig.* 1990, **78**, suppl. 1, 22 (38).

12 Rauws, E.A.J., Royen, E.A.V., Langenberg, W., Woensel, J.V., Vrij, A.A. & Tytgat, G.N. ^{14}C-urea breath test in *C. pylori* gastritis. *Gut* 1989, **30**, 798–803.

13 Klein, P.D. & Graham, D.Y. 1989. Detection of *Campylobacter pylori* by the ^{13}C-urea breath test. In Rathbone, B.J. & Heatley, R.V. (eds) *Campylobacter pylori and Gastroduodenal Disease.* Blackwell Scientific Publications, Oxford, pp. 94–105.

14 Heinrich, H.C. & Gabbe, E.E. The on-line ^{14}C-urea-^{14}CO$_2$ conversion test as a marker for the efficacy of treatment of *Campylobacter pylori* infection with bismuth compounds $\pm$ antibiotics. *Klin. Wochenschr.* 1989, **67**, suppl. 18, 22.

15 Logan, R.P.H., Gummett, P.A., Misiewicz, J.J., Walker, M.M., Karim, O.N. & Baron, J.H. The urease activity of *H. pylori* before, during and after treatment with omeprazole. *Gastroenterology* 1991, **100**, A112.

16 Cacoulis, F., Batten, J., Logan, R.P.H., Baron, J.H.B. & Karim, N.Q. Quantifying the extent of *H. pylori* with the ^{13}C-urea breath test. *Gut* 1991, **32**, A565.

17 Sharp, J., Logan, R.P.H., Walker, M.M., Gummett, P.A., Misiewicz, J.J. & Baron, J.H. The effect of omeprazole on *Helicobacter pylori. Gut* 1991, **32**, A565.

18 Craig, H. Isotopic standards for carbon and oxygen and correction factors for mass spectrometric analysis of carbon dioxide. *Geochim. Cosmochim. Acta* 1957, **12** 133–49.

19 Brookes, S.T., Prosser, S.J., Harrison, G., Powell, K. & Bell, G.D. Rapid analysis of ^{13}CO$_2$ for ^{13}C-urea breath test. Proceedings of the III Workshop of the European *Helicobacter pylori* Study Group. *Rev. Esp. Enf. Dig.* 1990, **78**, suppl. 1, 22 (38).

20 Barthel, J.S. & Everett, E.D. Diagnosis of *Campylobacter pylori* infections: the 'gold standard' and the alternatives. *Rev. Infect. Dis.* 1990, **12**, S107–S114.

21 Meyer, B., Werth, B., Beglinger, C. *et al. Helicobacter pylori* infection in healthy people: a dynamic process? *Gut* 1991, **32**, 351–4.

22 Reiff, A., Jacobs, E. & Kist, M. Seroepidemiological study of the immune response to *Campylobacter pylori* in potential risk groups. *Eur. J. Clin. Microbiol. Infect. Dis.* 1989, **8**, 592–6.

23 Marshall, B.J., Goodwin, C.S., Warren, J.R. *et al.* A

prospective double-blind trial of duodenal ulcer relapse after eradication of *Campylobacter pylori*. *Lancet* 1988, **2**, 1437–42.

24 Coghlan, J.G., Humphries, H., Dooley, C. *et al. Campylobacter pylori* and recurrence of duodenal ulcers – a 12-month follow-up study. *Lancet* 1987, **ii**, 1109–11.

25 Tytgat, G.N.J., Axon, A.T.R., Dixon, M.F., Graham, D.Y., Lee, A. & Marshall, B.J. *Helicobacter pylori*: causal agent in peptic ulcer disease? World Congress of Gastroenterology Working Party report. *J. Gastroenterol. Hepatol.* 1991 (in press).

26 Logan, R.P.H., Polson, R.J., Baron, J.H. & Misiewicz, J.J. Follow-up after anti-*Helicobacter pylori* treatment. *Lancet* 1991, **337**, 562–3.

27 Hirsch, A.M., Rathbone, B.J., Wyatt, J.I., Berger, J. & Rotter, M.L. Comparison of ELISA antigen preparations in serodiagnosis of *Helicobacter pylori* infections. *J. Clin. Pathol.* 1990, **43**, 511–13.

11 Epidemiology of Helicobacter pylori Infection

F.MEGRAUD

Some epidemiological characteristics concerning *Helicobacter pylori* infection are now well established, and we now know the magnitude of this infection. It has a worldwide distribution and virtually all populations are affected. The infection appears to be lifelong once established. Obviously, because the bacterium was only recently discovered, we do not have a long time-span to evaluate, but current data suggest this evolutionary pattern [1]. As a consequence, the most useful measure will be the prevalence of the infection.

The first epidemiological data gathered concerned the prevalence of the infection in general populations from different countries and the influence of classical parameters such as age, gender, etc. Most of the studies have focused on this area in the past. Other studies concern the possible source and route of infection and this area still lacks substantial results.

Prevalence and incidence studies

Methods used to establish the diagnosis

The reference technique for determining the *H. pylori* status of a subject is to perform an endoscopy with biopsy sampling, which then allows the detection of both the organism and possible gastric lesions. Obviously, this approach cannot be used in most epidemiological studies, for ethical and practical reasons. However, it has been carried out in a few volunteer studies, permitting the validation of other techniques, in particular, serology (Table 11.1) [2–9]. Morris *et al.* [10] studied human stomach obtained at postmortem. This revealed the distribution of *H.*

pylori in different areas of the stomach, and its relation to gastritis, which was widespread in 80% of the cases [10].

The breath test has been used in some studies [11, 12]. We do not favour this technique over serology for epidemiological studies. The breath test is more time-consuming and costly. Moreover, an overgrowth of intestinal bacteria could falsify the results (unpublished personal data), especially in malnourished children from developing countries.

Serology is the most suitable technique for epidemiological studies. The availability of kits using purified antigens instead of home-made crude antigens has been a real advance in terms of sensitivity and specificity. However, erroneous results did not occur in studies performed with these crude antigens. For example, the high prevalence of infection observed in Africa using serological techniques was confirmed by endoscopy [7, 8]. The technique of absorption of sera with intestinal campylobacters before testing them with a crude antigen [13] is not advisable. It is not known if the absorbed antibodies may include anti-*H. pylori* antibodies. The prevalence obtained has a high specificity but a ridiculously low sensitivity. We agree with Perez-Perez *et al.* [14] that, if purified antigens are not available, a better alternative is to use a low concentration of unwashed and centrifuged antigen and a higher serum dilution. However, immunoblotting seems to be a more adequate way of studying such a complex reaction.

Prevalence in developed countries

It is obviously difficult to compare the results

Table 11.1 *Helicobacter pylori* infection in healthy volunteers studied by endoscopy and biopsy examination.

References	n	Mean age (years)	H. pylori +ve (%)	Gastritis in H. pylori +ve (%)	Correlation with serology
North America					
Dooley et al. [2]	113	48	32	100	Exc.
Gregson et al. [3]	54	28	11	98	ND
Barthel et al. [4] Westblom et al. [5]	20	29	20	100	Exc.
Dehesa et al. [6]	58	41	79	98	Exc.
Africa					
Lachlan et al. [7]	14	22	93	100	ND
Holcombe et al. [8]	23	23	78	94	
Asia					
Raedsch et al. [9]	194	20	85.6	96	ND

Exc. excellent; ND: not done.

obtained in different studies because, in addition to the variety of methods used, different groups of healthy people have been concerned: blood donors, volunteers recruited in diverse ways, individuals presenting themselves in health centres for check-ups, etc., and, for children, usually patients referred to hospitals for diseases other than those related to the digestive tract.

In endoscopic studies performed on volunteers, in addition to confirming the results of the serological methods used, it has been noted that gastritis was almost always present when *H. pylori* was detected and most cases of gastritis were accompanied by *H. pylori*. Therefore, the epidemiological data obtained in the past for gastritis can be paralleled to those for *H. pylori* infection. A group of Finnish investigators has conducted population-based studies on the prevalence of gastritis by using biopsy material obtained either blindly in Finland [15] or by endoscopy in Estonia [16]. They were able to gather data on the prevalence of chronic gastritis and the evolution of chronic gastritis towards atrophy, using mathematical models. When biopsies were recently re-examined, *H. pylori* was present in approximately 80% of the cases of chronic gastritis [17].

It was also recognized by these authors that chronic gastritis is a premalignant condition which favours the development of gastric cancer.

The overall results of several studies [18–30], presented in Table 11.2, give an outline of the situation and allow us to draw at least two conclusions: the infection is seldom found in children and is rather common in adults. The situation seems comparable in all the countries cited except Greece, which seems to have a higher prevalence.

Prevalence in developing countries

Data from different countries in Africa and Asia have been obtained and are in agreement. In contrast to developed countries, the prevalence in adults is very high and ranges from 60 to 90% (Table 11.3) [14, 22, 31–36]. One can extrapolate that in some places the entire population will eventually be infected. Moreover, children become infected early in life. Again, gastritis is a constant consequence of *H. pylori* infection.

Factors influencing the prevalence rate of H. pylori infection

Age. The first paper presenting prevalence studies stratified by age was by Marshall *et al.* [37] and their findings were later confirmed in all developed countries. There is a progressive increase in the prevalence rate of *H. pylori* infec-

Table 11.2 Seroepidemiology of *Helicobacter pylori* based on IgG determination in developed countries.

References	Population studied	Antigen	Number tested	H. pylori-+ve (%)	Age (years) <20	21–30	31–40	41–50	51–60	61–70	71–80	81–90
Europe												
Austria [18]	BD	Sonicate	282	26.2	18[a] (100)[b]	22 (59)	37 (56)	47 (44)	60 (23)			
England [19]	Health Screening Clinic	Whole cell	771	34	22 (160)	27 (146)	30 (137)	41 (150)	51 (178)			
[20]	BD	GE	498	25	6 (151)	19 (64)	19 (53)	16 (37)	40 (28)	49 (43)	49 (69)	41 (53)
Finland [21]	BD	GE	500	36	10 (100)	31 (100)	39 (100)	40 (100)	60 (100)			
France [22]	Health Screening Clinic	Sonicate	1086	30.4	16 (98)	25 (105)	26 (229)	33 (285)	37 (324)	33 (45)		
Greece [23]	Military and Vaccination Clinic	Sonicate	414	54.5	39 (188)	67 (226)						
Ireland [24]	Military	Sonicate	130	38		35 (89)	47 (32)	45 (9)				
Italy [25]	BD	Sonicate	545	37	11 (71)	19 (53)	29 (131)	40 (153)	49 (129)	49 (61)		
Netherlands [26]	BD	Sonicate	396	35.8		19 (53)	27 (127)	39 (136)	52 (68)	58 (12)		
Oceania												
Australia [27]	BD (whites)	Sonicate	144	15	10.5 (19)	0 (32)	12.5 (24)	7 (36)	30 (33)			
New Zealand [28]	BD	Whole cell	480	36	32 (175)	32 (165)	45 (93)	54 (35)	33 (12)			
America US												
Denver [29]	Healthy population	Sonicate	126	30	15 (30)	10 (37)			50 (18)		50 (41)	
Houston [30]		Purified antigen	351		14	14	39	40	55	67		

Data adapted from the references cited.
[a] % *H. pylori*-positive; [b] number tested.
BD: blood donors; GE: glycine extract.

Table 11.3 Seroepidemiology of *Helicobacter pylori* infection based on IgG determination or urea breath test in developing countries.

References	Population studied	Antigen	Number tested	H. pylori-+ve (%)	Age (years)							
					0–10	11–20	21–30	31–40	41–50	51–60	61–70	>70
Africa												
Algeria [22]	BD	Sonicate	277	78	45[a] (42)[b]	73 (59)	84 (83)	88 (49)	96 (27)	88 (17)		
Ivory Coast [22]	Random sample	Sonicate	363	69	55 (116)	75 (100)	75 (78)	82 (40)	77 (22)	71 (7)		
Gambia [31]		Whole cell	353		31 (353)							
Nigeria [32]		?	72		50 (72)							
Zaire [33]		UBT	143	79	79 (24)	73 (22)	81 (59)	82 (22)	87 (8)	66 (9)		
Asia												
Saudi Arabia [34]	Random sample	Purified antigen	551	66	40 (66)	50 (137)	75 (103)	73 (87)	75 (65)	85 (53)	80 (32)	80 (14)
Thailand [14]	General population	Sonicate	161	58.1	10 (41)	50 (20)	60 (20)	80 (20)	90 (20)	80 (30)	70 (10)	
Vietnam [22]	BD	Sonicate	353	60	13.1 (61)	46.5 (43)	74 (92)	77.7 (72)	86 (50)	52 (21)	57 (14)	
China [35]	General population	Sonicate	1019	60			46 (35)	64 (99)	60 (359)	60 (407)	58 (100)	79 (19)
South America												
Peru [36]	General population	GE	361	65	40 (89)	71 (87)	70 (117)		75 (47)		95 (21)	

Data adapted from the references cited.
[a] % *H. pylori*-positive; [b] number tested.
BD: blood donors; UBT: urea breath test; GE: glycine extract.

tion from childhood to 50 years of age (Table 11.2). This phenomenon can be explained by two hypotheses:

1 The chance of becoming infected has remained the same for the last 50 years (or more) and the yearly occurrence of new cases has been constant, i.e. approximately 1% annually, as was noted by Graham *et al.* [38]. The curve obtained by Loffeld *et al.* [26] illustrates this hypothesis.

2 The chance of becoming infected has changed relative to the past. It can be postulated that, during the nineteenth century, the prevalence rate of *H. pylori* infection was close to what is actually observed in developing countries (80–90%). It would have gradually decreased since then to a prevalence rate of 50–60% due to improvements in hygiene. In the 1950s, the introduction of antibiotics would have decreased the prevalence rate to approximately 20%. These speculations are based on the assumption that *H. pylori* infection is mainly acquired at a young age and is lifelong. It has been described as a cohort phenomenon. The shape of curves obtained in some studies [29, 39] are in agreement with this second hypothesis. Newell *et al.* [40], studying subjects from different areas of the UK, also noted that differences appeared to be due to the earlier infection of young persons.

In developing countries, the prevalence rate of *H. pylori* infection is constant during adulthood (Table 11.3). Children can acquire the infection as early as in the first year of life, as was shown in Peru [41].

A common point in all the age prevalence curves is the slight decrease in the prevalence rate in the older age-groups. This can be explained by the fact that, after many years of gastritis, atrophy occurs and *H. pylori* progressively disappears from the lesions that they contributed to. When biopsies have been performed in elderly persons, a discordance between serology and culture has been noted because of this atrophy.

Socio-economic status. The most important factor with regard to *H. pylori* infection besides age seems to be the socio-economic status. The poor-

er a population is, the sooner in life it will become infected and the higher the cumulative infection rate will be. The best illustration is seen when comparing the difference in infection rates between developed and developing countries. But this difference can also exist within a country. In an isolated territory such as Reunion Island in the Indian Ocean, the prevalence curves for individuals from high and low socio-economic status are as different as those from developed and developing countries (unpublished data). Dehesa *et al.* [6], who studied Hispanics, both immigrants and US-born, living in California, also observed a very high infection rate relative to the Caucasians.

Vietnamese immigrants in Australia, who are usually in the highest socio-economic class, have a lower infection rate than Vietnamese blood donors of the same age in Ho Chi Minh City, living under very difficult conditions ($2\,m^2$ living space/persons) [22, 27].

In Saudi Arabia, *H. pylori* infection occurs with significantly less frequency in adults with a high socio-economic status as measured by the educational level (college level) [34].

In a study [42] performed in the US, epidemiological data were gathered for 247 healthy children and young adults aged 3–21 years. The socio-economic status was measured by the family income and happened to be a very important risk factor: the rate of infection in those families with incomes of less than $5000 per year was double that of families earning more than $75 000 per year [42].

It can be assumed that promiscuity and hygiene standards, for example, are not the same in poor families as in rich families; therefore, the risk of transmission increases.

Ethnic background. It is difficult to claim that some ethnic groups have a particular susceptibility to *H. pylori* infection. As was mentioned previously, the socio-economic conditions are an enormous source of bias. Comparisons must be made using subjects with the same socio-economic status in the same environment and, in addition, the socio-economic status of the subjects' parents should also be taken into account since the infection is likely to have been acquired during youth. Such a comparative study has not yet been attempted.

Some studies have led us to believe that blacks have a particular predisposition to infection. In the study of Fiedorek *et al.* [42], after controlling for age and socio-economic status, *H. pylori* infection was still more prevalent in young blacks (*P* < 0.05). Also, on Reunion Island, blacks showed a higher prevalence rate than poor Caucasians but the difference was not statistically significant [43]. A sociologic approach could probably tell us if particular customs followed in black families are responsible for this difference rather than genetic predispositions.

Early results concerning the higher prevalence rate of *H. pylori* infection in ethnic groups living in New Zealand (Maori, Samoan and Tongan) in comparison with random blood donor sera should be interpreted cautiously since the socio-economic status was not taken into consideration [28].

A very interesting finding is the lack of *H. pylori* infection and ulcers in Australian Aborigines who live in settlements with little contact with white Australians [44]. It is known that, when Aborigines become westernized, they have a high incidence of *H. pylori* infection and ulcers, reflecting their poor economic status, so they are not genetically protected from this infection. It may be possible to explain the lack of *H. pylori* infection in Aborigines by the geographical isolation of these tribes from the rest of the world during thousands of years.

Gender. It is generally accepted that males and females have the same risk of becoming infected in all age-groups considered (Fig. 11.1) [22, 34].

Living conditions. Nowottny & Heilmann [45] found no difference between the prevalence rates of *H. pylori* infection in urban and rural populations after controlling for socio-economic status.

Alcohol consumption and cigarette-smoking are not risk factors for *H. pylori* infection. Associations have been found in some studies but they were below the level of statistical significance when corrected for socio-economic status.

Vegetarians were compared with meat-eaters in two studies and no association with *H. pylori* infection could be found [46, 47]. Some investigators have found that milk consumption may be a possible risk factor. This could be explained by the buffering role of milk, which would permit the infection, but more careful studies must be carried out.

Incidence

The prevalence of *H. pylori* infection is determined by performing a test at a given time. The incidence is not so easily defined, since it is necessary to follow the population during a given time period in order to obtain the number of newly infected persons. No assumptions can be made from the prevalence rate since we do not know the duration of the infection. Few studies have been performed and most have been done retrospectively, using stored sera.

Eldridge & Jones [48] studied the sera of 329 English schoolchildren aged 17–18 years; 10 (3.3%) were *H. pylori*-positive as determined by serology. Six out of the 10 children already had antibodies by the age of 11 and four (1.2%) were considered to have acquired the infection between the ages of 11 and 18. However, nine sera gave equivocal results and therefore the incidence could be greater [48].

Parsonnet *et al.* [49] were able to obtain serum samples from 355 (46%) of 766 Epidemiology Intelligence Service alumni who had previously given serum to the Centres for Disease Control blood bank. *H. pylori* immunoglobulin G (IgG) was detected in 73 (21%) of the more recent serum samples. The age-related infection rate was consistent with a cohort phenomenon, with a break in the curve at the age of 40. Sixteen (4.5%) of the *H. pylori*-positive alumni were infected during the follow-up period [49].

In Finland, Rautelin *et al.* [50] followed 152 students. During the 2-year follow-up period, two new students became infected (1.3%) [50].

These scanty data lead us to believe that, in the 1990s in developed countries and in young

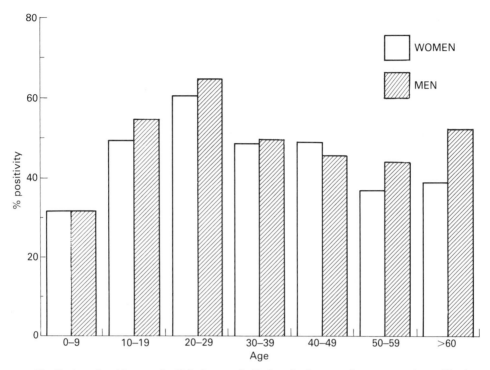

Fig. 11.1 Distribution of positive sera for *Helicobacter pylori* IgG antibodies according to age and sex. (The data are pooled from different studies and cannot be interpreted for age prevalence.)

people, the yearly incidence rate is very low and much less than 1%. It would be interesting to have access to stored serum samples from serum banks to clarify the picture of the past.

Moreover, because of this low incidence rate and the design of the studies, it was not possible to find any symptom associated with seroconversion.

Transmission studies

Reservoir

Current data suggest that *H. pylori* is a bacterium restricted to humans and other primates. *H. pylori* lives in a restricted niche – the stomach. This fact can be explained by adapted colonizing factors: urease to resist the acidic environment by buffering a microenvironment around the organism [51], motility to move in the mucus lying on the gastric mucosa [52], and adherence to specific receptors, e.g. glycolipids

present on the antral epithelial cell [53, 54]. The antral cell can be considered as the target cell of *H. pylori*. However, antral cells can also be found outside the antrum and therefore *H. pylori* is also to be found in other settings, e.g. fundus, duodenum, oesophagus and even the rectum [55].

A number of isolates have been recovered from non-human primates. Newell *et al.* [56] reported the isolation of *H. pylori* from four of seven rhesus monkeys (*Macaca mulatta*), aged 2–8 years and autopsied. This observation was also made by Reed & Berridge [57], but the organisms were not cultured. Dubois *et al.* [58] found four out of 16 rhesus monkeys to be infected by *H. pylori* after gastroscopy and three were cultured. When the organisms obtained from *Macaca mulatta* were compared with human organisms, besides colony size, there was no difference in morphology, enzymatic and fatty acid content [59], protein profile and antigenic properties; unfortunately, hybridization data are not available to confirm that they are the same species as in humans.

Bronsdon & Schoenknecht [60] also found *H. pylori* in six of 24 pigtailed macaques (*Macaca nemestrina*). By using a semi-quantitative hybridization technique they concluded that they were indeed *H. pylori* [60].

Strains of *H. pylori* have also been isolated in a *Cynomolgus* monkey (1/23) [61] and in baboons [62].

Considering the little contact between non-human primates and humans and the magnitude of human infection, it is highly probable that primate *H. pylori* do not play a significant role in human contamination and that the infection in primates has evolved in parallel to human infection. Precise hybridization data are needed. The data obtained by comparing human isolates have shown great variability [63], some strains being at the limit of the species definition [64]. It is possible that new species (< 70% deoxyribonucleic acid (DNA)–DNA homology) will emerge from such comparative studies.

Epidemiological markers

In order to follow the route of transmission of an organism, epidemiological markers are needed. These markers give a 'fingerprint' of the isolates found in different specimens.

Traditional markers used in clinical bacteriology are serogrouping, biotyping and phagetyping. These markers have been of little help in the epidemiology of *H. pylori* infection. Attempts were made by Lior *et al.* [65] to serogroup *H. pylori* by using heat-labile antigens. Four groups were defined but, since most of the strains fell into the same group, this technique had no discriminatory role [65]. Concerning biotyping, variability was found in the enzymatic content but weak reactions and reproducibility problems made it difficult to use this as a routine procedure [66]. Recently, some attempts have been made with the strip APIzym [67, 68].

Lectin-typing [69] and haemagglutination profiles [70] have been studied, and now molecular fingerprinting methods are being developed. Those based on proteins include: one-dimensional polyacrylamide gel electrophoresis protein pattern [71], immunoblot fingerprinting [72], outer membrane protein profile [73] and multilocus enzyme analysis [74]. However, the technique which attracted the most interest is restriction endonuclease DNA analysis, following the work of Langenberg *et al.* [75]. After extraction, the DNA is digested by a restriction enzyme and the DNA fragments are separated on an agarose gel. The endonuclease commonly used is Hind III [75–78] but Hae III can also give satisfactory results [77]. The association of two enzymes, Hind III and Bst EII, has been proposed [78]. With this technique, virtually all infected subjects harbour a different strain and so, if the same pattern is found in different cases, it means that the strains originate from the same clone. However, Majewski & Goodwin [76] described differences in the patterns of *H. pylori* isolates from subsequent biopsy specimens in half of the cases, suggesting this marker's lack of stability. Oudbier *et al.* [79] showed that such differences, usually restricted to one or two bands, were not artefacts but were due to the coexistence in the stomach of subpopulations of *H. pylori* with slightly different chromosomal DNA, probably caused by mutation *in vivo*. They were able to obtain this mutation *in vitro* by subculturing the organism [79].

When different specimens obtained from the same patient at the same time were tested by this technique, it was possible to assess the multicontamination of some patients. For example, Beji *et al.* [80] found three multicontaminated cases among 22 patients tested.

It would be of interest to undertake a large study testing many clones of the same patient's specimen – also using other markers – and to have a follow-up in order to determine the frequency of contamination.

Transmission in gastroscopy units

Gastroscopy units can be considered a privileged area for the transmission of *H. pylori* because of access to the stomach and possible regurgitation of gastric juice. The careful follow-up of patients performed by an Amsterdam group enabled them to detect, in three instances, subclinical reinfections with *H. pylori* in two successfully treated patients. The reinfections occurred 1 month and 21 months after antibacterial treatment for the first patient and 32 months for the second patient. The transmission was proved by restriction enzyme analysis of bacterial DNA. In both cases, the isolate was identical to the isolate of the patient, who had had a preceding gastroscopy. The cleaning procedure included a mechanical treatment using a detergent and a brush to clean the shaft tip and channels of the endoscope as well as the valves, followed by rinsing with sterile water, treatment with 70% ethanol and a final rinsing. The risk of gastroscopic cross-infection with *H. pylori* was estimated by retrospective analysis of the data of 281 negative examinations and was found to be 1.1% [81]. This would clearly have been higher if the procedure was not as carefully performed as in this study. Cleaning of the biopsy forceps is an essential part of decontamination but it is not always sufficient to eliminate *H. pylori*, as was observed in the study of Karim *et al.* [82]. Disinfection or sterilization is necessary.

The outbreak of epidemic gastritis with hypochlorhydria described by Ramsey *et al.* [83], in which 17 of 37 healthy volunteers became infected after endoscopy for a study on acid secretion, was probably the consequence of cross-infection. However, at the time, *H. pylori* had not yet been discovered and therefore the strains are not available for comparison. *H. pylori* was only observed on histological preparations [83].

Seroepidemiological data also highlight the risk of contamination for gastroenterologists. Mitchell *et al.* [84] found that the prevalence of *H. pylori* infection in gastroenterologists, determined by an IgG enzyme-linked immunosorbent assay (ELISA), was significantly higher than the prevalence of age-matched blood donors ($P < 0.01$) and the prevalence observed in general practitioners and gastroenterology nurses. The discrepancy with the latter group could be explained by the fact that 9% of the gastroenterologists wore gloves compared with 72% of the nurses [84].

When endoscopy staff members in Germany were compared with age-matched controls for the combined presence of IgG and IgA by immunoblot test, a statistically significant difference was noted ($P = 0.004$, odds ratio (OR) 2.8), while no difference existed with the dental staff [85].

However, in studies by Rawles *et al.* [86] and Morris *et al.* [87], no significant difference was found between the endoscopy staff and the controls.

Transmission in open communities

Animal sources. The existence of an animal reservoir of *H. pylori* besides primates is still hypothetical. The only firm data available describe one strain isolated by Jones & Eldridge [88] from a laboratory pig, which was indistinguishable from human strains. In fact, the particular conditions of its isolation raised the possibility that the laboratory pig had been contaminated by a human strain. Experimentally, it is possible to infect gnotobiotic [89] and barrier-born [90] newborn pigs. Vaira *et al.* [91] were able to detect spiral bacteria reacting with *H. pylori* monoclonal antibodies in the stomach of abattoir pigs and rabbits, but the organisms were not cultured. Other spiral organisms, such as *Gastrospirillum* species, can be found in the stomach of animals and these organisms sometimes cross-react with *H. pylori* [92]; *G. suis*, which has been isolated from the stomach of pigs in Brazil [93], could be the cause of such cross-reactions.

A seroepidemiological study by Vaira *et al.* [94] favoured the transmission route from animals to humans. This study was performed on abattoir workers in Bologna. There is no doubt about the high frequency of *H. pylori* infection in this particular group, but the workers were not compared with a group of the same socio-economic level and therefore a bias exists, suggesting that the workers, from a low socio-economic level, were already *H. pylori*-positive when they were employed.

The bacteria must be able to survive in the external environment in order to be significant, if one believes that an animal source exists. By

Table 12.1 *Helicobacter pylori* and activity in chronic gastritis.

Study group	Active			Inactive		
	n	*H. pylori* + ve	%	*n*	*H. pylori* + ve	%
Goodwin *et al.* (1986) [8] Perth, Western Australia	51	47	92	23	8	35
Morris *et al.* (1986) [9] Auckland, New Zealand	28	23	82	7	1	14
Rawles *et al.* (1986) [10] Baltimore, USA	23	16	70	47	7	15
Wyatt *et al.* (1986) [11] Leeds, UK	109	95	87	35	13	37
Andersen *et al.* (1987) [12] Hillerod, Denmark	74	67	91	16	2	13
Fiocca *et al.* (1987) [13] Pavia, Italy	239	213	89	124	91	73
Jiang *et al.* (1987) [14] Shanghai, China	49	44	90	72	36	50

the antrum showed chronic gastritis. The most plausible conclusions to draw from these studies are that *H. pylori* does not have a role in the pathogenesis of autoimmune gastritis and that the finding of antral gastritis in these patients does not represent coincidental infection. Nevertheless, it remains a possibility that the hypochlorhydric stomach is hostile to *H. pylori* so that along with the development of severe atrophy helicobacters previously present in the stomach have been eliminated.

'New' forms of gastritis

Lymphocytic gastritis

The finding that the vast majority of cases of active chronic gastritis are *H. pylori*-positive led us to review negative cases to determine whether or not there were any distinctive features. This review brought to light several cases where the surface and foveolar epithelium was infiltrated by unusually large numbers of lymphocytes – so-called 'lymphocytic gastritis' [17]. Lymphocytic gastritis has a characteristic endoscopic appearance, frequently described as 'varioliform' and displaying nodular prominence of the gastric mucosa, the nodules being surmounted by shallow aphthoid erosions. This striking appearance is usually confined to the corpus of the stomach but can be diffuse.

In contrast to predominantly antral chronic gastritis, lymphocytic gastritis shows a far lower prevalence of *H. pylori* positivity [18]. Haot and

Table 12.2 Characteristics of patients with chronic gastritis with and without atrophy.

Condition	*n*	Active	*H. pylori* +ve	Inactive	*H. pylori* +ve
Chronic gastritis without atrophy	98	69	68 (99%)	29	25 (86%)
Chronic gastritis with:					
Mild atrophy	58	50	50	8	6
Moderate atrophy	19	18	18	1	1
Severe atrophy	3	1	1	2	0
	80	69	69 (100%)	11	7 (64%)

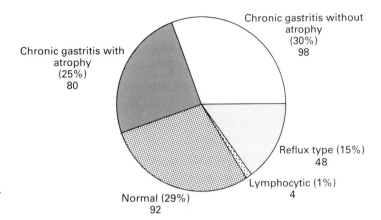

Fig. 12.2 Histological diagnoses in 322 consecutive patients undergoing oesophagogastroscopy for dyspeptic symptoms.

co-workers (who first recognized this entity) found only 8% positivity amongst 102 cases of lymphocytic gastritis [19]. However, this does not rule out a role for *H. pylori* in this condition; some of our negative cases exhibited serological evidence of previous *H. pylori* infection [18], and Flejou *et al.* [20] found on follow-up of *H. pylori*-positive patients that two of those who became negative revealed the histological picture of lymphocytic gastritis.

We have previously demonstrated that the intra-epithelial lymphocytes in lymphocytic gastritis are almost exclusively T cells [18]. More recently, using frozen material, we have established that these are CD8-positive T cells (personal observation). These findings suggested to us that the condition might arise from a perturbed immune response in the gastric mucosa analogous to that found in the small intestine in coeliac disease [18]. Subsequent to this speculation, others have examined gastric biopsies from coeliac patients and found high intra-epithelial lymphocyte counts consistent with lymphocytic gastritis in 15–45% of cases [21, 22]. These authors concluded that lymphocytic gastritis may occur as a manifestation of coeliac disease.

Reflux gastritis

Increasing familiarity with biopsies from the

postoperative stomach led us to distinguish a further type of chronic gastritis, related to enterogastric reflux [23]. This 'reflux gastritis' results from persistent injury to the surface epithelium and is characterized by compensatory foveolar hyperplasia and a vascular and exudative response, evidenced by capillary dilatation and congestion and lamina propria oedema. There is no notable increase in inflammatory cells. At a later stage, increased numbers of smooth muscle fibres and collagen bundles appear in the lamina propria.

The pathogenesis of reflux gastritis involves damage to the surface epithelium by bile acids and lysolecithin, resulting in disruption of the mucous barrier and cell exfoliation [24]. Access of bile constituents to the mucosa leads to degranulation of mast cells and a histamine-mediated vascular response [25]. Further damage to the surface epithelium ensues – possibly mediated by depressed prostaglandin synthesis, and back-diffusion of hydrogen ions may contribute to the mucosal injury.

Although we initially described the histological appearances in reflux as 'distinctive', this is only true in the sense that they characterize chemical injury to the stomach. Identical appearances can be seen in repeated injury by salicylates and other non-steroid anti-inflammatory drugs (NSAIDs) [26], and it is possible that alcohol could produce a similar response. Thus there is a need for a less restrictive term than 'reflux' to describe these appearances, and we have suggested that the designation chemical (type C) gastritis would be an appropriate and useful omnibus term for this category. However, the term 'chemical' with its connotations of exogenous corrosive or irritant injury has not met with wide acceptance and alternative terminology has been sought. The Sydney Working Party [27] settled on 'reactive' gastritis, but even this term has its shortcomings.

Reflux gastritis is essentially *H. pylori*-negative. However, in the postoperative stomach one is not dealing with enterogastric reflux in isolation. Prior to peptic ulcer surgery, all (or almost all) of these patients will have a *H. pylori*-positive chronic gastritis. Following operations which lead to reflux, this form of chronic gastritis will gradually give way to an *H. pylori*-negative reflux gastritis, which will only be seen in a 'pure' form some years after surgery [28]. In the intact stomach, the reflux (or reactive) picture can only be recognized in *H. pylori*-negative patients. In *H. pylori*-positive cases the chronic gastritis associated with bacterial infection will dominate the histological appearances. It might be that *H. pylori*-positive patients who also have duodenogastric reflux or take NSAIDs exhibit more foveolar hyperplasia, oedema and congestion than those with pure *H. pylori* gastritis. Such 'mixed' cases will be difficult to distinguish and might only be revealed by detailed morphometry. We have recently compared a group of patients whose biopsies revealed a reflux picture with a group of normals taken from the same overall population [29]. Those with 'reflux gastritis' had a significantly higher prevalence of associated peptic ulceration and of NSAID use. There was also a trend towards a higher alcohol consumption. Surprisingly, on testing fasting gastric juice for bile acids, only one patient in this group of relatively young dyspeptics (mean age = 37 years) had bile reflux, but in another series comprised of older patients (mean age = 58 years) we have shown that even in the intact stomach there is a significant association between bile reflux and the 'distinctive' histological picture previously recognized in postoperative patients [30].

Morphological aspects of H. pylori-associated gastritis

Acute inflammation

The acute phase of *Helicobacter* infection is rarely encountered in gastric biopsies because the illness which accompanies it is transient and vague in its symptomatology. The few descriptions in the literature are derived from human ingestion studies [31, 32] or from 'natural' infection in endoscopy personnel [33]. The acute gastritis is characterized by marked neutrophil polymorph infiltration of the mucosa with exudation at the surface. This contrasts with the more frequently seen acute haemorrhagic gastritis found with NSAID use or alcohol injury, where there is epithelial exfoliation, oedema and haemorrhage into the lamina propria but little or no polymorph response.

Chronic inflammation

The histological appearances in chronic gastritis are well known, but there are some aspects which are worth emphasizing. For instance, it is conventional to think that infiltration of the superficial lamina propria by lymphocytes and plasma cells represents the earliest stage of chronic gastritis. However, in cases where there is only mild inflammatory cell infiltration (therefore presumed to be early chronic inflammation), one frequently sees a midzonal infiltrate with sparing of the superficial lamina propria (Fig. 12.3). As far as polymorph infiltration is concerned, this has been borne out by morphometric methods, which have confirmed maximal activity centred on the pit–isthmus region [34]. Interestingly, Correa [5], in the pre-*H. pylori* era, wrote that 'a rather chracteristic focal necrosis and acute inflammation of the glandular neck area is observed' in environmental chronic gastritis. In attempting to link the polymorph response to *H. pylori* colonization, this concentration in the foveolar neck region represents something of a paradox in that, when the density of organisms is assessed in routine histological preparations, they appear to decline steadily from surface to neck. When the mucus

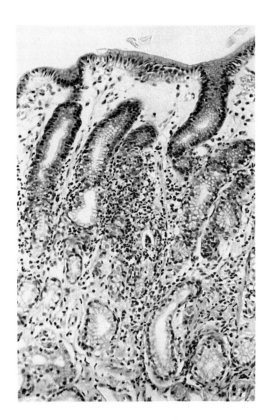

Fig. 12.3 'Early' chronic gastritis showing predominantly midzonal infiltration by lymphocytes and polymorphs centred on the pit–isthmus region. There is no increase of cells in the superficial lamina propria.

gel is stabilized prior to processing, however, the surface gel contains dispersed bacteria and the site of maximum density and epithelial contact is within the pits [35]. Thus, exposure to bacterial cytotoxins and ammonia is also likely to be maximal in the gastric pits. On the other hand, it might be that the immature foveolar epithelium just above the isthmic proliferative zone is more permeable to leucotactic factors, such as complement products generated following activation by *H. pylori*.

Lymphoid follicles

A further aspect of note is the finding of lymphoid follicles. These are more frequently seen when the inflammatory cell infiltrate extends through the full thickness of the mucosa and, by

separating the glandular elements, may give a false impression of atrophy [36]. It is not widely appreciated that the finding of reactive lymphoid follicles is virtually confined to *H. pylori*-positive gastritis [37] (Fig. 12.4), and their prevalence in antral mucosa is dependent on the degree and activity of the gastritis [38]. Lymphoid follicles form a prominent feature of *H. pylori* gastritis in children and may give rise to a characteristic endoscopic picture [39].

Atrophy

Atrophy is recognized by glandular loss and separation of the remaining glands by fibrous tissue. While the release of proteases by polymorphs and the production of other cytotoxic factors in the inflammatory and immune response could lead to glandular destruction, the role of *H. pylori* in the progression to diffuse antral and corporal atrophy is not clear-cut. Indeed Correa [6] has denied a role for *H. pylori* in the pathogenesis of multifocal atrophic gastritis, and Paull & Yardley [40] claim that their analogous metaplastic atrophic gastritis is not a sequel to *H. pylori* infection but is a result of 'poorly defined dietary habits and/or exposure to environmental agents'. In their follow-up study of chronic gastritis and *H. pylori* positivity, Villako *et al.* [41] found that progression from superficial (i.e. non-atrophic) to atrophic gastritis was always associated with the presence of *H pylori* but claimed that the later progression of atrophic gastritis is determined by other factors. Based on serological evidence, Faisal *et al.* [42] found an equal prevalence of positive *H. pylori* antibody titres in people with chronic superficial gastritis and those with atrophic gastritis. Although such findings do not prove an aetiological role for *H. pylori* in the development of atrophy, these studies indicate that *H. pylori*-associated gastritis is a frequent and immediate precursor of atrophic gastritis. It is true that *H. pylori* positivity (as detected histologically) declines with increasing atrophy, but this can be explained by the intragastric milieu becoming 'hostile' to the organism. Possible antagonistic factors involved in the elimination or suppres-

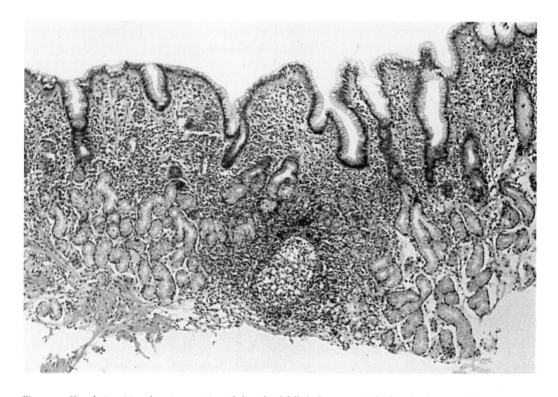

Fig. 12.4 *H. pylori*-positive chronic gastritis with lymphoid follicle formation. Whether this has resulted in separation of glands or is in an area of glandular atrophy is debatable and underlines the difficulties involved in categorizing biopsies as atrophic or not.

sion of *H. pylori* are the intestinal-type mucus secreted by metaplastic epithelium blocking bacterial penetration and attachment, and competition by the mixed bacterial flora colonizing the hypochlorhydric stomach [43]. Thus, despite originating from an *H. pylori*-positive gastritis, chronic gastritis with severe atrophy and IM is frequently *H. pylori*-negative. In keeping with this, the inflammatory response subsides, giving rise to a histological picture of 'quiescent' gastritis with atrophy where there are very few inflammatory cells. While progression from *H. pylori*-associated gastritis represents the major route whereby atrophy is produced, there is also a contribution from autoimmune gastritis and long-standing reflux or reactive gastritis which could have been *H. pylori*-negative from the outset. Thus atrophy is the end result of more than one form of gastritis, and these interrelations are illustrated in Fig. 12.5.

Intestinal metaplasia

Persistent chronic inflammation in the stomach eventually leads to IM. There are those authors who claim that atrophy and metaplasia are inextricably bound together [40]. Many histopathologists use metaplasia as a criterion for the diagnosis of atrophy, invoking as justification the poor inter-observer agreement that obtains in the recognition of minor degrees of atrophy. If glandular atrophy is sought as an independent feature, however, it is apparent that a substantial proportion of cases exhibit atrophy in the absence of metaplasia. Kekki *et al.* [43] found that 50% of subjects showing loss of antral and body glands lacked IM. Furthermore, cohort follow-up studies reveal progression from chronic gastritis with atrophy to IM [44].

Three main types of IM are recognized: an 'incomplete' small-intestinal type in which goblet cells secreting acidic sialomucins appear

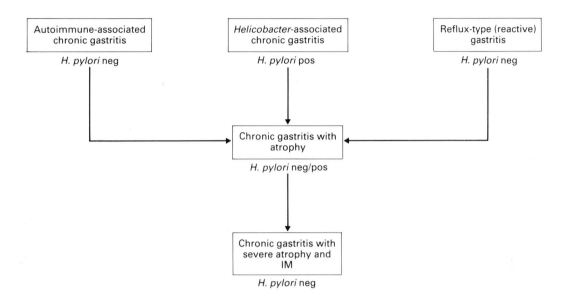

Fig. 12.5 Routes of development of atrophy in chronic gastritis.

interspersed between normal neutral mucin-secreting gastric epithelial cells (type II metaplasia); a 'complete' small-intestinal type where the intervening cells are absorptive in character, Paneth cells appear and there is villous transformation (type I metaplasia); and thirdly an 'incomplete' large-intestinal type where the mucosa takes on 'colonic' characteristics in that both the goblet cells and the non-absorptive intervening cells secrete sulphomucins (type III). *H. pylori* do not adhere to normal intestinal epithelium and, in keeping with this, organisms are not found on areas of IM in the stomach (Fig. 12.6). It has been suggested that this could explain the low prevalence of *H. pylori* in autoimmune gastritis [45], but metaplasia is rarely sufficiently widespread to preclude colonization.

With regard to the biological significance of IM, the conventional view is that it represents 'faulty regeneration' of the gastric mucosa and that the change in differentiation, particularly with regard to type III metaplasia, reflects a premalignant condition [46]. However, it is equally plausible that such metaplasia is an adaptive response to an altered microenvironment. Thus one can speculate that the develop-

ment of small-intestinal-type epithelium could confer a biological advantage either by preventing the adhesion of *H. pylori*, or, in the context of reflux gastritis, by rendering the mucosa more resistant to bile. Similarly the acquisition of colonic characteristics could be a response to the proliferation of 'faecal' organisms in the hypochlorhydric stomach consequent upon severe glandular atrophy. Therefore, in regard to *H. pylori* infection, type I metaplasia can be viewed as a relatively short-term (and potentially reversible) consequence of chronic inflammation, whereas type III metaplasia develops in the longer term in an atrophic mucosa in which *H. pylori* may no longer be detectable histologically. This explanation is consistent with the age distribution of subtypes of IM, in that patients with sulphomucin-positive IM (largely type III) are significantly older than sulphomucin-negative (types I and II) patients [47]. Furthermore, type I IM is generally found in association with moderate or severe chronic inflammation, while type III IM is usually seen in the absence of inflammation [48]. These findings can be explained by persistence of *H. pylori* where there is mild or moderate atrophy and type I metaplasia

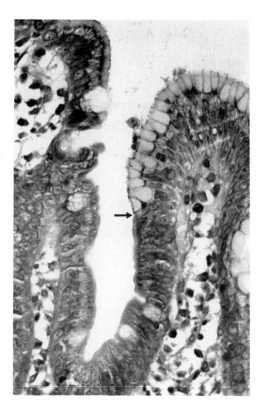

Fig. 12.6 Chronic gastritis with intestinal metaplasia. The heavy colonization of the normal gastric epithelium ends abruptly (at the arrow) with the change to intestinal-type epithelium composed of absorptive cells and goblet cells (complete IM – type I).

but disappearance of this organism from severely atrophic stomachs exibiting type III metaplasia.

Intestinal metaplasia can be viewed therefore as a 'defence response' which could be an epi-phenomenon with respect to the development of carcinoma [47]. This particularly applies to type I metaplasia, in which regression following gastric ulcer treatment has been documented [48]. The intragastric conditions which appear to induce type III intestinal metaplasia also predispose to the formation of carcinogens, so that carcinoma more frequently follows in the train of this type of metaplasia. We found that sulphomucin-positive IM, including type III metaplasia, lacks specificity for the subsequent development of gastric cancer [47], but other authors claim that the detection of type III IM may be useful in the identification of a 'higher-risk' group for surveillance [48, 49].

When malignancy develops in the *H. pylori*-positive stomach, the areas of high-grade dysplasia and intramucosal carcinoma are not colonized [14], presumably because of changes in the surface membrane characteristics of the malignant cells with loss of the specific glycoprotein responsible for binding the organism.

Distribution and density of H. pylori

On the basis of paired gastric biopsy specimens taken from 10 sites from 50 patients, Bayerdörffer *et al.* [50] established that all patients with active chronic gastritis at one or more sites were *H. pylori*-positive. A quarter of their patients showed patchy distribution of gastritis, however, and they calculated that four or five random biopsies would be required to detect active chronic gastritis with a high level (>95%) of confidence.

With regard to the relationship between the distribution and density of *H. pylori* and the severity of gastritis, Stolte *et al.* [51] have demonstrated a highly significant association between the degree of colonization and the severity and activity of gastritis in both the antrum and corpus from 1265 patients with *H. pylori*-associated gastritis. They found that the degree of colonization was identical in corpus and antrum in 49%; the antrum was more markedly colonized in 39% and the corpus in 12%. The degree and activity of gastritis, however, was much more pronounced in the antrum than in the corpus, even when the latter was equally colonized. Other authors using more sophisticated morphometric techniques have also found a significant correlation between bacterial colonization density and the degree of inflammation in antral biopsies [52, 53].

Ultrastructure

Ultrastructural studies on *H. pylori* in chronic gastritis lend support to its pathogenic role in that degenerative changes are frequently encountered in epithelial cells in close proximity to bacteria. Abundant phagolysosomes and depleted mucin content in cells have been observed in cells showing intimate contact with *H. pylori* [54]. Tricottet *et al.* [55] observed focal cell necrosis and partially digested organisms in heterophagosomes in foveolar cells. Both studies revealed patchy loss of microvilli in regions of bacterial attachment, and bacteria were seen within widened intercellular gaps and in the canaliculi of parietal cells. Controversy surrounds the finding of *H. pylori* within epithelial cells but a recent study in which intracellular organisms were identified seems convincing [56].

An early ultrastructural observation was the finding of so-called adhesion 'pedestals' at the site of *H. pylori* attachment to epithelial cells. These pedestals are similar to those marking the sites of attachment of enteropathogenic *Escherichia coli* to intestinal epithelium [57]. Our observations indicate that proximity of *H. pylori* to the surface epithelium results in loss of microvilli from the plasma membrane. Initial adhesion follows the development of an electron-dense 'fuzzy' or fibrillar layer between the organism and the membrane, and ruthenium red staining would support this being a glycoprotein ligand. The organism comes to abut the membrane, which extrudes to form an elevated plateau and subsequently 'cups' the bacterium to form a fully developed pedestal. In our study the proportion of organisms exhibiting adhesion sites in *H. pylori*-positive antral gastritis varied from 0 to 41% (mean = 19%) and those showing full pedestal formation from 0 to 21% (mean = 3.4%) [58]. The proportion of attached *H. pylori* was significantly correlated with the finding of degenerative changes in the surface epithelium seen on histological examination of parallel antral biopsies, but not with other indicators of disease activity, such as polymorph infiltration, mononuclear cell response and mucin depletion. It must be conceded, however, that the numbers of bacteria found in close apposition to the plasma membrane will have been exaggerated by contraction of the mucus layer during fixation and processing [35].

The Sydney System

The multiplicity of classifications of gastritis and the attendant confusion, together with a growing conviction that *H. pylori* was the major cause of chronic gastritis, prompted the organizers of the World Congresses of Gastroenterology in Sydney to set up a working party with the object of devising a new and universally acceptable classification of gastritis. The result of their deliberations was the Sydney System [27].

In order to be widely accepted the classification aimed to be simple, easy to apply, flexible and comprehensive. It has two major divisions, the histological and the endoscopic (Fig. 12.7).

The histological division is based on adequate sampling of both antrum and corpus, but it can be applied in a less complete form to single biopsies from either site. The system is centred on a core comprising a morphological summary and the topographical distribution of the gastritis. The major morphological changes are added as a suffix, and the aetiology and/or pathogenic associations are added as a prefix.

The morphological summary indicates whether the gastritis is acute, chronic or a special form (see overall classification in Table 12.3). On the basis of the pattern of involvement of the stomach, the gastritis is classified as affecting the antrum, or the corpus, or both in a so-called pangastritis. If there is widespread involvement but the severity is much more marked in one mucosal region than the other, then the terms antrum predominant and corpus predominant are employed.

The major morphological features are graded as nil, mild, moderate and severe, and when present are added as a suffix. Thus chronic inflammation, activity, atrophy, IM and the density of helicobacters are all graded. Other nonspecific features, such as mucin depletion, oedema and foveolar hyperplasia, should be commented upon if present but it was felt that these need not be graded in a routine report. Specific features, such as granulomas, lymphocytic infiltration of the surface epithelium, eosinophilic infiltration, or other infectious

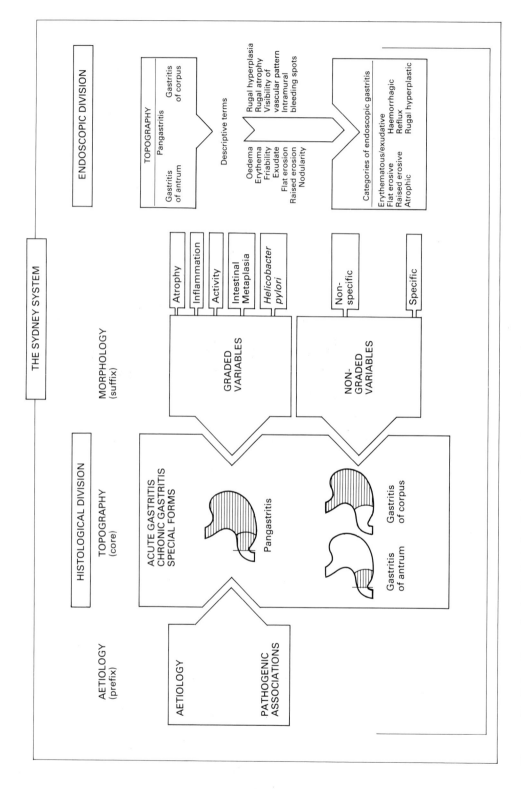

Fig. 12.7 The Sydney System for the histological and endoscopic classification of gastritis from Misiewicz *et al.* 1990 [27].

Table 12.3 Diagnostic categories of gastritis.

---

1 Aetiology or pathogenic associations of gastritis
H. pylori-associated
Autoimmune-associated
Drug-associated or other known gastric irritants
Infective (excluding *H. pylori*)
    Bacterial
    Viral
    Parasitic
    Fungal
Idiopathic

2 'Special' forms of gastritis
Eosinophilic gastritis
Lymphocytic gastritis
Granulomatous gastritis
    Crohn's-associated
    Sarcoid
    Idiopathic
Reactive (reflux-type) gastritis
Radiation-associated
Phlegmonous gastritis

---

agents (e.g. *'Gastrospirillum hominis'*), determine the nature of the special forms of gastritis.

Where the aetiology (or the most likely aetiological association) is known, this is shown as a prefix: for example *Helicobacter*-associated, NSAID-associated or autoimmune-associated chronic gastritis. The final diagnosis might therefore appear as '*Helicobacter*-associated chronic gastritis of the antrum with moderate activity' or 'autoimmune-associated chronic gastritis of the corpus with severe atrophy and moderate intestinal metaplasia'.

The Sydney System is adaptable to new data, and the other classifications can be translated into it. If widely adopted, it would standardize histopathological reporting at a higher level than has generally applied hitherto, and the system would provide sufficient detail for most clinicopathological research.

Patterns of gastritis and ulcer risk

It has been known for many years that patients with DU or GU exhibit an associated chronic gastritis, but the pattern of inflammation is different for the two ulcer sites.

The gastritis associated with DU predominantly affects the antrum. Conventionally, it is stated that there is little or no involvement of corpus mucosa [59]. More recent work suggests, however, that there is usually mild or moderate chronic inflammation, albeit with much less activity than is found in the antrum [60]. Glandular atrophy is absent or mild and IM is infrequent. Prepyloric GU are also accompanied by this pattern of gastritis, and it is now appreciated that this is invariably an *H. pylori*-associated gastritis. Organisms are usually plentiful on the actively inflamed antral mucosa but can also be found on the corpus mucosa, at a correspondingly lower density.

Proximal GU are associated with involvement of corpus and antral mucosa in a pangastritis. Glandular atrophy and IM are consistent findings, their degree and extent increasing with advancing age [61]. Atrophy commences in the antrum and extends along the lesser curvature into the corpus mucosa [62]. Further foci of atrophy and metaplasia appear in the anterior and posterior walls, producing a multifocal atrophic gastritis, and these gradually enlarge and coalesce so that much of the corpus mucosa shows an antrophic picture [63]. Although, as discussed above, *H. pylori* can disappear from the severely atrophic stomach, most patients with GU are *H. pylori*-positive, particularly if patients with known causes of ulceration, such as NSAIDs, are eliminated [64].

The two apparently distinct patterns of gastritis found in association with DU and GU are both therefore attributable to *H. pylori* infection. The fact that in the former category the gastritis is much more pronounced in the antrum may be a result of 'protection' of the corpus by the intrinsically higher acid production found in DU patients. Stolte, Eidt & Ohnsmann [51] invoked this mechanism in explaining the discrepancy between the distribution of organisms and the absence or mild degree of gastritis in the corpus. In so far as the reduced inflammatory reaction is only partly explicable by an acid-induced lowering of *H. pylori* colonization, these authors postulated that acid affected the production of cytotoxins, ammonia or leucotactic substances by organisms overlying corpus mucosa. This hypothesis is supported firstly by the linear increase in the density of colonization in the corpus in parallel with increasing age [51], as it is known that acid production falls with ageing, and secondly by the relatively low level of *H. pylori* infection in the stomachs of patients with the Zollinger–Ellison syndrome [65].

Further evidence that the corpus is more resistant to gastritis in DU patients is provided by the observation that the rate of extension from the antrum and progression of gastritis in such patients is much slower than in non-ulcer controls with chronic gastritis [66]. That there is no permanent barrier to inflammation is indicated by the finding of rapid extension of inflammation into the corpus after vagotomy [67] and a 'normal' rate of progression of gastritis in the corpus of DU patients following antrectomy [68].

Viewed from a functional standpoint, the pattern of gastritis found in DU patients – a diffuse antral gastritis with relative sparing of the corpus – means that the parietal cell mass is unaffected by atrophy and permits normal or even increased acid production. In contrast, GU patients exhibit multifocal atrophy in both antral and corpus mucosa, which results in diminished acid and pepsin production but renders the gastric mucosa more susceptible to ulceration. Thus patients with predominantly antral gastritis are at much increased risk of duodenal and prepyloric ulcers compared with normals, whereas those with involvement of both antrum and corpus by atrophic mucosa are unlikely to develop DU but there remains an increased risk of GU [69]. Patients with severe degrees of atrophy in corpus mucosa will have such low acid levels that even with a vulnerable mucosa the ulcer risk is very low; this is in keeping with the 'no-acid, no-ulcer' dictum.

Natural history

There have been very few longitudinal histological studies which examine the evolution of *H. pylori* infection. Our own serendipitous study of infection in a gastroenterologist revealed progression from an acute neutrophilic gastritis to chronic gastritis over the course of 2.5 months [33]. While epidemiological evidence points to such progression being a frequent event, the ingestion experiment by Marshall *et al.* [31] demonstrates that spontaneous clearance of infection with resolution of the inflammatory reaction is possible.

The evolution of *Helicobacter*-associated chronic gastritis has not been adequately documented. We can assume, however, that the plethora of studies conducted in the pre-*H. pylori* era which examined the progress of chronic superficial gastritis are valid examples of the behaviour of *H. pylori* gastritis.

The conclusion to be drawn from these epidemiological studies is that there are various levels of genetic predisposition to gastritis mediated through mucosal defence and immunological mechanisms. This emphasizes that the response to *H. pylori* infection is not uniform and will vary according to genetic susceptibility. This partly explains why some people exposed to infection will suffer a mild and self-limiting acute gastritis, in which the organisms are eliminated and the inflammatory response resolves, while the majority of individuals are unable to eliminate the organism and a chronic gastritis ensues.

Although, once established, *H. pylori* infection is diffusely present in the stomach, the degree of colonization is maximal in the antrum and inflammation varies accordingly [38]. The variation between antrum and corpus is particularly marked in the small proportion of inviduals who have a large parietal cell mass and therefore have a DU diathesis, and one can speculate that protection of the corpus by increased acid production results in predominantly antral inflammation [70]. The majority of individuals, however, will develop diffuse chronic inflammation. Whether or not *H. pylori*-related inflammation of itself leads to multifocal atrophy and IM is controversial. The balance of evidence points to a very close association with *H. pylori*, if not a direct aetiological role, but the subsequent progression of the atrophy is more likely to be influenced by environmental factors. The precise nature of these factors is unknown, but differences in diet, water supply and socio-economic conditions may in some measure explain the

marked variation in the incidence of chronic gastritis and atrophy between countries [5]. An alternative explanation, however, might be that these same factors influence the age at which *H. pylori* infection is acquired, and onset in childhood would allow greater time for the progression from non-atrophic to atrophic chronic gastritis to occur. How much the pattern and evolution of chronic gastritis is influenced by the virulence of the infecting strain of *H. pylori* has yet to be determined.

It seems unlikely that *H. pylori* has any role in producing the severe corpus atrophy of pernicious anaemia. The epidemiological data remain consistent with the view that this is a distinct autoimmune gastritis, occurring in people who are predisposed by the inheritance of a dominant genetic abnormality but the possibilities that the disease is triggered by *H. pylori* infection [71] or that pernicious anaemia is the end result of *H. pylori*-induced atrophy [72] cannot be excluded.

References

1 Motteram, R. A biopsy study of chronic gastritis and gastric atrophy. *J. Pathol. Bacteriol.* 1951, **63**, 389–94.

2 Cheli, R., Santi, L., Ciancameria, G. & Canciani, G. A clinical and statistical follow-up study of atrophic gastritis. *Dig. Dis.* 1973, **18**, 1061–6.

3 Strickland, R.G. & Mackay, I.R. A reappraisal of the nature and significance of chronic atrophic gastritis. *Dig. Dis.* 1973, **18**, 426–40.

4 Glass, G.B.J. & Pitchumoni, C.S. Atrophic gastritis. *Hum. Pathol.* 1975, **6**, 219–50.

5 Correa, P. The epidemiology and pathogenesis of chronic gastritis: three etiologic entities. *Front Gastrointest. Res.* 1980, **6**, 98–108.

6 Correa, P. Chronic gastritis: a clinico-pathological classification. *Am. J. Gastroenterol.* 1988, **83**, 504–9.

7 Warren, J.R. & Marshall, B. Unidentified curved bacilli on gastric epithelium in active chronic gastritis. *Lancet* 1983, **i**, 1273–5.

8 Goodwin, C.S., Armstrong, J.A. & Marshall, B.J. *Campylobacter pyloridis*, gastritis and peptic ulceration. *J. Clin. Pathol.* 1986, **39**, 353–65.

9 Morris, A., Arthur, J. & Nicholson, G. *Campylobacter pyloridis* infection in Auckland patients with gastritis. *NZ Med. J.* 1986, **99**, 353–5.

10 Rawles, J.W., Paull, G., Yardley, J.H., Hendrix, T.R., Rayich, W.J., Walters, L.L., Dick, J.D. & Margolis, A. Gastric *Campylobacter*-like organisms in a U.S. hospital population. *Gastroenterology* 1986, **91**, 1599A.

11 Wyatt, J.I., Rathbone, B.J. & Heatley, R.V. Local immune response to gastric *Campylobacter* in non-ulcer dyspepsia. *J. Clin. Pathol.* 1986, **39**, 863–70.

12 Andersen, L.P., Holck, S., Povlsen, C.O., Elsborg, L. & Justensen, T. *Campylobacter pyloridis* in peptic ulcer disease. *Scand. J. Gastroenterol.* 1987, **22**, 219–24.

13 Fiocca, R., Vallani, L., Turpini, R. & Solcia, E. High incidence of *Campylobacter* like organisms in endoscopic biopsies from patients with gastritis, with or without peptic ulcer. *Digestion* 1987, **38**, 234–44.

14 Jiang, S.J., Liu, W.Z., Zhang, D.Z., Shi, Y., Xiao, S.D., Zhang, Z.H. & Lu, D.Y. *Campylobacter* like organisms in chronic gastritis, peptic ulcer and gastric carcinoma. *Scand. J. Gastroenterol.* 1987, **22**, 553–8.

15 O'Connor, H.J., Axon, A.T.R. & Dixon, M.F. *Campylobacter*-like organisms unusual in type A (pernicious anaemia) gastritis. *Lancet* 1984, **ii**, 1091.

16 Flejou, P.F., Bahame, P., Smith, A., Stockbrugger, R.W., Rode, J. & Price, A.B. Pernicious anaemia and *Campylobacter* like organisms: is the gastric antrum resistant to colonization? *Gut* 1989, **30**, 60–4.

17 Haot, J., Delos, M., Wallez, L., Hardy, N., Lensen, B. & Jouret-Mourin, A. Intraepithelial lymphocytes in inflammatory gastric pathology. *Acta Endoscop.* 1986, **16**, 61–7.

18 Dixon, M.F., Wyatt, J.I., Burke, D.A. & Rathbone, B.J. Lymphocytic gastritis – relationship to *Campylobacter pylori* infection. *J. Pathol.* 1988, **154**, 125–32.

19 Wallez, L., Weynaud, B. & Haot, J. Evaluation histologique de la présence d'organismes de type *Campylobacter* dans les gastrite lymphocytaires. *Acta Endoscop.* 1987, **17**, 41–50.

20 Flejou, J.F., Price, A.B. & Smith, A.C. A natural history of *Campylobacter pylori* in the stomach: a follow-up biopsy study. *Gastroenterol. Int.* 1988, 1085A.

21 Karttunen, T. & Niemala, S. Lymphocytic gastritis and coeliac disease. *J. Clin. Pathol.* 1990, **43**, 436.

22 Wolber, R., Owen, D., DelBuono, L., Appelman, H. & Freeman, H. Lymphocytic gastritis in patients with celiac sprue or sprue-like intestinal disease. *Gastroenterology* 1990, **98**, 310–15.

23 Dixon, M.F., O'Connor, H.J., Axon, A.T.R., King, R.F.J.G. & Johnston, D. Reflux gastritis: distinct histopathological entity? *J. Clin. Pathol.* 1986, **39**, 524–30.

24 Eastwood, G.L. Effect of pH on bile salt injury to mouse gastric mucosa: a light and electron microscope study. *Gastroenterology* 1975, **68**, 1456–65.

25 Rees, W. & Rhodes, J. Bile reflux in gastro-oesophageal disease. *Clin. Gastroenterol.* 1977, **6**, 179–200.

26 Laine, L., Marin-Sorensen, M. & Weinstein, W.M. The histology of gastric erosions in patients taking non-steroidal anti-inflammatory drug (NSAIDs): a prospective study. *Gastroenterology* 1988, **94**, A247.

27 Misiewicz, J.J., Tytgat, G.N.J., Goodwin, C.S., Price, A.B., Sipponen, P., Strickland, R.G. & Cheli, R. 1990. The Sydney System: a new classification of gastritis. In *Working Party Reports of the World Congresses of*

Gastroenterology. Blackwell Scientific Publications, Melbourne, pp. 1–10.

28 O'Connor, H.J., Dixon, M.F., Wyatt, J.J., Axon, A.T.R., Ward, D.C., Dewar, E.P. & Johnston, D. Effect of duodenal ulcer surgery and enterogastric reflux on *Campylobacter pyloridis. Lancet* 1986, ii, 1178–81.

29 Sobala, G.M., King, R.F.G., Axon, A.T.R. & Dixon, M.F. Reflux gastritis in the intact stomach. *Gut* 1990, 43, 303–6.

30 Sobala, G.M., Dixon, M.F., Pignatelli, B. *et al.* Levels of nitrate, nitrate, N-nitrosocompounds, ascorbic acid and total bile acids in gastric juice of patients with and without pre-cancerous conditions of the stomach. *Carcinogenesis* 1991, 12, 193–8.

31 Marshall, B., Armstrong, J., McGechie, D. & Glancy, R. Attempt to fulfil Koch's postulates for pyloric *Campylobacter. Med. J. Aust.* 1985, 142, 436–9.

32 Morris, A. & Nicholson, G. Ingestion of *Campylobacter pyloridis* causes gastritis and raised fasting gastric pH. *Am. J. Gastroenterol.* 1987, 82, 192–9.

33 Sobala, G.M., Crabtree, J., Dixon, M.F., Schorah, C.J., Taylor, J.D., Rathbone, B.J., Heatley, R.V. & Axon, A.T.R. Acute *Helicobacter pylori* infection: clinical features, local and systemic immune response, gastric mucosal histology and gastric juice ascorbic acid concentrations. *Gut* 1991, 32, 1415–18.

34 Hopwood, D. A histometric analysis of gastric biopsies from patients treated with Gastritex: a new drug active against acute or chronic gastritis. *J. Pathol.* 1988, 154, 86A.

35 Thomsen, L.L., Gavin, J.B. & Tasman-Jones, C. Relation of *Helicobacter pylori* to the human gastric mucosa in chronic gastritis of the antrum. *Gut* 1990, 31, 1230–6.

36 Wyatt, J.I. & Dixon, M.F. Chronic gastritis – a pathogenetic approach. *J. Pathol.* 1988, 154, 113–24.

37 Wyatt, J.I. & Rathbone, B.J. Immune response of the gastric mucosa to *Campylobacter pylori. Scand. J. Gastroenterol.* 1988, 23, suppl. 142, 44–9.

38 Stolte, M. & Eidt, S. Lymphoid follicles in antral mucosa: immune response to *Campylobacter pylori? J. Clin. Pathol.* 1989, 42, 1269–71.

39 Mahony, M.J., Wyatt, J.I. & Littlewood, J.M. *Campylobacter pylori* gastrits. *Arch. Dis. Child.* 1988, 63, 654–5.

40 Paull, G. & Yardley, J.H. 1989. Pathology of *C. pylori*-associated gastric and eosophageal lesions. In Blaser, M.J. (ed.) *Campylobacter pylori in Gastritis and Peptic Ulcer Disease.* Igaku-Shoin, New York, pp. 73–97.

41 Villako, K., Maards, H., Tammur, R., Keevallik R., Reetsalu, M., Sipponen, P., Kekki, M. & Siurala, M. *Helicobacter (Campylobacter) pylori* infestation and the development and progression of chronic gastritis: results of long-term follow-up examinations of a random sample. *Endoscopy* 1990, 22, 114–17.

42 Faisal, M.A., Russell, R.M., Samloff, I.M. & Holt, P.R. *Helicobacter pylori* infection and atrophic gastritis in the elderly. *Gastroenterology* 1990, 99, 1543–4.

43 Kekki, M., Siurala, M., Varis, K., Sipponen, P., Sistonen, P. & Nevanlinna, H.R. Classification principles and genetics of chronic gastritis. *Scand. J. Gastroenterol.* 1987, 22, suppl. 141, 1–28.

44 Correa, P., Haenszel, W., Cuello, C., Zavala, D., Fontham, E., Zarama, G., Tannenbaum, S., Collazos, T. & Ruiz, B. Gastric precancerous process in a high risk population: cohort follow-up. *Cancer Res.* 1990, 50, 4737–40.

45 Thomas, J.M. *Campylobacter*-like organisms in gastritis. *Lancet* 1984, ii, 1217.

46 Sugimara, T., Matsukura, N. & Sato, S. Intestinal metaplasia of the stomach as a precancerous stage. *IARC Sci. Pub.* 1982, 39, 515–30.

47 Ectors, N. & Dixon, M.F. The prognostic value of sulphomucin positive intestinal metaplasia in the development of gastric cancer. *Histopathology* 1986, 10, 1271–7.

48 Silva, S., Filipe, M.I. & Pinho, A. Variants of intestinal metaplasia in the evolution of chronic atrophic gastritis and gastric ulcer. A follow-up study. *Gut* 1990, 31, 1097–104.

49 Filipe, M.I. & Jass, J.R. 1986. Intestinal metaplasia subtypes and cancer risk. In Filipe, M.I. & Jass, J.R. (eds) *Current Problems in Tumour Pathology: Gastric Carcinoma.* Churchill Livingstone, Edinburgh, pp. 87–115.

50 Bayerdörffer, E., Oertel, H., Lehn, N., Kasper, G., Mannes, G.A., Sauerbruch, T. & Stolte, M. Topographic association between active gastritis and *Campylobacter pylori* colonisation. *J. Clin. Pathol.* 1989, 42, 834–9.

51 Stolte, M., Eidt, S. & Ohnsmann, A. Differences in *Helicobacter pylori*, associated gastritis in the antrum and body of the stomach. *Z. Gastroenterol.* 1990, 28, 229–33.

52 Steininger, H., Schneider, U., Bartz, K. & Simmler, B. *Campylobacter pylori* und Gastritis – Besiedelungsdichte und Grad der Entzündung. Semiquantitative und morphometrische Untersuchung. *Leber Magen Darm* 1989, 19, 70–8.

53 Collins, J.S.A., Sloan, J.M., Hamilton, P.W., Watt, P.C.H. & Love, A.H.G. Investigation of the relationship between gastric antral inflammation and *Campylobacter pylori* using graphic tablet planimetry. *J. Pathol.* 1989, 159, 281–5.

54 Chen, X.G., Correa, P., Offerhaus, J., Rodriguez, E., Janney, F., Hoffmann, E., Fox, J., Hunter, F. & Diavolitsis, S. Ultrastructure of the gastric mucosa harbouring *Campylobacter*-like organisms. *Am. J. Clin. Pathol.* 1986, 86, 575–82.

55 Tricottet, V., Bruneval, P., Vire, O. & Camilleri, J.P. *Campylobacter*-like organisms and surface epithelium abnormalities in active, chronic gastritis in humans: an ultrastructural study. *Ultrastruct. Pathol.* 1986, 10, 113–22.

56 Kazi, J.L., Sinniah, R., Zaman, V., Ng, M.L., Jafarey, N.A., Alam, S.M., Zuberi, S.J. & Kazi, A.M., Ultrastructural study of *Helicobacter pylori*-associated gastritis. *J. Pathol.* 1990, **161**, 65–70.

57 Cantey, J.R., Lushbaugh, W.B. & Inman, L.R. Attachment of bacteria to intestinal epithelial cells in diarrhoea caused by *E. coli* strain RDEC-1 in the rabbit: stages and role of capsule. *J. Infect. Dis.* 1981, **143**, 219–30.

58 Hessey, S.J., Wyatt, J.I., Axon, A.T.R., Sobala, G., Rathbone, B.J. & Dixon, M.F. The relationship between adhesion sites and disease activity in *C. pylori* associated gastritis. *Gut* 1990, **31**, 134–8.

59 Trier, J.S., Morphology of the gastric mucosa in patients with ulcer diseases. *Am. J. Dig. Dis.* 1976, **21**, 138–40.

60 Eidt, S. & Stolte, M. 1990. Differences between *Helicobacter pylori* associated gastritis in patients with duodenal ulcer, pyloric ulcer, other gastric ulcer, and gastritis without ulcer. In Malfertheiner, P. & Ditschuneit, H. (eds) *Helicobacter pylori, Gastritis and Peptic Ulcer.* Springer-Verlag, Berlin, pp. 228–36.

61 Maaroos, H.I., Salupere, V., Uibo, R., Kekki, M. & Sipponen, P. Seven year follow-up study of chronic gastritis in gastric ulcer patients. *Scand. J. Gastroenterol.* 1985, **20**, 198–204.

62 Kimura, K., Chronological transition of the fundic–pyloric border determined by stepwise biopsy of the lesser and greater curvatures of the stomach. *Gastroenterology* 1972, **63**, 584–92.

63 Fujishima, K., Misumi, A. & Akagi, M. Histopathologic study on development and extension of atrophic change in the gastric mucosa. *Gastroenterol. Jap.* 1984, **19**, 9–17.

64 Shallcross, T.M., Rathbone, B.J., Wyatt, J.I. & Heatley, R.V. *Helicobacter pylori* associated chronic gastritis and peptic ulceration in patients taking nonsteroidal anti-inflammatory drugs. *Aliment. Pharmacol. Ther.* 1990, **4**, 515–22.

65 Talley, N.J. 1990. Is *Helicobacter pylori* negative duodenal ulcer a separate disease? In Malfertheiner, P. & Ditschuneit, H. (eds) *Helicobacter pylori, Gastritis and Peptic Ulcer.* Springer-Verlag, Berlin, pp. 340–4.

66 Kekki, M., Sipponen, P. & Siurala, M. Progression of antral and body gastritis in patients with active and healed duodenal ulcer and duodentis. *Scand. J. Gastroenterol.* 1984, **19**, 382–8.

67 Meikle, D.D., Taylor, K.B., Truelove, S.C. & Whitehead, R. Gastritis, duodenitis, and circulating levels of gastrin in duodenal ulcer before and after vagotomy. *Gut* 1976, **17**, 719–28.

68 Kekki, M., Saukkonen, M., Sipponen, P., Varis, K. & Siurala, M. Dynamics of chronic gastritis in the remnant after partial gastrectomy for duodenal ulcer. *Scand. J. Gastroenterol.* 1980, **15**, 509–12.

69 Sipponen, P., Seppälä, K., Aarynen, M., Helske, T. & Kettunen, P. Chronic gastritis and gastroduodenal ulcer: a case control study on risk of coexisting duodenal or gastric ulcer in patients with gastritis. *Gut* 1989, **30**, 922–9.

70 Dixon, M.F. *Helicobacter pylori* and peptic ulceration: Histopathological aspects. *J. Gastroenterol. Hepatol.* 1991, **6**, 125–30.

71 Negrini, R., Lisato, L., Zanella, I., Cavazzini, L., Gullini, S., Villanacci, V., Poiesi, C., Albertini, A. & Ghielmi, S. *Helicobacter pylori* infection induces antibodies cross-reacting with human gastric mucosa. *Gastroenterology* 1991, **101**, 437–45.

72 de Luca, V.A. *Helicobacter pylori* gastric atrophy and pernicious anemia. *Gastroenterology* 1992, **102**, 744–5.

13 Helicobacter pylori, Duodenitis and Duodenal Ulceration

J.I.WYATT

Introduction

'Peptic duodenitis', characterized by inflammation of the duodenal mucosa with polymorph infiltration and surface gastric metaplasia [1], is commonly seen in biopsies from the margin of duodenal ulcers, and also occurs in the absence of duodenal ulceration. Most workers believe that duodenitis and duodenal ulcer belong to the same pathophysiological spectrum [1, 2]. However, since duodenal biopsies are not often routinely taken, duodenitis has received less attention than gastritis.

It has been recognized for some time that patients with duodenal ulcer have chronic gastritis which diffusely involves the antral mucosa, often with mucosal lymphoid follicles. The body-type mucosa is normal or only mildly inflamed, and does not show any atrophy of acid-secreting glands [3]. This is the diffuse antral (previously 'hypersecretory') pattern of gastritis, described by Correa [3], which we now know to be very closely associated with *Helicobacter pylori* colonization [4]. The proportion of *H. pylori*-positive patients who have this pattern of gastritis varies, but in our experience in Leeds is at least 35%. The maintenance of the integrity of the corpus mucosa is important in preserving acid-secretory capacity; *H. pylori*-positive patients with atrophic gastritis of the corpus and consequent loss of the acid-secreting glands are not at increased risk of duodenal ulcer [5]. Sipponen *et al.* [6] have recently confirmed that the gastritis precedes the development of peptic ulceration, and not vice versa. The importance of the role of *H. pylori* in the aetiology of duodenal ulcer is most convincingly demonstrated by the absence of ulcer relapse in patients from whom *H. pylori* has been eradicated, an effect which is independent of any mucosal protective effect of bismuth agents [7].

H. pylori in patients with duodenal ulcer and duodenitis

The association between duodenal ulcer and *H. pylori* gastritis is very strong (Table 13.1) [8–17]. In our experience, 95% of duodenal ulcer patients have *Helicobacter*-associated gastritis; others have found that in the few *H. pylori*-negative patients with duodenal ulcer there is usually some different aetiological factor, such as use of non-steroidal anti-inflammatory agents or pancreatitis to account for the duodenal ulcer [8, 18].

H. pylori is now implicated in the pathogenesis of duodenal ulcer in two ways: firstly, by directly infecting the duodenal mucosa in patients who have areas of gastric epithelium in the duodenum, resulting in inflammation of the duodenal mucosa (Fig. 13.1); and, secondly, the presence of *Helicobacter*-associated gastritis is associated with alterations in gastric physiology, such as elevation of serum gastrin, which are characteristic of the population at risk of duodenal ulcer, and which may predispose to ulceration. Therefore the association with duodenal ulcer may have two components – firstly, that *H. pylori* plays a direct role in causing the mucosal damage in the duodenum which may lead to ulceration and, secondly, that *H. pylori* gastritis is associated with the pathophysiological disturbances present in duodenal ulcer patients.

Various pathogenic mechanisms have been

Table 13.1 Prevalence of *H. pylori* in patients with duodenal ulcer.

Patients studied	Number (%) with *H. pylori*	References
70	63 (90%)	Marshall *et al.* 1985 [8]
21	17 (80%)	Price *et al.* 1985 [9]
32	25 (78%)	Booth *et al.* 1986 [10]
36	35 (97%)	O'Connor *et al.* 1986 [11]
37	28 (76%)	Marcheggiano *et al.* 1987 [12]
14	12 (86%)	Jiang *et al.* 1987 [13]
17	12 (70%)	Raskov *et al.* 1987 [14]
66	61 (93%)	Coghlan *et al.* 1987 [15]
36	36 (100%)	Rauws *et al.* 1988 [16]
107	100 (93%)	Goodwin *et al.* 1988 [17]

proposed for *H. pylori* and their relative importance *in vivo* is not yet clear. However, these require that the bacterium is closely associated with the mucosal surface for damage to occur. If *H. pylori* is to have a direct role in duodenal mucosal damage, colonization of the duodenal mucosa is necessary. We have recently confirmed that the inflammatory infiltrate in duodenitis includes cells involved in the local humoral response to *H. pylori*-specific antigens, in the same way as has been shown in the gastric mucosa [19].

Several groups have shown that *H. pylori* is found in the duodenum in patients with duodenitis and duodenal ulcer. In all these

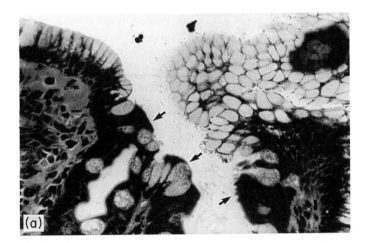

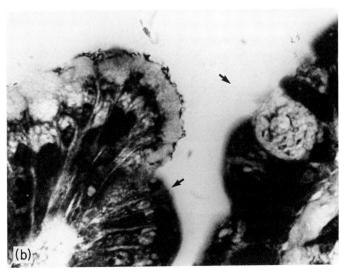

Fig. 13.1 Gastric mucosa with *H. pylori* colonization; the foci of intestinal metaplasia (arrows) are not colonized by bacteria. Magnification: (a) × 80; (b) × 198. Modified Giemsa stain.

Table 13.2 Frequency of *H. pylori* in duodenal biopsies from patients with duodenal ulcer and duodenitis.

H. pylori + ve/total duodenal ulcer	*H. pylori* + ve/total duodenitis	*H. pylori* + ve/total normal	Reference
8/11	–	–	Steer 1984 [20]
45/53	36/39	0/58	Johnson *et al.* 1986 [18]
8/13	11/21	0/256	Wyatt *et al.* 1987 [21]
7/24	–	–	Bode *et al.* 1987 [22]
14/14	5/16	–	Caselli *et al.* 1988 [23]

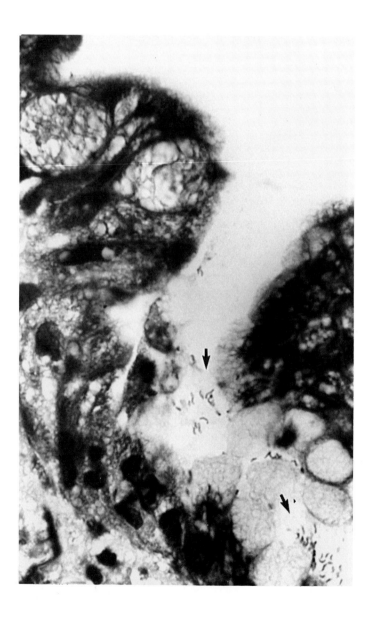

Fig. 13.2 *H. pylori* in the duodenum in a patient with duodenitis; bacteria are found only on areas of intestinal metaplasia (arrows). Modified Giemsa stain, × 225.

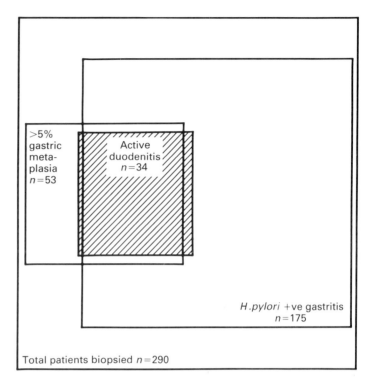

Fig. 13.3 Active duodenitis, gastric metaplasia in the duodenum and *Helicobacter*-associated gastritis in 290 dyspeptic patients. Reproduced with permission of the *Journal of Clinical Pathology* [21].

reports, *H. pylori* is only found in duodenal mucosa showing active inflammation, with areas of gastric-type surface epithelium. The reported frequency of this finding is between 29% and 100%, as shown in Table 13.2 [18, 20–23]. *H. pylori* is unable to colonize small-intestinal epithelium, as demonstrated by the sparing of intestinal metaplasia in chronic gastritis (Fig. 13.1) [24, 25]. In the same way, the distribution of *H. pylori* in the duodenum is restricted to foci of gastric epithelium in the duodenal mucosa (Fig. 13.2) [18, 20–23].

We studied histologically the relationship between *Helicobacter*-associated gastritis, gastric metaplasia in the duodenum, and duodenal inflammation in 290 dyspeptic patients [21]. The proportion of the surface epithelium of the duodenal biopsies showing gastric metaplasia was subjectively graded. The relationship between duodenal inflammation and gastric metaplasia is shown in Table 13.3. Active ('peptic') duodenitis was associated with gastric metaplasia and increased in frequency with

increasing extent of metaplasia. However, a proportion of biopsies with metaplasia showed no inflammation.

The relationship between gastric metaplasia, *H. pylori* and active duodenitis is shown in Fig. 13.3; duodenitis developed specifically in the group of patients who were *H. pylori*-positive and had gastric metaplasia in the duodenum. Morphological studies therefore strongly favour a direct local role for bacterial infection of this metaplastic epithelium in causing active duodenitis.

In this series, *H. pylori* were observed in the duodenal biopsies in 55% of patients with duodenitis. This frequency is considerably lower than is seen in chronic gastritis (although reports vary; see Table 13.2) [18, 20–23]. This may be for two reasons: unlike gastritis, duodenitis is a patchy lesion in the mucosa [26], and so sampling error will be important; and, secondly, *H. pylori* are sparser and smaller in the duodenum, often appearing coccoid [23, 27], and are thus less easily detected by histology.

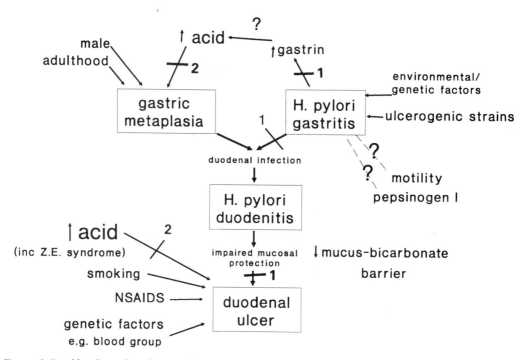

Fig. 13.6 Possible relationship of various factors related to duodenal ulcer pathogenesis (modified from ref. 48). 1, Effect of eradication of *H. pylori*. 2, Effect of reducing acid.

Ellison syndrome [43]. It is not found in patients with atrophic gastritis and intestinal metaplasia affecting the acid-secreting corpus mucosa [35], and appears to be reduced after highly selective vagotomy [21, 44]. It is significantly more common in males than females, which may be related to their higher acid secretory capacity [35]. It is not specifically a response to acid injury, since it is also occasionally seen in Crohn's disease and ulcerative jejunitis [45, 46], but, in the proximal duodenum, high acid load represents the most frequent potential cause of mucosal injury. Of the other factors which may be related to duodenal mucosal injury, gastric metaplasia shows no correlation with use of NSAIDs or with smoking [29, 35], but may be more common in heavy alcohol drinkers [47]. We found that gastric metaplasia is no more frequent in patients with *Helicobacter*-associated gastritis than in those with normal gastric mucosa, but the foci tend to be larger in patients infected by the organism [35]. Possibly in these patients the mucosal damage incurred during duodenitis

itself provides an additional stimulus to the formation of gastric metaplasia.

Effect of H. pylori on gastric pathophysiology

There has been much recent interest in the association between *Helicobacter*-associated gastritis and a number of alterations in gastroduodenal physiology, some of which were recognized as characteristic of duodenal ulcer patients before their association with *H. pylori* was known. These include changes in serum gastrin, possible effects on gastroduodenal motility and altered pepsinogen secretion [48]. To what extent these contribute to the pathogenesis of duodenal ulcer is currently unclear. For example, serum gastrin has a trophic effect on the parietal cells, and may increase parietal cell mass in patients with gastritis who do not develop atrophic gastritis of the corpus mucosa. Other changes may contribute to duodenal acid load, and thus will tend to cause duodenal mucosal damage directly and promote the formation of gastric metaplasia.

The higher serum gastrin levels in patients with *H. pylori* have received most attention. This elevation is a characteristic of both patients with duodenal ulcer and *H. pylori* [49] and normal volunteers who are *H. pylori*-positive [50]. The effect is reversed on eradication of *H. pylori* [51], but since it does not appear to be accompanied by changes in acid output [51] it may not be of direct importance in duodenal ulcer pathogenesis.

Duodenal ulcer is a multifactorial condition, and its pathogenesis will depend on the interplay of *H. pylori* with many other factors. These may potentially act at three levels – in the development of gastric metaplasia, in determining host susceptibility to *H. pylori* and in causing ulceration of the inflamed duodenum. Figure 13.6 summarizes the possible relationship between *H. pylori* and other factors involved in the pathogenesis of duodenitis and duodenal ulcer. Whether a subject infected with *H. pylori* will develop a duodenal ulcer may be affected but the strain of organism [52], the host's genetic factors, and other environmental factors such as smoking.

The significance of different factors can be tested by studying the effects of *H. pylori* eradication. For example, serum gastrin levels return to normal after eradication of *H. pylori* [51], showing that gastrin elevation is related to the bacteria or gastritis, and is not an independent (genetic?) factor in predisposing patients to duodenal ulcer. Smoking is associated with duodenal ulcer relapse only in patients who remain *H. pylori*-positive [53]. Blood group status shows no association with *H. pylori* [54, 55] and presumably represents an independent, genetic factor in duodenal ulcer pathogenesis. The distribution of chronic gastritis – whether it affects the antrum only or is associated with atrophic gastritis in the corpus as well – may also be dependent on genetic or environmental factors [56]. Finally, non-steroidal anti-inflammatory agents are associated with duodenal ulceration independently of any effect of *H. pylori* or gastric metaplasia [57, 58], while a very high acid output, as in patients with Zollinger–Ellison syndrome, is sufficient to cause ulceration without the additional factor of *H. pylori* [59]. Further studies may clarify the interaction of these factors within a unifying concept of duodenal ulcer pathogenesis.

References

1 Joffe, S.N., Lee, F.D. & Blumgart, L.H. Duodenitis. *Clin. Gastroenterol.* 1978, 7, 635–50.
2 Thompson, W.O., Joffe, S.N., Robertson, A.G. *et al.* Is duodenitis a dyspeptic myth? *Lancet* 1977, ii, 1197–8.
3 Correa, P. Chronic gastritis: a clinico-pathological classification. *Am. J. Gastroenterol.* 1988, 83, 504–9.
4 Chen, X.G., Correa, P., Offerhaus, J. *et al.* Ultrastructure of the gastric mucosa harbouring campylobacter-like organisms. *Am. J. Clin. Pathol.* 1986, 86, 575–52.
5 Sipponen, P., Seppala, K., Aarynen, M. & Kettunen, P. Chronic gastritis and gastroduodenal ulcer: a case-control study on risk of coexisting duodenal or gastric ulcer in patients with gastritis. *Gut* 1989, 30, 922–9.
6 Sipponen, P., Maris, K., Fraki, O. *et al.* Cumulative 10-year risk of symptomatic duodenal and gastric ulcer in patients with or without chronic gastritis. *Scand. J. Gastroenterol.* 1990, 25, 966–73.
7 Rauws, E.A. & Tytgat, G.N. Cure of duodenal ulcer associated with eradication of *Helicobacter pylori*. *Lancet* 1990, ii, 1233–5.
8 Marshall, B.J., McGechie, D.B., Rogers, P.A. *et al.* Pyloric *Campylobacter* infection and gastroduodenal disease. *Med. J. Aust.* 1985, 142, 439–44.
9 Price, A.B., Levi, J., Dolby, J.M. *et al. Campylobacter pyloridis* in peptic ulcer disease: microbiology, pathology and scanning electron microscopy. *Gut* 1985, 21, 1183–8.
10 Booth, L., Holdstock, G., MacBride, H. *et al.* Clinical importance of *Campylobacter pyloridis* and associated serum IgG and IgA antibody responses in patients undergoing upper gastrointestinal endoscopy. *J. Clin. Pathol.* 1986, 39, 215–19.
11 O'Connor, H.J., Dixon, M.F., Wyatt, J.I. *et al.* Effect of duodenal ulcer surgery and enterogastric reflux on *Campylobacter pyloridis*. *Lancet* 1986, ii, 1178–81.
12 Marcheggiano, A., Kannoni, C., Agnello, M. *et al. Campylobacter*-like organisms on the human gastric mucosa. Relation to type and extent of gastritis in different clinical groups. *Gastroenterol. Clin. Biol.* 1987, 11, 376–81.
13 Jiang, S.J., Liu, W.Z., Zhang, D.Z. *et al. Campylobacter*-like organisms in chronic gastritis, peptic ulcer, and gastric carcinoma. *Scand. J. Gastroenterol.* 1987, 22, 553–8.
14 Raskov, H., Lanng, K., Gaarslev, B. *et al.* Screening

for *Campylobacter pyloridis* in patients with upper dyspepsia and the relation to inflammation of the human gastric antrum. *Scand. J. Gastroenterol.* 1987, **22**, 568–72.

15 Coghlan, J.G., Gilligan, D., Humphries, H. *et al. Campylobacter pylori* and recurrence of duodenal ulcers – a 12 month follow-up study. *Lancet* 1987, **ii**, 1109–11.

16 Rauws, E.A.J., Langenberg, W., Houthoff, H.J. *et al. Campylobacter pyloridis*-associated chronic active antral gastritis: a prospective study of its prevalence and the effects of antibacterial and antiulcer treatment. *Gastroenterology* 1988, **94**, 33–40.

17 Goodwin, C.S., Marshall, B.J., Blincow, E.D. *et al.* Prevention of nitroimidazole resistance in *Campylobacter pylori* by co-administration of colloidal bismuth subcitrate: clinical and *in vitro* studies. *J. Clin. Pathol.* 1988, **41**, 207–10.

18 Johnson, B.J., Reed, P.I. & Ali, M.H. *Campylobacter* like organisms in duodenal and antral endoscopic biopsies: relationship to inflammation. *Gut* 1986, **27**, 1132–7.

19 Crabtree, J.E., Shallcross, T.M., Wyatt, J.I. *et al.* Mucosal humoral immune response to *Helicobacter pylori* in patients with duodenitis. *Dig. Dis. Sci.* (in press).

20 Steer, H.W., Surface morphology of the gastroduodenal mucosa in duodenal ulceration. *Gut* 1984, **25**, 1203–10.

21 Wyatt, J.I., Rathbone, B.J., Dixon, M.F. *et al. Campylobacter pyloridis* and acid-induced gastric metaplasia in the pathogenesis of duodenitis. *J. Clin. Pathol.* 1987, **40**, 841–8.

22 Bode, G., Malfertheiner, P. & Ditschuneit, H. Pathogenetic implications of ultrastructural findings in *Campylobacter pylori* related gastroduodenal disease. *Scand. J. Gastroenterol.* 1987, **23**, suppl. 142, 25–39.

23 Caselli, M., Bovolenta, M.R., Aleotti, A. *et al.* Epithelial morphology of duodenal bulb and *Campylobacter*-like organisms. *J. Submicrosc. Cytol. Pathol.* 1988, **20**, 237–42.

24 Thomas, J.M. *Campylobacter*-like organisms in gastritis. *Lancet* 1984, **ii**, 1217.

25 Wyatt, J.I. & Dixon, M.F. Chronic gastritis – a pathogenetic approach. *J. Pathol.* 1988, **154**, 113–24.

26 Hasan, M., Sircus, W. & Ferguson, A. Duodenal mucosal architecture in non-specific and ulcer-associated duodenitis. *Gut* 1981, **22**, 637–41.

27 Delmee, M., Debongnie, J.C., Warzee, P. *et al.* Une méthode originale de prélèvement bactériologique pour l'étude de '*Campylobacter pylori*' dans l'ulcère duodénale. *Gastroenterol. Clin. Biol.* 1987, **11**, 550–3.

28 Shousha, S., Spiller, R.C. & Parkins, R.A. The endoscopically abnormal duodenum in patients with dyspepsia: biopsy findings in 60 cases. *Histopathology* 1983, **7**, 23–34.

29 Carrick, J., Lee, A., Hazell, S. *et al. Campylobacter*

pylori, duodenal ulcer, and gastric metaplasia: possible role of functional heterotopic tissue in ulcerogenesis. *Gut* 1989, **30**, 790–7.

30 Kreuning, J., Bosman, F.T., Kuiper, G. *et al.* Gastric and duodenal mucosa in 'healthy' individuals. An endoscopic and histopathological study of 50 volunteers. *J. Clin. Pathol.* 1978, **31**, 69–77.

31 James, A.H. Gastric epithelium in the duodenum. *Gut* 1964, **5**, 285.

32 Morrissey, S.M., Ward, P.M., Jayari, A.P. *et al.* Histochemical changes in mucosa in duodenal ulceration. *Gut* 1983, **24**, 909–13.

33 Gregory, M.A. & Spitaels, J.M. Variations in the morphology of villous epithelial cells within 8 mm of untreated duodenal ulcers. *J. Pathol.* 1987, **53**, 109–19.

34 Pajares, J.M., Blanco, M., Moreno, M.J. & Jimenez, M.L. Is gastric metaplasia a factor in relapsing duodenal ulcer? *Rev. Esp. Enf. Dig.* 1990, **78**, suppl. 1, 72.

35 Wyatt, J.I., Rathbone, B.J., Sobala, G.M. *et al.* Gastric epithelium in the duodenum: its association with *Helicobacter pylori* and inflammation. *J. Clin. Pathol.* 1990, **43**, 981–6.

36 Florey, H.W. & Harding, H.E. The healing of artificial defects of the duodenal mucosa. *J. Pathol.* 1935, **40**, 211–18.

37 Florey, H.W., Jennings, M.A., Jennings, D.A. *et al.* The reactions of the intestine of the pig to gastric juice. *J. Pathol. Bacteriol.* 1939, **49**, 105–23.

38 Rhodes, J. Experimental production of gastric epithelium in the duodenum. *Gut* 1964, **5**, 454–8.

39 Gaskin, R.J., Gad, A., Barros, A.A.J. *et al.* Natural history and morphology of secretagogue-induced ulcers in rats. *Gastroenterology* 1975, **69**, 903–10.

40 Natelson, B., Dubois, A. & Sodetz, F.J. Effect of multiple-stress procedures on monkey gastroduodenal mucosa, serum gastrin and hydrogen ion kinetics. *Dig. Dis. Sci.* 1977, **22**, 888–97.

41 Tatsuta, M., Ishii, H., Yamamura, H. *et al.* Enhancement by tetragastrin of experimental induction of gastric epithelium in the duodenum. *Gut.* 1989, **30**, 311–15.

42 Patrick, W.J.A., Denham, D. & Forrest, A.P.M. Mucous change in the human duodenum: a light and electron microscopic study and correlation. *Gut.* 1974, **15**, 767–76.

43 Parrish, J.A. & Rawlins, D.C. Intestinal mucosa in the Zollinger–Ellison syndrome. *Gut* 1965, **6**, 286–9.

44 Wyatt, J.I., Dyke, G.W. & Hall, R. *Helicobacter pylori* status and histology of the gastroduodenal mucosa after vagotomy for duodenal ulcer: a follow-up study after 5–30 years. *Rev. Esp. Enf. Dig.* 1990, **78**, suppl. 1, 73.

45 Lee, F.D. & Toner, P.G. 1980 *Biopsy Pathology of the Small Intestine.* Chapman and Hall, London.

46 Whitehead, R. 1984. *Mucosal Biopsy of the Gastroin-*

testinal Tract, 3rd edn. W.B. Saunders, Philadelphia.

47 Lev, R., Thomas, E. & Paul, F.F. Pathological and histomorphometric study of the effects of alcohol on the human duodenum. *Digestion* 1980, **20**, 207–13.

48 1990. *Helicobacter pylori* in duodenal ulcer pathogenesis. In Malfertheiner, P. & Ditschuneit, H. (eds) *Helicobacter pylori, Gastritis and Peptic Ulcer*. Springer-Verlag, Berlin, pp. 271–35.

49 Levi, S., Beardshall, K., Haddad, G. *et al. Campylobacter pylori* and duodenal ulcers: the gastrin link. *Lancet* 1989, **i**, 1167–8.

50 Smith, J.T., Pounder, R.E., Nwokolo, C.U. *et al.* Inappropriate hypergastrinaemia in asymptomatic healthy subjects infected with *Helicobacter pylori*. *Gut* 1990, **31**, 522–5.

51 Graham, D.Y., Opekun, A., Lew, G.M. *et al.* Ablation of exaggerated meal-stimulated gastrin release in duodenal ulcer patients after clearance of *Helicobacter (Campylobacter) pylori* infection. *Am. J. Gastroenterol.* 1990, **85**, 394–8.

52 Cover, T.I., Dooley, C.P. & Blaser, M.J. Characterisation of and human serological responses to proteins in *H. pylori* broth culture supernatants with vacuolising cytotoxin activity. *Infect. Immun.* 1990, **58**, 603–10.

53 Marshall, B.J., Warren, J.R., Blincow, E.D. *et al.* Pros-pective double-blind trial of duodenal ulcer relapse after eradication of *Campylobacter pylori*. *Lancet* 1988, **ii**, 1437–41.

54 Hook-Nikanne, J., Sistonen, P., Kosunen, T.U. Effect of ABO blood group and secretor status on the frequency of *Helicobacter pylori* antibodies. *Scand. J. Gastroenterol.* 1990, **25**, 815–18.

55 Sipponen, P., Aarynen, M., Kaariainen, I. *et al.* Chronic antral gastritis, Lewis a+ phenotype, and male sex as factors in predicting coexisting duodenal ulcer. *Scand. J. Gastroenterol.* 1989, **24**, 581–8.

56 Sipponen, P. Chronic gastritis and ulcer risk. *Scand. J. Gastroenterol.* 1990, **25**, 193–6.

57 Shallcross, T.M., Rathbone, B.J., Wyatt, J.I. & Heatley, R.V. *Helicobacter pylori* associated chronic gastritis and peptic ulceration in patients taking non-steroidal anti-inflammatory drugs. *Aliment. Pharmacol. Ther.* 1990, **4**, 515–22.

58 Martin, D.N., Montgomery, E., Dobek, A.S. *et al. Campylobacter pylori*, non-steroidal anti-inflammatory drugs and smoking: risk factors for peptic ulcer disease. *Am. J. Gastroenterol.* 1989, **84**, 1268–72.

59 Talley, N.J. 1990. Is *Helicobacter pylori* negative duodenal ulcer a separate disease? In Malfertheiner, P. & Ditschuneit, H. (eds) *Helicobacter pylori Gastritis and Peptic Ulcer*. Springer-Verlag, Berlin, pp. 340–4.

14 Helicobacter pylori, Gastric Ulceration and the Postoperative Stomach

G.M.SOBALA AND A.T.R.AXON

Helicobacter pylori and gastric ulcer

In spite of a proliferating literature on *Helicobacter pylori* and duodenal ulcer, relatively few studies have examined its role in gastric ulcer disease. The existing data are inconclusive and on occasions misleading. It is therefore appropriate to consider briefly the relationship between chronic gastritis and gastric ulceration, before turning to *H. pylori* itself.

Chronic gastritis and gastric ulceration

The close association between chronic gastritis and gastric ulceration was appreciated long before *H. pylori* was isolated [1]. For example, Gear *et al.* [2] performed biopsies according to a standardized protocol and found that, of 35 patients with untreated gastric ulcers, 28 had atrophic chronic gastritis and the other seven superficial gastritis. None had completely normal mucosa. In a much larger recent study, Sipponen *et al.* [3] biopsied 186 patients with gastric ulcer and found that 96.6% had antral gastritis and 87.0% had body gastritis.

Gastritis is a primary phenomenon, not merely secondary to the ulcer. Gear *et al.* [2] found that successful medical treatment of the gastric ulcer was not accompanied by any improvement in the degree of gastritis. Indeed, in many cases it became more severe. Sipponen *et al.* [4] followed for 10 years 454 consecutive patients free of peptic ulceration who had undergone endoscopy and biopsy and found that all 11 gastric ulcers (and all but one of the 24 pyloroduodenal ulcers) that were detected in the follow-up period occurred in individuals who had initially had gastritis. The gastritis therefore precedes the ulcer.

The position of the gastric ulcer is related to the distribution of gastritis. Gear *et al.* [2] found that more proximally situated ulcers were associated with a greater proximal extent of the gastritis, and it has been a consistent finding that most gastric ulcers occur in the boundary zone between inflamed, antral, non-acid-secreting mucosa and body-type, acid-secreting mucosa [1, 5–8]. In patients with gastritis this boundary moves slowly proximally, especially along the lesser curve of the stomach, and thus even ulcers halfway along the lesser curve fall into this boundary zone. This area of mucosa may be most at risk, its integrity being compromised because the inflamed epithelium is immediately adjacent to acid-secreting mucosa.

A small proportion of gastric ulcers occur much more proximally in the body of the stomach, but these too may occur at a boundary, this time between body-type and cardia-type mucosa [5].

Gastric ulceration is associated with a particular pattern of gastritis. Tatsuta *et al.* [8] found that antral ulcers that coexisted with duodenal ulcers showed a pattern of gastritis similar to that in duodenal ulcer disease, with extensive, relatively normal, acid-secreting areas associated with an antral atrophic gastritis. Proximally situated gastric ulcers were associated with severely atrophic antral gastritis and extensive gastritis in the corpus as well. They concluded that increasingly atrophic antral gastritis in duodenal ulcer patients predicted the development of coexisting gastric ulceration. These findings have recently been confirmed in

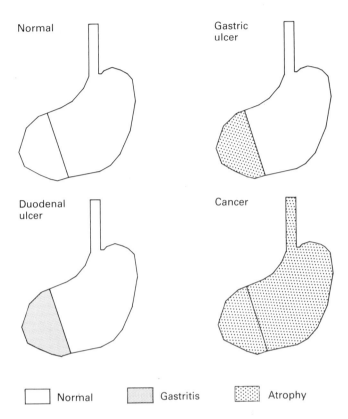

Fig. 14.1 Association between different patterns of *H. pylori*-associated gastritis and gastroduodenal pathology.

☐ Normal   ▨ Gastritis   ▨ Atrophy

a large study by Sipponen *et al.* [4]. They biopsied 571 patients with peptic ulcer, including 186 with gastric ulcer, and 1074 non-ulcer controls. They found that the relative risk for gastric ulceration was 32.2 in men and 24.4 in women in the presence of atrophic antral gastritis, as compared with individuals with normal antral mucosa. Ulceration was more likely in the presence of severe antral atrophy, but less likely as body atrophy progressed.

Figure 14.1 is a simple hypothetical summary of how different patterns of gastritis may relate to different gastroduodenal diseases. A key research goal should be to determine the factors that govern the differentiation of gastritis along a particular pathway, especially as it is increasingly likely that all these patterns are associated with *H. pylori*.

Prevalence of H. pylori in gastric ulcer disease
Table 14.1 is a summary of studies [9–22] reporting the prevalence of *H. pylori* infection in

at least 25 patients with gastric ulcer. As a summary of such studies, a rough estimate of 70% is often quoted [23, 24] and unfortunately seems to have passed into general gastroenterological folklore. This prevalence is markedly lower than that of chronic gastritis in the same condition, and this would appear to suggest that the chronic gastritis of gastric ulcer disease is often different from the *H. pylori*-associated gastritis that has been so much researched recently. However, there are good reasons to suspect that the true prevalence of *H. pylori* in gastric ulcer disease is much higher than 70%, and is the same as the prevalence of chronic gastritis.

Firstly, not all studies on the prevalence of *H. pylori* in gastric ulceration have used the same criteria. The definition of an ulcer, as opposed to an erosion, is likely to vary from centre to centre. Prevalence has been estimated from antral biopsies, antral and body biopsies, biopsies of the ulcer itself and even biopsies of the scar after

Table 14.1 Studies reporting incidence of *H. pylori* in at least 25 gastric ulcer (GU) patients.

Author	Year	Number of GU patients	Prevalence of *H. pylori* (%)	Biopsy site	Detection method	Reference number
Marshall *et al.*	1985	40	68	a	h(c)	9
Niemala *et al.*	1987	33	58	abu	h	10
O'Connor *et al.*	1987	54	72	a	h	11
Hui *et al.*	1987	61	77	abu	hc	12
Rauws *et al.*	1988	27	96	a	hc	13
Kalogeropoulos & Whitehead	1988	102	56	u	h	14
Feng & Wang	1988	28	86	a	hcu	15
Gad *et al.*	1989	146	87	abu	h	16
Inouye *et al.*	1989	25	96	ab	hc	17
Yoshida *et al.*	1989	99	91	ab	hcu	18
Kolarski *et al.*	1989	28	86	?	h	19
Wagner *et al.*	1989	40	70	a	h(cu)	20
Koch *et al.*	1990	134	66 (84)	ab	h(u)	21
Tessaro *et al.*	1990	51	56	a	u	22
Sobala, G.M.	1990	46	91	a(b)	h or s	Unpublished

Biopsy site: a = antrum, b = body, u = ulcer. Detection method: h = histology, c = culture, u = urease test, s = serology.

healing. For example, Kalogeropoulos & Whitehead [14] found *Helicobacter*-like organisms in only 56% of 102 gastric ulcer patients. This was a study performed on archival histological material, and it would appear that the samples examined originated from the region of the ulcer itself rather than from uninvolved antral mucosa. Many of the studies report results based on only a single method of detection of *H. pylori*, and are thus likely to underestimate the prevalence. Koch *et al.* [21] reported a prevalence of 66% based on histology, but it is evident from the published data that an additional 18% of patients negative for *H. pylori* by histology had a positive biopsy urease test.

Secondly, a number of the recently reported low prevalences of *H. pylori* in gastric ulcer disease have come from centres which are perhaps still on a learning curve as how best to detect this organism. It is noteworthy that a centre that has developed great experience in this field reported 26 (96%) of 27 gastric ulcers to be *H. pylori*-positive [13]. In two very careful Japanese studies, in which multiple biopsies were taken of several areas of the stomach and at least two different diagnostic tests for *H. pylori*

were used, high prevalences of *H. pylori* were recorded: 96% in 25 patients [17] and 91% in 99 patients [18]. These findings are in line with our own recent experience: 42 (91%) of 46 gastric ulcer patients were positive for *H. pylori*, sought for by histology in 29 and serology in 17.

Thirdly, *H. pylori* is hard to find in association with increasing degrees of mucosal atrophy [25]. In gastric ulcer disease there is often severe antral atrophy and intestinal metaplasia and a most thorough search for *H. pylori* may be required. Treatment with H_2 receptor antagonists may decrease the numbers of *H. pylori* in gastric ulcer patients further still [26]. Therefore, although *H. pylori* infection may still be the initiating factor for the chronic gastritis of gastric ulcer disease, as atrophic changes and intestinal metaplasia develop the intensity of colonization may fall.

Finally, O'Connor *et al.* [11] reported that eight of 14 *H. pylori*-negative patients with gastric ulcer did not have chronic gastritis, but had the histological condition 'reflux gastritis'. A significant proportion of patients in this study had previously undergone gastric surgery. 'Reflux gastritis' has now been retermed 'reactive gastritis' under the Sydney classification [27] and is known to be correlated, not only with duodenogastric bile reflux [28], but also with the use of non-steroid anti-inflammatory drugs (NSAIDs) [29]. The use of these drugs has increased since 1975, when Gear et al. [2] reported a 100% incidence of chronic gastritis in patients with gastric ulcer, and it is likely that in the 1990s a larger proportion of gastric ulcers are secondary to NSAID-associated reactive gastritis rather than H. pylori-associated chronic gastritis. Thus Marshall et al. [9] reported that 30% of gastric ulcers were not associated with chronic gastritis, and that 75% of these patients were taking NSAIDs.

Helicobacter pylori and gastric ulcer: cause and effect?

We conclude that H. pylori is frequently associated with gastric ulcer. Does it play a pathogenic role? A number of hypotheses have been proposed as to how it may do so. Hazell & Lee [30] suggested that the ammonia produced by the action of the H. pylori urease leads to alterations in the milieu of the gastric epithelium, preventing the normal passage of hydrogen ions through the mucus and thus leading to peptic mucosal damage. The occurrence of frank ulceration would depend on other contributing factors. This hypothesis seems to miss the point that gastric ulcers occur in antral-type, non-acid-secreting mucosa [1, 6]. Sidebotham & Baron [31] proposed that the ammonia leads to structural changes in the mucus layer of the stomach, facilitating colonization by H. pylori and potentiating other ulcerogenic effects of the organism, such as somatostatin inhibition, vagal stimulation and endotoxin release. Neither of these hypotheses explains how gastric ulcer, a focal lesion, occurs as a result of H. pylori-associated gastritis, a diffuse one. Ormand & Talley [32] have suggested a possible mechanism. H. pylori colonization is not uniform. They propose that the mucus layer is degraded at the areas of densest H. pylori colonization and hydrogen ion back-diffusion occurs. The change in mucosal pH stimulates the organisms to migrate else-

where. The balance between healing and noxious factors at the injured site determines whether focal ulceration occurs. This is intuitively appealing, and could account for the known facts about atrophy and topography in gastric ulcerogenesis. Atrophic mucosa may be less able to recover when damaged, and hydrogen ion load is likely to be greatest in those areas of mucosa directly adjacent to acid-secreting areas.

Thus hypotheses abound whilst hard evidence for a role for H. pylori in gastric ulcer is lacking. Studies similar to those performed in duodenal ulcer disease are needed, in which relapse is prevented by eradication of the organism. Such studies are more difficult in gastric ulcer disease: it is a less common condition, the patients are older and likely to be less suitable for clinical trials, and the natural relapse rate is lower. A properly designed study has not yet been reported. There are suggestions, but no more, that we shall eventually see similar results to those obtained in duodenal ulcer disease. In two studies performed in China whilst still in ignorance of H. pylori, an antibiotic, furazolidone, was shown to heal gastric ulcers [33] and to reduce the relapse rate at 4 years from 33% to 10% [34]. Tatsuta et al. [35] showed in 35 patients that 2 weeks of cefixime 100 mg daily reduced the relapse rate, at 12 weeks, of gastric ulcers healed with cimetidine from 47% to 17%. However, the cefixime usually just suppressed H. pylori and only successfully eradicated it in four of 17 patients, and by 24 weeks' follow-up there was no difference in relapse rates between the two treatment groups.

Helicobacter pylori and the postoperative stomach

Research on H. pylori and chronic gastritis has clarified thinking on other forms of gastritis. It is now accepted that there is a quite distinct histological entity, 'reactive gastritis' [27], characterized by foveolar hyperplasia, vasodilatation, capillary congestion, lamina propria oedema and a paucity of inflammatory cells (Fig. 14.2). This is associated with duodenogastric reflux of

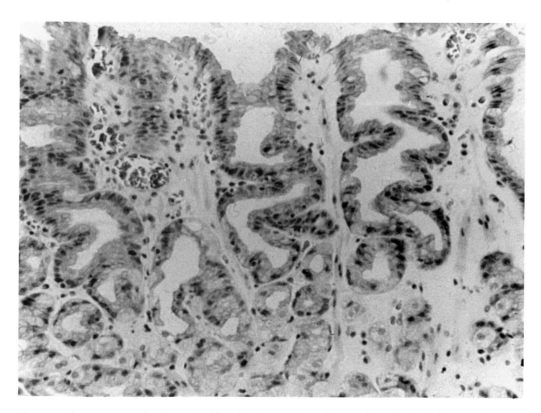

Fig. 14.2 Biopsy specimen showing marked foveolar hyperplasia, moderate oedema in the lamina propria, severe capillary congestion and a paucity of chronic inflammatory cells and polymorphs: reactive gastritis.

bile in the postoperative stomach [28] and NSAID consumption in the intact stomach [29].

O'Connor *et al.* [36] showed that, in a heterogenous group of patients, some with intact stomachs and some postoperative, *H. pylori* infection was negatively associated both with the histological picture of reflux gastritis and also with intragastric bile acid concentrations.

O'Connor *et al.* [37] went on to examine the role of surgery on *H. pylori* colonization more closely. They studied a group of unoperated and postoperative duodenal ulcer patients. They found that, whilst 97% of the unoperated patients and 94% of the patients who had undergone highly selective vagotomy without any drainage procedure were *H. pylori*-positive, only 50% of the patients with truncal vagotomy and gastroenterostomy, 47% of those with Billroth II partial gastrectomy and 22% with Billroth I partial gastrectomy were still positive.

Furthermore, the longer the time interval between operation and endoscopic assessment in these latter groups, the lower the colonization rate. 'Reflux gastritis' was common in these groups, as was biochemical evidence of bile reflux. Thus bile reflux, occurring as a consequence of these operations, leads to the clearance of *H. pylori* and the replacement of *H. pylori*-associated chronic gastritis with bile-induced reactive gastritis. This was confirmed in a further study in which 24 patients with previous partial gastrectomy or drainage procedure were endoscoped and biopsied before and after Roux-en-Y biliary diversion [38]. The prevalence of *H. pylori* infection rose from 54% before diversion to 92% after diversion, and this increase was accompanied by a decrease in a 'histological reflux score'. This raises the suspicion that bile reflux merely suppresses *H. pylori* rather than eradicates it: once bile is removed,

H. pylori can flourish again. Indeed, Loffeld *et al.* [39] found that *H. pylori* was more commonly found high in the gastric remnant rather than in the peristomal area in patients who had undergone partial gastrectomy. If postoperative patients are only assessed by peristomal biopsies, as in the studies by O'Connor *et al.* [36–38], *H. pylori* prevalence may be underestimated.

Roux-en-Y diversion was further studied by Offerhaus *et al.* [40], who prospectively assigned 17 peptic ulcer patients to either Billroth II partial gastrectomy or partial gastrectomy with Roux-en-Y diversion. After Billroth II, bile acid reflux was greater than after Roux-en-Y. All patients were *H. pylori*-positive before surgery, and all eight undergoing Roux-en-Y remained so. Four of the patients who underwent Billroth II gastrectomy cleared their *H. pylori* infection and developed changes of reactive gastritis around the stoma.

It should be stressed that the clearance of *H. pylori* by bile reflux caused by surgery should not be considered a 'good thing' in the same sense that eradication of *H. pylori* by drug treatment is good in duodenal ulcer disease. Firstly, it is unlikely to have much to do with the success of the surgery. Highly selective vagotomy is an efficacious anti-ulcer operation, despite little action on *H. pylori*. Secondly, the bile reflux caused by operations such as Billroth I- and II-type partial gastrectomies on to already compromised mucosa has been implicated as a cause of the increased incidence of gastric cancer described 20 years post-surgery [41].

The relationship between *H. pylori* and bile reflux in the intact stomach is less clear. Raedsch *et al.* [42] described significantly lower intragastric bile acid concentrations in patients with gastritis when *H. pylori* was present, and Tewari *et al.* [43] noted a lower prevalence of *H. pylori* in gastritis in individuals with endoscopic evidence of bile reflux. Niemala *et al.* [44], on the other hand, found no association in 107 patients between *H. pylori* numbers and either gastric juice bile acid concentrations or externally measured bile reflux. This is in line with our recent experience. We have measured fasting gastric bile acid concentrations in 135 patients

Table 14.2 Fasting gastric juice bile acid concentrations according to histological assessment of antral *H. pylori* density in 135 patients with intact stomachs. Spearman correlation coefficient = −0.08, not significant.

Antral *H. pylori* density	Number of patients	Median bile acid concentration (μmol/l)	Interquartile range
None	59	0.03	0.00–0.17
Low	14	0.07	0.00–0.27
Moderate	37	0.04	0.00–0.27
High	25	0.02	0.00–0.40

with intact stomachs. There were no significant correlations between bile acid concentrations and histologically assessed *H. pylori* density on antral biopsies (Table 14.2). Probably bile reflux is insufficiently severe in most patients with unoperated stomachs to dislodge *H. pylori*, and the histological appearance of *H. pylori*-associated gastritis masks those of reactive gastritis.

Conclusions

At least 85% of gastric ulcers are accompanied by *H. pylori*-positive chronic gastritis. Most of the remainder are secondary to NSAID usage and are not associated with *H. pylori* or chronic gastritis. It is still unknown whether eradication of *H. pylori* can prevent gastric ulcer relapse.

Surgically induced bile reflux can suppress *H. pylori* and convert the histological appearance of chronic gastritis to that of reactive gastritis. However, this may simply represent suppression rather than eradication, and *H. pylori* infection can recur after biliary diversion.

References

1 Magnus, H.A. The pathology of peptic ulceration. *Postgrad. Med. J.* 1954, **30**, 131–6.
2 Gear, M.W.L., Truelove, S.C. & Whitehead, R. Gastric ulcer and gastritis. *Gut* 1971, **12**, 639–45.
3 Sipponen, P., Seppala, K., Aarynen, M., Helske, T. & Kettunen, P. Chronic gastritis and gastroduodenal ulcer: a case control study on risk of coexisting duodenal or gastric ulcer in patients with gastritis. *Gut* 1989, **30**, 922–9.
4 Sipponen, P., Varis, K., Fraki, O., Korri, U-M., Seppala, K. & Siurala, M. Cumulative 10-year risk of

15 Helicobacter pylori and Gastric Cancer

P.CORREA AND B.RUIZ

Introduction

Multidisciplinary research carried out over several decades by teams of investigators in many countries has led to the hypothesis that most gastric cancers in humans are the end result of events related to multiple consecutive regressive phenotypic changes in the gastric epithelium [1]. In most human situations, many years elapse between the initial stages of the process and the final invasion and spread of the tumour.

Most of the information available on this precancerous process was obtained before *Helicobacter pylori* was recognized as a factor in gastric disease. Only recently have attempts been made to understand the relationship between *H. pylori* and the precancerous process [2]. This relationship is explored in this chapter, based on published material and personal experiences of the authors.

Types of gastric cancer and their precursors

Biologically, gastric carcinoma is not a homogeneous entity and considerable differences in the aetiological forces involved have been identified for the several types so far recognized. For one of the types, the 'diffuse' or 'infiltrative' type of gastric carcinoma, our knowledge of the precursor stages is so meagre as to make it impossible to describe them in any meaningful way [3, 4]. For the other types of gastric cancer, specific precancerous lesions have been characterized.

Gastric carcinoma associated with the pernicious anaemia syndrome is preceded by diffuse corporal (type A) atrophic gastritis [5], which appears to be unrelated to *H. pylori*.

In patients with previous gastrectomy, the 'stump carcinoma' is observed. Characteristically these patients manifest 'reflux' gastritis, again apparently unrelated to *Helicobacter pylori* [6]. The precursor of stump carcinoma is gastritis cystica polyposa, present only at the anastomosis site itself and not observed away from it, where reflux gastritis is ubiquitous [7]. There are no grounds to implicate *Helicobacter pylori* in the pathogenesis of this disease complex.

In the region of the gastro-oesophageal junction, adenocarcinomas arise from either the cardiac gastric glands or the glands of Barrett's oesophagus. In some cases the exact site of origin is obscure. The precursors of carcinoma of the gastric cardiac glands have not been characterized. The precursors of carcinoma arising in Barrett's oesophagus have been fairly well characterized as metaplastic and dysplastic changes essentially identical to those described below for the 'epidemic' or 'intestinal' type of carcinoma. It should be noted that both the cardiac region of the stomach and the epithelium in Barrett's oesophagus are frequently colonized by *H. pylori*.

In most human populations displaying high gastric cancer risk, the types of gastric cancer mentioned above are the least frequent. Most gastric carcinomas are morphologically of the 'intestinal' or 'expansive' type and have epidemiological characteristics which have made them deserve the label 'epidemic' type. Such carcinomas make their appearance in the midst of a precursor lesion called multifocal chronic atrophic gastritis (MAG), sometimes also called 'environmental' or 'type B' [5].

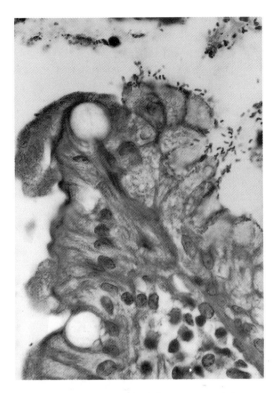

Fig. 15.1 Microphotograph of the area around the limit between a focus of intestinal metaplasia (left) and gastric mucosa lined by foveolar cells (right). Abundant *Helicobacter* organisms are seen on and between foveolar cells but not near the goblet cells or enterocytes of the metaplastic epithelium. Warthin–Starry stain, × 715.

Multifocal chronic atrophic gastritis as a cancer precursor

MAG as a nosological entity covers a broad morphological spectrum as it involves progressively more extensive areas of the gastric mucosa. It has a characteristic topographical distribution and pattern of progression: in younger individuals, it appears around the area of the incisura angularis, the lesser curvature and the corpus–antrum junction as independent foci which coalesce and extend to the antrum and corpus. Atrophy of glands appears, preceded by chronic inflammatory infiltrate in the superficial portion of the lamina propria and around groups of gastric glands, especially in the antrum. Focal acute inflammation (poly-morphonuclear infiltrate) is occasionally seen in and around the epithelium of the foveolae and the gland necks.

Intestinal-type epithelium replaces the glands lost in the atrophic process, first resembling small intestine (type I intestinal metaplasia) and later resembling colonic epithelium (types II and III). In more advanced lesions, mature intestinal phenotypes are replaced by immature types, which display the histological pattern of dysplasia, a lesion considered precancerous [8–10].

Epidemiological and experimental studies have identified aetiological factors which play a role in the precancerous process, either initiating and promoting its progress or retarding and blocking it. Factors which inhibit the precancerous process are mainly antioxidants such as vitamin C, vitamin E and β-carotene. Factors which aggravate the process are mostly irritants, such as excessive salt in foods [1]. These irritants not only induce gastric inflammation but also potentiate the effect of gastric carcinogens such as MNNG [11] by some poorly understood mechanism. The precancerous role of gastric irritants is substantiated by abundant epidemiological and experimental literature [1].

The role of Helicobacter in MAG

The association between *H. pylori* and chronic gastritis has been reported in many countries but frequently the heterogeneity of chronic gastritis is not recognized and no indication is given as to the type of gastritis being reported. Table 15.1 shows the prevalence of *H. pylori* reported in case series [12–21] specifically mentioning atrophic gastritis.

The reports show clearly that *H. pylori* is frequently associated with atrophic gastritis. It is well known that *H. pylori* does not colonize metaplastic epithelium, as shown in Fig. 15.1, in which the bacteria are very abundant around foveolar epithelial cells but are absent in the immediate vicinity of cells of intestinal phenotype.

Epithelial cell damage is associated with *H. pylori* colonization, as seen in Fig. 15.2, in which a marked decrease of cytoplasmic mucin is seen

Table 15.1 Reported prevalence of *H. pylori* in atrophic gastritis.

Author	%	Number of cases
Fiocca *et al.* [12]	89.5	38
Le Bodic *et al.* [13]	5.0	12
Barbosa *et al.* [14]	71.4	7
Booth *et al.* [15]	70.6	34
Menge *et al.* [16]	67.7	31
Andersen *et al.* [17]	64.7	17
Price *et al.* [18]	61.5	13
Jones *et al.* [19]	52.9	17
Chen *et al.* [20]	46.7	30
Sethi *et al.* [21]	43.5	23

where colonization is severe. Cell damage is followed by cell repair, as seen in Fig. 15.3, in which the presence of the bacteria is associated with increase in size and number of nuclei as well as their displacement to upper portions of the cytoplasm. A certain degree of irregular polarity is also observed in the nuclei of Fig. 15.2. From epidemiological and histopathological evidence, it is therefore clear that *H. pylori* is very much a part of the chronic atrophic gastritis spectrum.

MAG correlates very closely with the risk of gastric cancer; its prevalence is higher in populations at high cancer risk. We studied two series of gastric biopsies from subjects of high-risk communities [22]. In Nariño, Colombia, the risk is extremely high (over 100/100 000 per year) and MAG is the predominant type of gastritis. In the city of Cali, the cancer rate is approximately 50/100 000 per year. In the New Orleans black community, the risk is lower, but still relatively high (around 20/100 000 compared with the risk in whites under 10/100 000), and MAG is also frequent, followed by diffuse antral gastritis.

The prevalence of *H. pylori* in these populations as evaluated by the Warthin–Starry stain is seen in Table 15.2. In the MAG complex (chronic atrophic gastritis and intestinal metaplasia), the prevalence is around 94% in Nariño, compared with 72% in Cali and 64% in New Orleans [23]. The higher rate in Nariño is significant, when compared with New Orleans. It should also be noted that, although small in number, all cases of dysplasia were colonized by *H. pylori* in the areas of remaining gastric foveolar epithelium.

In populations of low gastric cancer risk, MAG is very rare or non-existent. In such populations diffuse antral gastritis is usually predominant.

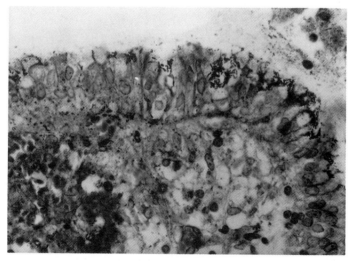

Fig. 15.2 Microphotograph of the gastric mucosa with acute and chronic inflammation associated with marked colonization by *Helicobacter pylori*. The bacteria are between foveolar cells, which have lost much of their normal cytoplasmic mucin. The nuclei are somewhat enlarged and irregular in location and orientation. Warthin–Starry stain, × 500.

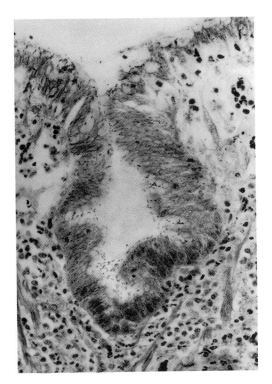

Fig. 15.3 Microphotograph of a gastric foveola with acute and chronic inflammation associated with *Helicobacter pylori* infection. Abundant organisms are seen in the foveolar lumen in the immediate vicinity of the epithelial cells. Cellular hyperplasia is manifested by increase in size and number of the nuclei of the foveolar cells. Warthin–Starry stain × 285.

This type of gastritis, however, is not known to be associated with increased gastric cancer risk. *H. pylori* is known to play a dominant role in diffuse antral gastritis. *H. pylori*, therefore, is not

Table 15.2 *H. pylori* in gastric biopsy material in two locations.

	Colombia		
Biopsy	Cali	Nariño	New Orleans
Normal	0	0	0
Superficial gastritis	55	87	86
Diffuse antral gastritis	70	100	85
Chronic atrophic gastritis	64	97	68
Intestinal metaplasia	86	93	58

Values represent the percentage of *H. pylori*-positive biopsies to the total biopsies in each case.

a sufficient cause of gastric cancer. Its role, if any, seems dependent on the previous existence of MAG.

Helicobacter and dysplasia

H. pylori is very frequently associated with gastric dysplasia [23]. Preliminary results of treatment of these patients with bismuth salts have reported dramatic histological and clinical improvement and drastic reduction in cellular regeneration, atypia and inflammatory infiltrate [24]. Although these results need confirmation, it appears that anti-*Helicobacter* therapy may play a role in reducing the intensity and perhaps reversing dysplastic changes.

Helicobacter and gastric carcinoma

There have been some reports of association of *H. pylori* with gastric carcinoma. It is well known that *H. pylori* does not colonize cancer cells and it follows that the prevalence in cancer cases represents colonization in the remaining foveolar epithelium of the stomach. A study of gastrectomy specimens from California found that the prevalence of *H. pylori* infection in the mucosa surrounding gastric carcinomas of the intestinal (or 'epidemic') type was 89%, compared with 32% for carcinomas of the 'diffuse' type. The difference was statistically highly significant [25]. This strong association of *H. pylori* infection with the intestinal type of gastric cancer, which greatly exceeds the prevalence normally seen in US populations, provides additional support for a role of *H. pylori* in the gastric carcinogenic process.

Epidemiological studies based on the detection of antibodies against *H. pylori* in serum samples have confirmed a high degree of correlation with gastric cancer rates. The prevalence of immunoglobulin G (IgG) antibodies against *H. pylori* in 1882 Chinese men was correlated with cancer mortality rates of the 46 rural counties they represented. No significant correlation was found between *H. pylori* antibodies and cancer rates, with the exception only of gastric cancer, for which a significant ($P = 0.02$) correlation

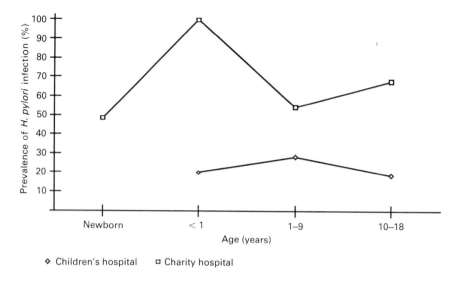

Fig. 15.4 Prevalence of *H. pylori* infection in black children attending Children's and Charity Hospitals in New Orleans by age-groups.

coefficient of 0.34 was found [26]. A retrospective cohort study in England has shown that the prevalence of IgG anti-*Helicobacter* antibodies was 69% in subjects who years later developed gastric cancer, compared with 47% in matched controls, yielding a statistically relative risk of 2.77 (D. Forman *et al.*, unpublished). Studies of seroepidemiology have consistently found that, in populations at high gastric cancer risk, the prevalence of the infection in children is higher than in populations at low risk [27]. Early infection with *H. pylori* may result from overcrowding. Housing patterns in childhood have been reported positively correlated with gastric cancer death rates, leading the authors to state that overcrowding at home during childhood 'might act by promoting the transmission of causative organisms' [28]. The influence of socio-economic factors on *H. pylori* infection in childhood is shown by a seroepidemiological study in New Orleans, where both cancer rates and *H. pylori* antibody prevalence are higher in blacks than in whites. As shown in Fig. 15.4, black children of low socio-economic status seen at the Charity Hospital have a much higher prevalence of infection than black children of higher socio-economic status seen at the Children's Hospital, a private institution [23]. Other factors, con-

comitant with *H. pylori*, may be needed to increase the rate of gastric cancer. This is suggested by the study of Costa Rican children, who had a very high prevalence of infection whether they live in a high- or low-risk area of gastric cancer (R. Sierra *et al.*, unpublished).

Helicobacter and the precancerous process

Agents involved in the aetiology of cancer are customarily classified mainly as either initiators or promoters. Initiators are genotoxic agents which may induce damage to deoxyribonucleic acid (DNA) on short-term exposure and which can be complete carcinogens when administered in multiple doses through a prolonged time period. *H. pylori* is present for many years in patients with chronic diffuse antral gastritis and probably plays a causal role in the disease. Since the condition has not been shown to increase the risk of gastric cancer, it follows that *H. pylori* should not be assigned the role of a complete carcinogen.

Promoters, on the other hand, effectively increase the risk of cancer only when applied repeatedly to cells which have been previously exposed to an initiator. Promoters may act by increasing cell replication, thereby making cells more vulnerable to the genotoxic effects of initiators, which require cell replication for their interaction with DNA. That type of role has been documented for other gastric irritants such as excessive salt [29]. As shown in Figs 15.2 and 15.3, glands in which *H. pylori* are present display increased nuclear activity. As an irritant of the gastric mucosa and as an inducer of excessive cell replication, it is plausible to assume that *H. pylori* may play the role of a cancer promoter. In the setting of diffuse antral gastritis, such promoting effect is not evident, presumably because of lack of initiators. In the setting of MAG, such irritation and excessive replication may result in promotion of the carcinogenesis process, presumably because genotoxic agents are also present.

Although a specific carcinogen responsible for gastric cancer has not been identified, it has been postulated that it may be formed or delivered *in situ* over a prolonged period of time [1]. The suggestion that nitroso compounds might be involved has found support in studies showing that the urinary excretion of nitrosoproline, adjusted for nitrate, is increased in patients with intestinal metaplasia [30]. Evidence has been provided recently indicating that the gastric mucosa possesses an antioxidant mechanism. Ascorbic acid, a potent antioxidant, is secreted into the gastric lumen by the gastric mucosa, which concentrates it from the blood supply [31]. Such concentrating and secretory capacity is impaired by chronic gastritis [32]. A previously normal individual lost his capacity to concentrate ascorbic acid into the gastric juice after an infection with *H. pylori*, resulting in gastritis [33]. It thus appears that *H. pylori* may impair naturally existing mechanisms of antioxidation which may be needed by the gastric mucosa to neutralize local carcinogens.

Acknowledgements

Work supported by Grants RO1-AI25590 and PO1-CA28842 of the National Institutes of Health.

References

1 Correa, P. A human model of gastric carcinogenesis. *Cancer Res.* 1988, **48**, 3554–60.

2 Rathbone, B. & Wyatt, J. 1988. *Campylobacter pylori* and precancerous lesions. In Reed, P.I. & Hill, M.J. (eds) *Gastric Carcinogenesis*. Excepta Medica, Amsterdam, pp. 132–44.

3 Lauren, P. The two main types of gastric carcinoma: diffuse and so-called intestinal type carcinoma. An attempt at a histoclinical classification. *Acta Pathol. Microbiol. Scand.* 1965, **64**, 31–49.

4 Ming, S.C. Gastric carcinoma. A pathologic classification. *Cancer* 1977, **39**, 2475–85.

5 Correa, P. Chronic gastritis: a clinico-pathologic classification. *Am. J. Gastroenterol.* 1988, **83**, 504–9.

6 O'Connor, H.J., Wyatt, J.I., Dixon, M.F. *et al. Campylobacter* like organisms and reflux gastritis. *J. Clin. Pathol.* 1986, **39**, 531–4.

7 Littler, E.R. & Gleibermann, E. Gastritis cystica polypsa: gastric mucosal polyposa at gastroenteroctomy site, with cysts and infiltrative epithelial hyperplasia. *Cancer* 1972, **29**, 205–9.

8 Heilman, K.K. & Hopker, W.W. Loss of differentiation in intestinal metaplasia in cancerous stomachs. A comparative study. *Pathol. Res. Pract.* 1979, **164**, 249–58.

9 Silva, S. & Filipe, M.I. Intestinal metaplasia and its variants in gastric carcinoma of Portuguese subjects: a comparative analysis of biopsy and gastrectomy material. *Hum. Pathol.* 1986, **17**, 988–95.

10 Cuello, C., Correa, P., Zarama, G. *et al.* Histopathology of gastric dysplasias. *Am. J. Surg. Pathol.* 1979, **3**, 491–500.

11 Takahashi, M., Kokuho, T., Furukawa, F. *et al.* Effect of high salt diet on rat gastric carcinogenesis induced by MNNG. *Gann* 1983, **74**, 28–34.

12 Fiocca, R., Villani, L., Turpini, R. & Salcia, E. High incidence of *Campylobacter*-like organisms in endoscopic biopsies from patients with gastritis with or without peptic ulcer. *Digestion* 1987, **38**, 234–44.

13 Le Bodic, M.F., Barre, P. & Freland, C. *Campylobacter pylori* et muqueuse gastrique: étude histologique, bactériologique et résultats préliminaires d'une enquête épidémiologique dans la région nantaise. *Gastroenterol. Clin. Biol.* 1987, **11**, 543–9.

14 Barbosa, A.J., Queiros, D.M., Mendes, E.N. *et al.* Immunocytochemical identification of *Campylobacter pylori* in gastritis and correlation with culture. *Arch. Pathol. Lab. Med.* 1988, **112**, 523–5.

15 Booth, L., Holdstock, G., MacBide, H. *et al.* Clinical importance of *Campylobacter pyloridis* and associated serum IgG and IgA antibody responses in patients undergoing upper gastrointestinal endoscopy. *J. Clin. Pathol.* 1986, **39**, 215–19.

16 Menge, H., Warrehman, M., Joy, V. *et al. Campylobacter pylori* in Magen, Duodenum und Kolon gastro-

often aided by other self-inflicted irritants such as alcohol, tobacco and spices. These supposedly cause inflammation of the gastric mucosa with resultant pain – hence the confusion of terminology between the 'touch of gastritis' blamed for acute upper gastrointestinal (GI) symptoms, the endoscopist's gastritis (varying from slight mucosal hyperaemia, to the florid picture of a red angry mucosa with haemorrhages and erosions), and the pathologist's classification based on cellular infiltrate and architectural changes. Many of the early writers attributed quite specific, though diverse, symptoms to gastritis [9], but unfortunately the simple concept that a red mucosa must be painful does not appear to hold true.

Because H. pylori has only been identified since 1983, earlier work on NUD cannot be applied directly to questions about the bacterium. However, the strong association between H. pylori and antral gastritis and duodenitis should allow some information to be gleaned from studies linking symptoms with gastric histology. Unfortunately, before the widespread availability of fibreoptic upper GI endoscopy, most gastric biopsies were taken using the Wood's tube or a similar device, producing untargeted biopsies mainly from the gastric body or fundus [10, 11]. Since gastritis of the body or fundus is much less sensitive and specific than antral gastritis as a predictor of H. pylori colonization, only studies using antral biopsies are of use in this context. Furthermore, 'gastritis' is often used to refer to the endoscopic appearance of the mucosa rather than to the histological change, which is unsatisfactory given the wide observer variation and lack of an accepted classification for the macroscopic features seen. Not surprisingly, just as H. pylori is present in an appreciable proportion of asymptomatic individuals, so is gastritis. Kreuning et al. [12] found antral gastritis in 36% of 50 normal volunteers (mean age 33 years), and chronic duodenitis in 12%. Cheli et al. [13] have shown antral or fundal gastritis in 46% and 73% of asymptomatic Italians and Hungarians respectively (two groups of 100 subjects, age range 20–79 years). Comparable results

have been reported in 10 medical students [14].

Comparative studies are hard to find, but neither Cheli et al. [15] nor Villako et al. [16] were able to show a significant association between gastritis and dyspepsia, whilst a study from Ethiopia [17] found gastritis in 98% of patients with dyspepsia and 100% of controls. Toukan et al. [18] compared the density of inflammatory infiltrate in gastroduodenal biopsies from 31 NUD patients with biopsies taken from a group of asymptomatic age-matched controls, and found the patients to have significantly higher neutrophil counts in the gastric body, antrum and duodenum than controls. Some workers have linked H. pylori with a neutrophil infiltrate [8, 19] but this finding is disputed by others [20].

Several groups have suggested a link between heartburn or reflux symptoms and gastritis. Earlam et al. [21], in a study of patients undergoing surgery for duodenal ulcer, found that all patients with heartburn also had gastritis, and 62% of those with gastritis had heartburn. However, as would be expected, 94% of the subjects had gastritis and, although the two without gastritis did not experience heartburn, this can hardly be considered significant. Fink et al. [22], in a study of 23 patients with gastro-oesophageal reflux (diagnosed by typical symptoms, positive Bernstein test and histology), found antral gastritis in 78%, compared with only 10% in a group of 20 normal volunteers. Unfortunately, the mean age of the patients was 53 years and that of the volunteers 29 years, the obvious conclusion being that both antral gastritis and reflux are more common with increasing age. However, the study did also show a significant correlation between the severity of gastritis judged histologically and the magnitude of delayed gastric emptying of a semisolid isotope-labelled meal, suggesting a link with symptoms.

One American group [23], in a study of 28 patients with NUD, showed a highly significant correlation between heartburn and the histological findings of chronic fundal gastritis, acute antral gastritis and chronic antral gastritis. The age difference between the two groups (heartburn and no heartburn) was less than 10 years.

Duodenitis is strongly linked with both antral gastritis and *H. pylori* [24, 25], and there is evidence that it may form part of a disease spectrum in which duodenal ulcer also occurs [26]. Opinion is divided as to whether duodenitis on its own can cause symptoms [27, 28], but more recently Collins *et al.* [29] have shown significantly higher inflammatory cell counts in duodenal biopsies from patients with NUD compared with controls, and a Swedish study [30] found a correlation between episodic pain and histological duodenitis.

Undoubtedly asymptomatic chronic gastritis is very common, but at present there is little hard evidence of a clear subgroup in which it causes symptoms, although there is some support for a link with heartburn. There is a little more support for a link between duodenitis and symptoms. These studies, however, cannot provide a definite answer to questions about the symptomatology of *H. pylori* infection.

Chronic H. pylori infection and non-ulcer dyspepsia

Most of the initial interest in *H. pylori* was directed at the association with gastritis and peptic ulcers. Consequently, little information concerning the symptoms found in *H. pylori*-positive and negative individuals was recorded. Subsequently, more attention has been paid to symptomatology, particularly with the availability of non-invasive tests to detect *H. pylori* infection, and also with fairly effective treatment which at least temporarily clears the organism from the gastric mucosa. In reviewing these studies, it is perhaps pertinent to address the three questions posed in the introduction to this chapter.

Is colonization by H. pylori more common in patients with NUD than in an asymptomatic population?

The majority of studies reporting the prevalence of *H. pylori* infection in different groups of patients have not included detailed symptomatic assessments. However, if *H. pylori* is responsible for many of the symptoms of NUD, then it should be possible to demonstrate a higher frequency of infection in these patients, compared with normal controls.

Unfortunately, there are considerable difficulties in making valid comparisons between NUD patients and asymptomatic controls. The prevalence of *H. pylori* infection, particularly in westernized populations, has been shown to rise steadily with increasing age, usually being present in less than 10% of people under 20 years of age, but rising to over 40% by the age of 50 years, and possibly much higher in old age [31–35]. The age profile of the control group is therefore of vital importance if comparable data are to be obtained. Not only is age important, but there are also marked ethnic variations in the frequency of infection in asymptomatic controls, with rates of 87% in Colombians of unspecified age [36], 79% in Africans aged 7–66 (mean 26) years [37], 60% in Chinese aged 20–39 years [32], 55% in Japanese aged 26–70 (mean 49) years [38] and 46% in Indians aged 20–29 years [39]. Rates varying between 60% [40] and 13% [41] have been reported in studies of young controls from Western countries, and in a serological study Forman *et al.* [42] have reported striking variations in prevalence within countries depending on both social and geographic factors. Endoscopic sampling techniques may also produce dramatically different results in the same population, Peterson *et al.* [43] reporting colonization rates of 39% in gastric antral biopsies, but 61% in biopsies from the fundus of 23 young volunteers.

Evidently, comparison of colonization rates between patients and controls in different studies is not likely to be meaningful. There are, however, a few reports [36, 38, 40, 41, 44–46] directly comparing NUD patients with controls, and these are summarized in Table 16.1. Not all of these studies specifically defined an NUD group, and some of the figures have been derived from larger groups so that accurate age data are not always available. Only the studies by Rokkas *et al.* [44] and Pettross *et al.* [41] reach statistical

Table 16.1 *H. pylori* colonization rates in endoscopic studies comparing NUD patients and normal volunteers.

Author	Country	Group	n	Mean age (years)	Range	% H. pylori + ve	Reference number
Rokkas *et al.*	UK	NUD	87	40.7	18–65	45.4	44
		Normal	15	39.5	24–72	13.3	
Pettross *et al.*	USA	NUD	32	47		47	41
		Normal	15	29		13	
Rauws & Tytgat	Netherlands	NUD	107		30–39	47	45
		Normal	44	34	19–71	27	
Inouye *et al.*	Japan	NUD	24			71	38
		Normal	20	49	26–70	55	
Guerre *et al.*	France	NUD	96	45.4		39.5	46
		Normal	26	52		34.6	
Gutlerrez *et al.*	Colombia	NUD	34			79.4	36
		Normal	15			86.6	
Collins *et al.*	Ireland	NUD	20	35.6	± 13.8	50	40
		Normal	9	31.8	± 5.6	60	

significance. It must be noted that in the second of these there is a difference of 18 years in the mean age of the NUD and control groups, together with an unusually low rate of colonization in the controls. Overall, there seems to be a trend towards higher rates of infection in the NUD groups, but this is far from conclusive. It must also be remembered that *H. pylori* colonization is common in the asymptomatic groups studied, making a strong link with NUD less likely.

Non-invasive population studies can now be carried out, using either serology or the ^{13}C or ^{14}C breath tests to screen large numbers of subjects for *H. pylori* infection and looking for a correlation with symptoms assessed by interview or self-administered questionnaire. Obviously, a firm diagnosis of NUD cannot be made by this method, since between 3% and 23% of the population can be expected to have peptic ulcers [47–50] and perhaps only 25% of people with 'dyspepsia' will have no other diagnosis after proper investigation [7]. Nevertheless, this type of study may yield useful information.

We have examined the age-related frequency of *H. pylori* determined histologically, in patients attending a dyspepsia clinic with NUD (defined as abdominal symptoms referable to the upper GI tract, in the absence of ulceration seen at

endoscopy, or other likely cause of the symptoms). These results have been compared with the frequency of infection determined serologically by enzyme-linked immunosorbent assay (ELISA), in a group of randomly selected blood donors from the same city (Fig. 16.1). Infection was more common in patients compared with blood donors at all ages, although this failed to reach significance in two of the groups.

Wyatt *et al.* [34], using a self-administered questionnaire to study 247 blood donors, found that only the occurrence of previous investigations for dyspepsia in those aged over 40 years was associated with *H. pylori* infection assessed serologically. Sixty-four per cent of those with positive serology gave no history of clinically significant dyspepsia.

Using a passive haemagglutination test, Marshall [51] studied 292 blood donors who had never been diagnosed as having had peptic ulcer disease. The frequency of positive *H. pylori* serology in subjects who had either been investigated for dyspepsia with a barium meal or endoscopy, or who had taken antacid in the preceding 7 days, was significantly higher than the frequency in the remainder of the group (28% vs. 14%).

Skoglund & Whalen [52] carried out a serological survey of 121 subjects, who also completed a self-assessment questionnaire

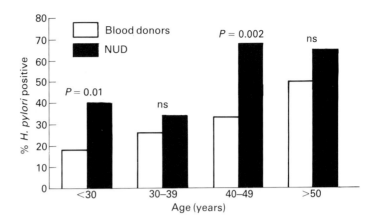

Fig. 16.1 Frequency of *H. pylori* in NUD patients and blood donors.

detailing antacid use. A strong positive correlation was shown between the quantity of antacid used and *H. pylori* colonization assessed by ELISA.

These reports do suggest some association between *H. pylori* infection and 'dyspepsia' using a broad definition, but cannot answer more specific questions about NUD. Detailed information will be hard to obtain using this non-invasive type of study without the use of substantial resources.

Are there specific symptoms or a symptom profile that typify NUD associated with H. pylori?

Marshall & Warren [8] in their original study of 100 patients found that the only symptom which correlated with the presence of *H. pylori* was 'burping', and this association remained even after exclusion of patients with peptic ulcers. Marshall subsequently suggested [53] that the most severe cases of 'nervous dyspepsia' (with symptoms including substernal and epigastric burning pain, reflux, burping, epigastric distension and periodic nausea) have *H. pylori* infection and gastritis, which respond to antibacterial therapy. However, this is anecdotal evidence only.

A number of other workers [8, 44, 46, 54–60] have attempted to define symptoms which distinguish *H. pylori*-positive and *H. pylori*-negative patients with NUD. These studies are summarized in Table 16.2. A number of the studies can be criticized because of differences

between the two groups in possible confounding factors such as use of ulcer-healing drugs or smoking, and one of the studies showed an unexpectedly high rate of *H. pylori*-positive normal gastric histology [59]. It must also be borne in mind that, when multiple symptoms are analysed, there is a high probability of some chance associations reaching statistical significance. The conclusion must be that, as yet, no clear symptom profile has emerged to separate *H. pylori*-related from *H. pylori*-unrelated NUD.

Does eradication of H. pylori lead to resolution or reduction of dyspeptic symptoms?

If *H. pylori* is a cause of NUD, then eradication of the organism from the gastric mucosa might be expected to result in an improvement in dyspeptic symptoms. Several double-blind placebo-controlled treatment studies evaluating changes in symptoms have now been published, and these can be broadly subdivided into those in which bismuth compounds have been used (either alone, or in conjunction with antibiotics) and those using antibiotics alone.

Studies including bismuth compounds in the treatment regimen. Eight studies using bismuth compounds have now been published. Four of these support a role for *H. pylori* in the aetiology of NUD, whilst four do not support this hypothesis.

Borody *et al.* [61] compared tripotassium dicitratobismuthate (TDB) with placebo in 43 *H. pylori*-positive patients with NUD, and showed significant improvement in the symptoms of

Table 16.2 Studies comparing symptoms in *H. pylori*-positive with negative NUD patients.

Author	No. of patients	Symptoms commoner in *H. pylori* + ve NUD	Reference number
Rathbone *et al.*	193	Oesophageal reflux symptoms	54
Vaira *et al.*	107	Postprandial bloating	55
Marshall & Warren	100	Burping	8
Rokkas *et al.*	55	Postprandial bloating	44
Andersen *et al.*	33	Symptoms present for more than 5 years	56
		Symptoms which varied throughout the year	
Sobala *et al.*	186	None	57
Borsch *et al.*	149	None	58
Loffeld *et al.*	109	None	59
Guerre *et al.*	96	None	46
Collins *et al.*	18	None	60

pain/burning, abdominal distension and nausea in the TDB-treated group during 4 weeks' treatment.

Rokkas *et al.* [62] treated 66 patients with colloidal bismuth subcitrate (CBS) for 8 weeks. Twelve patients in the treatment group and eight given placebo were *H. pylori*-positive. Overall symptom scores showed a significant improvement in the CBS group but not in the placebo group, and this difference remained when the *H. pylori*-positive subgroups were considered. Unlike most NUD treatment studies, however, no improvement in symptoms was seen in the placebo group and this must lead to questions about the validity of the study if applied to other populations of NUD patients. Also, seven of the 19 *H. pylori*-negative patients in the placebo group became *H. pylori*-positive during the study with a deterioration in symptoms (it seems likely that acute *H. pylori* infection can cause symptoms – see below).

Two further studies of CBS alone have shown a beneficial effect on symptoms. Lambert *et al.* [63] studied 82 NUD patients. Fifty (61%) were *H. pylori*-positive, and clearance of *H. pylori* was seen in 59% of those treated with CBS, in whom there was also a significant improvement in overall symptom score compared with those not cleared of bacteria. Improvement in overall symptom score was also shown in the *H. pylori*-negative group, but this did not reach significance. In a similar study of Kang *et al.* [64], 51 out of 73 patients completed the protocol.

Twenty-three of the 50 patients with adequate biopsies had histological antral gastritis (20 *H. pylori*-positive), and in this subgroup those treated with CBS were significantly more likely to report total relief of symptoms, and for the first 3 fortnights of the study used significantly fewer antacid tablets than those treated with placebo. Amongst those without gastritis, no significant differences were seen either in the numbers becoming symptom-free or in antacid use between CBS and placebo groups.

Conversely, Loffeld *et al.* [65], in a study of 55 NUD patients with *H. pylori*-associated gastritis treated with either CBS or placebo, could show no significant improvement in either overall subjective complaints or individual symptoms. Neither were McNulty *et al.* [66], in one of the earliest treatment studies, able to show any significant improvement in symptoms between active treatment and placebo groups in a study of 50 patients with NUD and *H. pylori*-associated gastritis. Interestingly, this protocol used two active treatment groups: bismuth salicylate or erythromycin ethylsuccinate.

Patchett *et al.* [67] were also unable to show a significant correlation between eradication of infection and improvement in symptom scores in a study of 84 patients with NUD and *H. pylori*-associated gastritis. Three treatment regimens were used (CBS alone, CBS plus amoxycillin plus metronidazole, and amoxycillin plus metronidazole) but with no placebo group. In a small but similar study, Bamford *et al.* [68]

reported no significant changes in symptom scores in 30 *H. pylori*-positive NUD patients who completed treatment with CBS or amoxycillin or placebo.

Studies using antibiotics but not bismuth. Two studies have been published in which antibiotics alone have been used to attempt eradication of *H. pylori*.

In a study of 106 Peruvian adults with *H. pylori*-associated gastritis and NUD, Morgan *et al.* [69] were unable to show significant differences in symptom improvement between the three treatment groups. Unfortunately, the trial was beset with problems; only 69 patients completed the protocol, 14 treated with furazolidine, 24 with nitrofurantoin, and 31 with placebo – most of the drop-outs were for protocol violations or adverse reactions. In the two antibiotic groups, good *H. pylori* clearance rates were attained (86% and 58% assessed by silver stain), but furazolidine was associated with vomiting and nitrofurantoin with nausea, thus confounding symptom assessment.

Glupczynski *et al.* [70] compared amoxycillin suspension with placebo in 45 patients with NUD and *H. pylori*-associated gastritis. Clearance of bacteria was seen in 91% of amoxycillin-treated patients but surprisingly also in 16% of the placebo group. No differences in symptom scores were seen between active and placebo groups, or between those cleared or not cleared of bacteria.

It is impossible to provide a clear consensus view from these studies about the role of *H. pylori* eradication in the treatment of NUD, and there are a number of reasons why this may be. Unfortunately, the use of bismuth as a therapeutic agent to eradicate *H. pylori* has some inherent problems. Although bismuth has been shown to have a bactericidal effect on *H. pylori in vitro* and is effective in clearing the bacteria from the gastric mucosa with a resultant improvement in gastritis, it also has a number of other local effects in the stomach which may be important either in improving symptoms or in healing gastritis. Bismuth binds to mucus glycoproteins and may reduce acid attack on the gastric mucosa [71]. It inhibits pepsin both *in vitro* and *in vivo* [72], stimulates prostaglandin synthesis by the gastric mucosa [73], inhibits peptic degradation of epidermal growth factor [74] and may increase mucosal bicarbonate secretion [75]. It is therefore possible that the bactericidal properties are of minor importance in its mode of action. There also remains the problem that a truly double-blind study is difficult to perform with an agent that produces such an obvious change in the stool. Antibiotics alone may also confound the assessment of symptom changes by producing upper GI symptoms of their own. In order to demonstrate conclusively that eradication of *H. pylori* alone can improve both gastritis and symptoms, studies using agents which produce effective long-term clearance of bacteria but have no direct effect either on the gastric mucosa or on symptoms are needed – at present no suitable compounds are available!

Even if suitable candidates are found for this role, there remain considerable methodological problems in the assessment of dyspeptic symptoms, and all of the studies published so far use a different method and so cannot be strictly comparable. It has been suggested by Nyren *et al.* [76] that absolute scoring systems may be more accurate than most of those currently used.

These studies do nevertheless provide at least some support for the idea that eradication of *H. pylori* using bismuth compounds will improve NUD symptoms in an as yet undefinable subgroup of patients.

H. pylori and non-steroidal anti-inflammatory drug-associated dyspepsia

Dyspepsia is common in patients taking non-steroid anti-inflammatory drugs (NSAIDs), but the reasons for this are unclear [77, 78]. Upadhyay *et al.* [79], in a study of 14 patients referred for endoscopy and 38 volunteers, all of whom were taking NSAIDs, found a significant positive correlation between the presence of *H. pylori* and the severity of dyspeptic symptoms. Five of the 26 bacteria-positive patients and three of the 26 negative patients had peptic ulcers. Symptomatic data, however, are not provided on these patients specifically, and so no definite conclusions about NUD can be drawn. A similar study from New Zealand [80] of 22 patients and 12 asymptomatic volunteers showed no correlation between symptoms and the presence of bacteria. However, only a small number of patients was studied, and only 41% experienced dyspepsia, making a significant result less likely.

We have carried out a survey of 97 randomly selected patients attending a rheumatology clinic. A structured questionnaire was completed at interview, and H. pylori colonization assessed by ELISA of anti-H. pylori antibodies in serum. Both current dyspepsia (defined as pain, discomfort or burning in the upper abdomen or lower chest) and a past history of dyspepsia were more common in the H. pylori-positive patients. This was observed taking the group as a whole, and also looking at the subgroups taking NSAIDs with or without rheumatoid arthritis, but the differences were not significant. Greater numbers might reveal a significant difference, although of course a diagnosis of NUD cannot be made by questionnaire, and peptic ulceration is common in these patients.

Acute infection and non-ulcer dyspepsia

There is now substantial evidence that acute infection with H. pylori can produce the clinical picture of a 'viral gastroenteritis' with marked upper abdominal symptoms. Both studies [81, 82], in which volunteers have ingested H. pylori, have reported short-lived upper abdominal symptoms such as epigastric pain, nausea, vomiting and epigastric fullness or bloating. However, the symptoms appear to have been self-limiting even though infection persisted in one case, with no suggestion that chronic dyspepsia has resulted.

Epidemic hypochlorhydria associated with acute active gastritis is now well documented [83–88], and in some cases H. pylori has been identified as the cause. In a number of these episodes a mild systemic illness accompanied by dyspeptic symptoms has been reported, but once

again these have been self-limiting and of short duration, and continuing dyspepsia has not been noted.

Interestingly, none of three children who presented with an acute H. pylori-positive gastritis and protein-losing enteropathy were noted to have had abdominal pain during the illness [89].

Conclusion

There seems little doubt that acute H. pylori infection can be symptomatic in some people, although it does not always cause symptoms. It is unlikely that many cases of acute infection will be encountered in hospital practice, and in general practice H. pylori will cause few problems. Certainly, there is no reason to attempt treatment of such patients at present.

Currently, there is little convincing evidence that H. pylori is a major factor in the pathogenesis of NUD, although the large number of reports showing some correlation do suggest that it has a role, at least in a subgroup of patients.

The high frequency of colonization by H. pylori in asymptomatic people, coupled with the considerable variations in the rate with age, ethnic group, geographical location and perhaps other, as yet unidentified, factors, have made the results of prevalence studies difficult to interpret and often of questionable value. The diverse actions of bismuth compounds make most of the treatment studies carried out so far of limited value in defining the role of H. pylori eradication in any symptomatic improvement.

There is a need for large studies of the prevalence of H. pylori in NUD patients, with careful definition of the selection criteria, and strict attention to the comparability of a control group. Such studies would of course always run the risk of subsequent invalidation by new information on the multiple factors leading to colonization. Carefully defined and controlled treatment studies seem more likely to provide a definitive answer, but at the moment these are hampered by the lack of a safe agent with specific anti-H. pylori efficacy, which will produce long-term eradication.

It must be concluded that at present there is no firm indication to treat *H. pylori*-associated dyspepsia with bismuth and/or antibacterial drugs, except within the confines of clinical trials. Nevertheless, many clinicians will feel convinced, from both anecdotal and personal experience (with some limited support from published studies), that there is a subgroup of non-ulcer dyspeptics whose problems are related to *H. pylori* and in whom specific therapy is both justifiable and effective.

References

1 Jones, R.H., Lydeard, S.E., Hobbs, F.D.R., Kenkre, J.E., Williams, E.I., Jones, S.J., Repper, J.A., Caldow, J.L., Dunwoodie, W.M.B. & Bottomley, J.M. Dyspepsia in England and Scotland. *Gut* 1990, **31**, 401–5.

2 Gear, M.W.L. & Barnes, R.J. Endoscopic studies of dyspepsia in a general practice. *Br. Med. J.* 1980, **280**, 1136–7.

3 Heatley, R.V. & Rathbone, B.J. Dyspepsia: a dilemma for doctors. *Lancet* 1987, **ii**, 779–82.

4 Adami, H.O., Agenas, I., Gustavsson, S., Loof, L., Nyberg, A., Nyren, O. & Tyllstrom, J. The clinical diagnosis of 'gastritis'. *Scand. J. Gastroenterol.* 1984, **19**, 216–19.

5 Knill-Jones, R.P. A formal approach to symptoms in dyspepsia. *Clin. Gastroenterol.* 1985, **14**, 517–29.

6 Anon. Management of dyspepsia: report of a working party. *Lancet* 1988, **i**, 576–9.

7 Talley, N.J. & Piper, D.W. The association between non-ulcer dyspepsia and other gastrointestinal disorders. *Scand. J. Gastroenterol.* 1985, **20**, 896–900.

8 Marshall, B.J. & Warren, J.R. Unidentified curved bacilli in the stomach of patients with gastritis and peptic ulceration. *Lancet* 1984, **i**, 1311–15.

9 Cheli, R., Perasso, A. & Giacosa, A. 1987. Symptomatology. In *Gastritis, a Critical Review*. Springer-Verlag, Berlin, Heidelberg, pp. 159–67.

10 Shiner, M. & Doniach, I. A study of X-ray negative dyspepsia with reference to histologic changes in the gastric mucosa. *Gastroenterology* 1957, **32**, 313–24.

11 Roberts, D.M. Chronic gastritis, alcohol, and non-ulcer dyspepsia. *Gut* 1972, **13**, 768–74.

12 Kreuning, J., Bosman, F.T., Kuiper, G., Van der Wal, A.M. & Lindeman, J. Gastric and duodenal mucosa in 'healthy' individuals. *J. Clin. Pathol.* 1978, **31**, 69–77.

13 Cheli, R., Simon, L., Aste, H., Figus, I.A., Nicold, G., Bajtai, A. & Puntoni, R. Atrophic gastritis and intestinal metaplasia in asymptomatic Hungarian and Italian populations. *Endoscopy* 1980, **12**, 105–8.

14 Myren, J. & Serck-Hanssen, A. Gastroscopic observations related to bioptical histology in healthy medical students. *Scand. J. Gastroenterol.* 1975, **10**, 353–5.

15 Cheli, R., Perasso, A. & Giacosa, A. Dyspepsia and chronic gastritis. *Hepato-gastroenterology* 1983, **30**, 21–3.

16 Villako, K., Ihamaki, T., Tamm, A. & Tammur, R. Upper abdominal complaints and gastritis. *Ann. Clin. Res.* 1984, **16**, 192–4.

17 Tsega, E., Manley, N. & Asfaw, T. A clinical and histological study of Ethiopian patients with non-ulcer dyspepsia. *E. Afr. Med. J.* 1985, **62**, 621–39.

18 Toukan, A.U., Kamal, M.F., Amr, S.S., Arnaout, M.A. & Abu-Romiyeh, A.S. Gastroduodenal inflammation in patients with nonulcer dyspepsia. A controlled endoscopic and morphometric study. *Dig. Dis. Sci.* 1985, **30**, 313–20.

19 Wyatt, J.I., Rathbone, B.J. & Heatley, R.V. Local immune response to gastric *Campylobacter* in non-ulcer dyspepsia. *J. Clin. Pathol.* 1986, **39**, 863–70.

20 Price, A.B. Histological aspects of *Campylobacter pylori* colonization and infection of gastric and duodenal mucosa. *Scand. J. Gastroenterol.* 1988, **23**, 21–4.

21 Earlam, R.J., Amerigo, J., Kakavoulis, T. & Pollock, D.J. Histological appearances of oesophagus, antrum and duodenum and their correlation with symptoms in patients with a duodenal ulcer. *Gut* 1985, **26**, 95–100.

22 Fink, S.M., Barwick, K.W., DeLuca, V., Sanders, F.J., Kandathil, M. & McCallum, R.W. The association of histologic gastritis with gastroesophageal reflux and delayed gastric emptying. *J. Clin. Gastroenterol.* 1984, **6**, 301–9.

23 Volpicelli, N.A., Yardley, J.H. & Hendrix, T.R. The association of heartburn with gastritis. *Dig. Dis.* 1977, **22**, 333–9.

24 Wyatt, J.I., Rathbone, B.J., Dixon, M.F. & Heatley, R.V. *Campylobacter pyloridis* and acid induced gastric metaplasia in the pathogenesis of duodenitis. *J. Clin. Pathol.* 1987, **40**, 841–8.

25 Johnston, B.J., Reed, P.I. & Ali, M.H. *Campylobacter* like organisms in duodenal and antral endoscopic biopsies: relationship to inflammation. *Gut* 1986, **27**, 1132–7.

26 Sircus, W. Duodenitis: a clinical, endoscopic and histopathologic study, *Quart. J. Med.* 1985, **56**, 593–600.

27 Greenlaw, R., Sheahan, D.G., DeLuca, V., Miller, D., Myerson, D. & Myerson, P. Gastroduodenitis, a broader concept of peptic ulcer disease. *Dig. Dis. Sci.* 1980, **25**, 660–72.

28 Thomson, W.O., Joffe, S.N., Robertson, A.G., Lee, F.D., Imrie, C.W. & Blumgart, L.H. Is duodenitis a dyspeptic myth? *Lancet* 1977, **i**, 1197–8.

29 Collins, J.S.A., Hamilton, P.W., Watt, P.C.H., Sloan, J.M. & Love, A.H.G. Quantitative histological study of mucosal inflammatory cell densities in endoscopic

duodenal biopsy specimens from dyspeptic patients using computer linked image analysis. *Gut* 1990, **31**, 858–61.

30 Jonsson, K.A., Gotthard, R., Bodemar, G. & Brodin, U. The clinical relevance of endoscopic and histologic inflammation of gastroduodenal mucosa in dyspepsia of unknown origin. *Scand. J. Gastroenterol.* 1989, **24**, 385–95.

31 Jones, D.M., Eldridge, J., Fox, A.J., Sethi, P. & Whorwell, P.J. Antibody to the gastric *Campylobacter*-like organism ('*Campylobacter pyloridis*') – clinical correlations and distribution in the normal population. *J. Med. Microbiol.* 1986, **22**, 57–62.

32 Graham, D.Y., Klein, P.D., Opekun, A.R. & Boutton, T.W. Effect of age on the frequency of active *Campylobacter pylori* infection diagnosed by the [^{13}C]Urea breath test in normal subjects and patients with peptic ulcer disease. *J. Infect. Dis.* 1988, **157**, 777–80.

33 Berkowicz, J. & Lee, A. Person-to-person transmission of *Campylobacter pylori* (letter). *Lancet* 1987, **ii**, 680–1.

34 Wyatt, J.I., Rathbone, B.J., Heatley, R.V. & Losowsky, M.S. *Campylobacter pylori* and history of dyspepsia in healthy blood donors. *Gut* 1988, **29**, A706–A707.

35 Dooley, C.P., Cohen, H., Fitzgibbons, P.L., Bauer, M., Appleman, M.D., Perez-Perez, G.I. and Blaser, M.J. Prevalence of *Helicobacter pylori* infection and histologic gastritis in asymptomatic persons. *N. Engl. J. Med.* 1989, **321**, 1562–6.

36 Gutlerrez, D., Sierra, F., Gomez, M.C. & Camargo, H. *Campylobacter pylori* in chronic environmental gastritis and duodenal ulcer patients. *Gastroenterology* 1988, **94**, A163.

37 Glupczynski, Y., Bourdeaus, L., Deprez, C., Devos, D., Molima, K., Balegmire, B., Hennart, P. & Butzler, J.P. *Campylobacter pylori*, gastritis and peptic ulcer: a prospective endoscopic study in rural Eastern Zaire. *Klin. Wochenschr.* 1989, **67**, suppl. XVIII, 23.

38 Inouye, H., Yamamoto, I., Tanida, N., Mikami, J., Tamura, K., Ohno, T., Kano, M. & Shimoyama, T. *Campylobacter pylori* in Japan: bacterological feature and prevalence in healthy subjects and patients with gastroduodenal disorders. *Gastroenterol. Jap.* 1989, **24**, 494–504.

39 Graham, D.Y., Klein, P.D., Opekun, A.R., Boutton, T.W., Evans, D.J. & Evans, D. Epidemiology of *Campylobacter pylori* infection: ethnic considerations. *Scand. J. Gastroenterol.* 1988, **S142**, 9–13.

40 Collins, J.S.A., Hamilton, P.W., Watt, P.C.H., Sloan, J.M. & Love, A.H.G. Superficial gastritis and *Campylobacter pylori* in dyspeptic patients – a quantitative study using computer-linked image analysis. *J. Pathol.* 1989, **158**, 303–10.

41 Pettross, C.W., Appleman, M.D., Cohen, H., Valenzuela, J.E. & Chandrasoma, P. Prevalence of *Campylobacter pylori* and association with antral mucosal histology in subjects with and without upper gastrointestinal symptoms. *Dig. Dis. Sci.* 1988, **33**, 649–53.

42 Forman, D., Sitas, F., Stacey, A., Newall, D., Yarnell, J., Burr, M., Elwood, P., Buiatti, E., Palli, D., Lachlan, G. & Chen, J. Epidemiology of *Campylobacter pylori*. *Klin. Wochenschr.* 1989, **67**, suppl. XVIII, 21.

43 Peterson, W.L., Lee, E. & Feldman, M. Relationship between *Campylobacter pylori* and gastritis in healthy humans after administration of placebo or indomethacin. *Gastroenterology* 1988, **95**, 1185–97.

44 Rokkas, T., Pursey, C., Uzoechina, E., Dorrington, L., Simmons, N.A. & Fillipe, M.I. *Campylobacter pylori* and non-ulcer dyspepsia. *Am. J. Gastroenterol.* 1987, **11**, 1149–52.

45 Rauws, E.A.J. & Tytgat, G.N.J. 1989. *Campylobacter pylori*. Gist-brocades Pharmaceuticals, Delft, The Netherlands, pp. 13–21.

46 Guerre, J., Berthe, Y., Chaussade, S., Merite, F., Gaudric, M., Tulliez, M., Deslignieres, S. & Zone, A. Has *Campylobacter pylori* gastritis a specific clinical symptomatology? *Klin. Wochenschr.* 1989, **67**, suppl. XVIII, 25.

47 Ihamaki, T., Varis, K. & Siurala, M. Morphological, functional and immunological state of the gastric mucosa in gastric carcinoma families. *Scand. J. Gastroenterol.* 1979, **14**, 801–12.

48 Araki, S. & Goto, Y. Peptic ulcer in male factory workers: a survey of prevalence, incidence, and aetiological factors. *J. Epidemiol. Commun. Health* 1985, **39**, 82–5.

49 Jorde, R. & Burhol, P.G. Asymptomatic peptic ulcer disease. *Scand. J. Gastroenterol.* 1987, **22**, 129–34.

50 Bernersen, B., Johnsen, R., Straume, B., Burhol, P.G., Jenssen, T.G., & Stakkevold, P.A. Towards a true prevalence of peptic ulcer: the Sorreisa gastrointestinal disorder study. *Gut* 1990, **31**, 989–92.

51 Marshall, B.J. 1988. *Campylobacter pylori*: addressing the controversies. In Menge, H., Gregor, M. & Tytgat, G.N.J. (eds) *Campylobacter pylori*. Springer-Verlag, Berlin, Heidelberg, pp. 235–45.

52 Skoglund, M.L. & Whalen, J.W. Correlation of *C. pylori* and upper GI symptoms. *Gastroenterology* 1988, **94**, A430.

53 Marshall, B.J. Nervous dyspepsia (letter). *Med. J. Aust.* 1985, **142**, 704.

54 Rathbone, B.J., Wyatt, J. & Heatley, R.V. Symptomatology in *C. pylori*-positive and -negative non-ulcer dyspepsia. *Gut* 1988, **29**, A1473.

55 Vaira, D., Holton, J., Osborn, J., Dowsett, J., McNeil, I. & Hatfield, A. Use of endoscopy in patients with dyspepsia. *Br. Med. J.* 1989, **299**, 237.

56 Andersen, L.P., Elsborg, L. & Justesen, T. *Campylobacter pylori* in peptic ulcer disease. III. Symptoms and paraclinical and epidemiologic findings. *Scand. J. Gastroenterol.* 1988, **23**, 347–50.

57 Sobala, G.M., Dixon, M.F. & Axon, A.T.R. *C. pylori* is

not associated with a distinct dyspeptic syndrome. *Gut* 1989, **30**, A733.

58 Borsch, G., Schmidt, G., Wegener, M., Sandmann, M., Adamek, R., Leverkus, F. & Reitemeyer, E. *Campylobacter pylori*: prospective analysis of clinical and histological factors associated with colonization of the upper gastrointestinal tract. *Eur. J. Clin. Invest.* 1988, **18**, 133–8.

59 Loffeld, R.J.L.F., Potters, H.V.P.J., Arends, J.W., Stobberingh, E. & Flendrig, J.A. *Campylobacter* associated gastritis in patients with non-ulcer dyspepsia. *J. Clin. Pathol.* 1988, **41**, 85–8.

60 Collins, J.S.A., Knill-Jones, R.P., Sloan, J.M., Watt, P.C.H., Hamilton, P.W., Crean, G.P. & Love, H.G. Comparison of symptoms between non-ulcer dyspepsia patients positive and negative for *Campylobacter pylori* using a single bias computer system for history taking. *Gut* 1989, **30**, A1475.

61 Borody, T., Daskalopoulos, G., Brandl, S., Carrick, J. & Hazell, S. Dyspeptic symptoms improve following eradication of gastric *Campylobacter pyloridis*. *Gastroenterology* 1987, **92**, 1324.

62 Rokkas, T., Pursey, C., Uzoechina, E., Dorrington, L., Simmons, N.A., Filipe, M.I. & Sladen, G.E. Non-ulcer dyspepsia and short term De-Nol therapy: a placebo controlled trial with particular reference to the role of *Campylobacter pylori*. *Gut* 1988, **29**, 1386–91.

63 Lambert, J.R., Dunn, K., Borromeo, M., Korman, M.G. & Hansky, J. *Campylobacter pylori* – a role in non-ulcer dyspepsia? *Scand. J. Gastroenterol.* 1989, **24**, suppl. 160, 7–13.

64 Kang, J.Y., Tay, H.H., Wee, A., Guan, R., Math, M.V. & Yap, I. Effect of colloidal bismuth subcitrate on symptoms and gastric histology in non-ulcer dyspepsia. A double blind placebo controlled study. *Gut* 1990, **31**, 476–80.

65 Loffeld, R.J.L.F., Potters, H.V.J.P., Stobberingh, E., Flendrig, J.A., Van Spreeuwel, J.P. & Arends, J.W. *Campylobacter* associated gastritis in patients with non-ulcer dyspepsia: a double blind placebo controlled trial with colloidal bismuth subcitrate. *Gut* 1989, **30**, 1206–12.

66 McNulty, C.A.M., Gearty, J.C., Crump, B., Davis, M., Donovan, I.A. & Melikian, V. *Campylobacter pyloridis* and associated gastritis: investigator blind, placebo controlled trial of bismuth salicylate and erythromycin ethylsuccinate. *Br. Med. J.* 1986, **293**, 645–9.

67 Patchett, S., Beattie, S., Leen, E., Keane, C. & O'Morain, C. A randomised controlled trial of eradication of *Helicobacter pylori* on the symptoms of non-ulcer dyspepsia. *Gut* 1990, **31**, A1178.

68 Bamford, K.M., Collins, J.S.A., Collins, B.J., Hughes, D.F., Porter, K.G. & Wilson, T.S. Amoxycillin and colloidal bismuth subcitrate improve associated gastritis but not symptoms in patients with non-ulcer

dyspepsia. *Klin. Wochenschr.* 1989, **67**, suppl. XVIII, 3.

69 Morgan, D., Kraft, W., Bender, M. & Pearson, A. Nitrofurantoins in the treatment of gastritis associated with *Campylobacter pylori*. *Gastroenterology* 1988, **95**, 1178–84.

70 Glupczynski, Y., Burette, A., Labbe, M., Deprez, C., De Reuck, M. & Deltenre, M. *Campylobacter pylori*-associated gastritis: a double blind placebo controlled trial with amoxycillin. *Am. J. Gastroenterol.* 1988, **83**, 365–72.

71 Tasman-Jones, C., Maher, C., Thomsen, L., Lee, S.P. & Vanderwee, M. Mucosal defences and gastroduodenal disease. *Digestion* 1987, **S2**, 1–7.

72 Rokkas, T. & Sladen, G.E. Bismuth: effects on gastritis and peptic ulcer. *Scand. J. Gastroenterol.* 1988, **S142**, 82–6.

73 Konturek, S.J., Brzozowski, T., Drozdowicz, D. & Bielanski, W. 1988. Gastroprotective and ulcer healing properties of bismuth salts. In Menge, H., Gregor, M., Tytgat, G.N.J. & Marshall, B.J. (eds) *Campylobacter pylori*. Springer-Verlag, Berlin, Heidelberg, pp. 184–94.

74 Slomiany, B.L., Bilski, J., Sarosiek, J., Liau, Y.H. & Slomiany, A. Coloidal bismuth subcitrate (De-nol) inhibits peptic degradation of epidermal growth factor. *Gastroenterology* 1988, **94**, A431.

75 Shorrock, C.J., Crampton, J.R., Gibbons, L.C. & Rees, W.D.W. Effect of bismuth subcitrate on amphibian gastroduodenal bicarbonate secretion. *Gut* 1989, **30**, 917–21.

76 Nyren, O., Adami, H.O., Bates, S., Bergstrom, R., Gustavsson, S., Loof, L. & Sjoden, P. Self-rating of pain in nonulcer dyspepsia. *J. Clin. Gastroenterol.* 1987, **9**, 408–14.

77 Larkai, E.N., Lacey-Smith, J., Lidsky, M.D. & Graham, D.Y. Gastroduodenal mucosa and dyspeptic symptoms in arthritic patients during chronic nonsteroidal anti-inflammatory drug use. *Am. J. Gastroenterol.* 1987, **82**, 1153–8.

78 Katzka, D.A., Sunshine, A.G. & Cohen, S. The effect of nonsteroidal anti-inflammatory drugs on upper gastrointestinal tract symptoms and mucosal integrity. *J. Clin. Gastroenterol.* 1987, **9**, 142–8.

79 Upadhyay, R., Howatson, A., McKinlay, A., Danesh, B.J.Z., Sturrock, R.D. & Russell, R. *Campylobacter pylori* associated gastritis in patients with rheumatoid arthritis taking nonsteroidal anti-inflammatory drugs. *Br. J. Rheumatol.* 1988, **27**, 113–16.

80 Doube, A. & Morris, A. Nonsteroidal anti-inflammatory drug-induced dyspepsia – is *Campylobacter pylori* implicated? *Br. J. Rheumatol.* 1988, **27**, 110–12.

81 Marshall, B.J., Amstrong, J.A., McGechie, J.A. & Glancy, R.J. Attempt to fulfil Koch's postulates for pyloric *Campylobacter*. *Med. J. Aust.* 1985, **142**, 436–9.

Table 18.1 Basal and peak acid outputs (mmol/hour) at 1, 8 and 18 months after onset of illness.

Case no.	Acid output	Months after onset of illness		
		1	8	18
1	Basal	0	2.6	2.6
	Peak	0.3	31.4	31.8
2	Basal	0	1.2	5.2
	Peak	8.8	29.4	35.2
3	Basal	0	0.8	a
	Peak	0	20.2	a
4	Basal	0	b	b
	Peak	1.2	b	b

[a] Refused further studies.
[b] Working overseas.

Schilling tests performed in three subjects at 8 months showed diminished retention of vitamin B_{12}.

All subjects had blood taken for viral serology 2 days and 2 weeks after the condition was recognized. Complement fixation tests were performed against the following antigens: influenza A, influenza B, adenovirus, cytomegalovirus and *Mycoplasma pneumoniae*. One month after the onset of hypochlorhydria, the patients were ad-

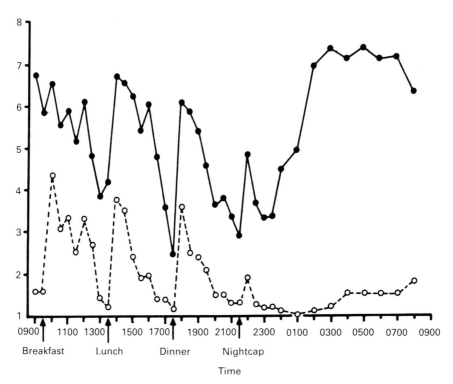

Fig. 18.1 Mean hourly pH values in four subjects who developed spontaneous hypochlorhydria (——) [46] and in eight subjects studied earlier (– – –).

mitted for 24 hours to study intragastric acidity (see Fig. 18.1), bacterial counts and concentrations of nitrite and N-nitroso compounds. Of the 48 samples of gastric juice examined, 47 had a bacterial growth of more than 10^5 organisms/ml, and 46 had a growth of nitrate-reducing bacteria of more than 10^5 organisms/ml. Mean intragastric nitrite concentrations were 10 times higher than in a group of eight healthy controls but both the mean total and the mean stable N-nitroso compound concentrations were not appreciably different from those of controls. Gastric juice was aspirated with a sterile syringe and transferred to a universal container sterilized with gas; mucus and food were broken up and bacteria dispersed by vortex mixing. Samples were placed inside an anaerobic chamber, where all subsequent manipulations were performed. The gastric juice was diluted $(10^1 - 10^{12})$ in prereduced brain/heart infusion broth, and added to indonitrite broth in microtitre plates. The total numbers of bacteria and nitrate-reducing bacteria were estimated by the most probable number method after anaerobic incubation at 36.5 °C for 5 days. In addition, one sample from each patient was examined to identify the individual bacterial species present. Haematological and biochemical screenings performed before and 2 weeks after the onset of illness showed unchanged results, and viral serology detected no rise in titres to influenza A and influenza B, adenovirus, cytomegalovirus or *M. pneumoniae*. Bacteria isolated by culture included *Neisseria, Corynebacterium, Streptococcus, Staphylococcus, Acinetobacter, Lactobacillus, Fusobacterium, Bacteroides, Veillonella* and *Bifidobacterium*, all of which are considered normal oral flora and had presumably been swallowed. Coliforms were not isolated.

Initial endoscopy in all subjects following illness showed a macroscopically normal stomach. However, histology showed active superficial gastritis in all subjects affected. The inflammatory response was most noticeable in the gastric antrum, and in some subjects clusters of polymorphs were present within the gastric glands. Cultures of gastric biopsy specimens in baboon kidney, HEP_2 and MRC_5 cell lines did not show

the presence of any virus. Endoscopy and biopsy were repeated after a further 8 months. Histology had returned to normal in one patient, although the three other subjects showed features of chronic gastritis, with plasma cell and lymphocytic infiltration replacing the polymorphs seen in the earlier specimens. A further patient still had active chronic gastritis after 18 months' follow-up. Thus, all patients in this study had superficial gastritis which became chronic in three, and in one patient moderate titres of parietal cell antibodies developed, suggesting that this condition might progress to atrophic gastritis.

Although community transmission was considered a possibility by these authors, serological screening and electron microscopy of gastric biopsy specimens failed to show an infective cause. Transmission of an unidentified enteric pathogen via a contaminated pH electrode was therefore suspected.

Spontaneous hypochlorhydria and Helicobacter pylori

The study reported by Gledhill *et al.* [46] was conducted between 1981 and 1982, at which time Warren [47] and Marshall [48] had not yet described the unidentified curved bacilli on the gastric epithelium of patients with active chronic gastritis, which has subsequently proved to be *Helicobacter pylori*.

The observation that hypo- or achlorhydria was associated with the voluntary ingestion of *H. pylori* in two otherwise healthy subjects [49, 50] suggests that *H. pylori* might have been the causative organism in the cluster studies reported by Ramsay *et al.* [45] and Gledhill *et al.* [46].

Subsequent to the discovery of *H. pylori*, Peterson *et al.* [51] tested serum samples taken during and after the illness in subjects reported by Ramsay *et al.* [45] for antibodies to *H. pylori*. They felt that the demonstration of organisms on mucosal biopsy would not be proof of infection because there is a high prevalence of *H. pylori* in normal fundic tissue of healthy subjects [52]. Acute and convalescent serum samples obtained at diagnosis and 6 months later from

12 patients were coded and assessed for the presence of immunoglobulin (IgG) antibody against *H. pylori*, using an enzyme-linked immunosorbent assay (ELISA). There was no significant difference between those subjects with gastritis and controls, although the convalescent gastritis sera showed a significant increase. Antibody titres to *H. pylori* rose during convalescence by at least one dilution in nine of the 12 patients with gastritis, suggesting that the organism played a role in the epidemic of gastritis.

Human ingestion studies

The reported documentation of alterations in gastric acid secretion in two volunteer ingestion studies with *H. pylori* [49, 50] is somewhat limited. When Marshall ingested *H. pylori*, no formal studies of basal or stimulated acid secretion were undertaken but the vomitus did not taste acidic and was not acid when tested with litmus paper [49]. In the study reported by Morris & Nicholson [50], basal acid pH was tested extensively before, during and subsequent to infection. Following ingestion of *H. pylori*, pH remained acidic until day 5 and by day 8 had risen to a pH of 7.6, which was maintained until day 27, following which the fasting gastric pH returned to 1.6 on day 29.

Two further carefully documented reports of *H. pylori* infection as a cause of epidemic hypochlorhydria have been reported [53, 54].

In the first [53], a 37-year-old, previously healthy, man had weekly gastric analyses with endoscopy and biopsies in a study of gastric adaptation to aspirin. In the second week of aspirin administration, he developed nausea and epigastric discomfort and aspirin was discontinued but gastric analyses and biopsies were continued as per the protocol. When compared with studies preceding the acute illness, there was a transient 7.4-fold increase in basal acid, a 3.6-fold increase in mucus secretion and a 12-fold increase in gastric bleeding. During the second week of infection basal acid secretion fell to zero and pepsin secretion was one-third of control. Endoscopy at the time of symptoms showed erosions in the gastric body and antrum, as well as numerous haemorrhages, and an acute ulcer was present in the antrum. Endoscopy 7 days later revealed that the gastric mucosa had almost completely recovered. Gastric biopsies were normal before and during the first 2 weeks of aspirin ingestion but at the time of the acute illness, when basal acid secretion was markedly increased, there was an acute inflammation of the antrum with many *H. pylori* present. At that time neither acute inflammation nor *H. pylori* was found in biopsies from the body of the stomach, but 1 week later biopsies showed acute inflammation in the gastric body and antrum. Within 1 week the features of chronic gastritis were present, and 2 years later persistent chronic gastritis with *H. pylori* was still present. This case showed that an increased basal acid and pepsin secretion occurred in response to the acute infection with *H. pylori* and this was followed by a phase of hypochlorhydria and subsequent recovery. Stimulated acid secretion in response to gastrin or histamine was not undertaken.

In the latest report [54], a 30-year-old gastroenterology research fellow was involved in handling many gastric juice samples. Two and a half years previously he had undergone a normal ^{14}C-urea breath test. He experienced a typical constellation of acute symptoms similar to those described above, which lasted some 5–7 days. Endoscopy on day 5 revealed erythema, and gastric juice pH was 7.0. The *Campylobacter*-like organism (CLO) test was negative at 1 hour but positive after 24 hours' incubation and *H. pylori* was successfully cultured, although growth was scanty. At day 14 the erythema was less pronounced but pH was still 7.5 and the CLO test and culture were both negative. At day 74 the endoscopic appearances were normal, gastric juice pH was 2 and *H. pylori* was successfully cultured. The ^{14}C-urea breath test was positive on day 94. Histology on day 5 confirmed an acute erosive gastritis with many polymorphs equally prominent in antrum and body. A few micro-organisms were seen but not convincing

Helicobacter were convincingly seen at this stage. At day 14 histology was essentially similar, with a few chronic inflammatory cells but again not convincing *H. pylori*. At day 74 a diffuse chronic gastritis with mild activity was seen and scanty *Helicobacter* confirmed. Further studies showed that the subject was seronegative on days 1, 5 and 14 but positive by day 74. Interestingly his ascorbic acid status was also examined since he had undergone normal studies previously. At day 37 ascorbic acid was scarcely detectable in gastric juice, which was still of neutral pH, either fasting or after intravenous injection of ascorbic acid. At day 161 he had regained acidity but both ascorbic acid and total vitamin C concentrations remained low and rose only slightly after intravenous injection.

Several aspects of this latter study [54] are especially interesting. A high incidence of *H. pylori* infection in endoscopy staff, as evidenced by positive serology, has been reported [55, 56] and it seems likely that this patient was infected in the environment of the gastroenterology unit.

The onset of the gastritis was acute, with similarity to that seen after alcohol or non-steroid anti-inflammatory drugs (NSAIDs) but with a conspicuous polymorph infiltration to distinguish *H. pylori* infection.

In this case it was difficult to clearly identify *H. pylori*, which may be related to the transient achlorhydria which occurs. *H. pylori* does not flourish when the gastric pH rises towards neutrality and there are several reports that *H. pylori* is infrequently found in patients taking omeprazole [57, 58].

Goldie *et al.* [59] have reported that high ascorbic acid concentrations inhibit *H. pylori*. There was a fall in ascorbic acid concentrations in the stomach of this subject and this reflected a failure of secretion of ascorbic acid across the gastric mucosa [54]. The decrease in ascorbic acid concentrations might favour the survival of *H. pylori*. Furthermore, the more speculative long-term implication would be a reduction in the antioxidant potential of gastric juice and removal of a factor considered to be protective against gastric cancer.

Acid secretion and serum gastrin

Acid secretion and serum gastrin levels have been evaluated in 36 individuals with *H. pylori* confirmed by Warthin–Starry stain [60]. Nineteen patients, 10 with gastric ulcer and nine with duodenal ulcer, had normal gastric secretion, and two patients with gastric ulcer were hypochlorhydric. Median basal acid output was higher for those with duodenal ulcer, at 38 mmol/hour, than for those with gastric ulcer, at 28 mmol/hour. *H. pylori* was found in six normogastrinaemic patients with elevated acid output and in one gastrinoma patient with marked acid hypersecretion. Histological chronic gastritis was present in all subjects and 29 had active chronic gastritis. While the authors conclude that *H. pylori* can survive in a wide range of acid conditions, this study gives no data to suggest prolonged hypochlorhydria in patients infected with *H. pylori*. Thus, if infection with *H. pylori* is indeed associated with diminished or absent acid secretion, the majority of patients appear to recover their acid secretory status.

However, inappropriate hypergastrinaemia has been observed in healthy subjects infected with *H. pylori* [61]. Eight of 95 apparently healthy volunteers had asymptomatic *H. pylori* infection at the time of simultaneous measurement of 24-hour intragastric acidity and plasma gastrin levels. There was no significant difference between the median integrated 24-hour acidity but the 24-hour plasma gastrin concentrations were significantly higher in the infected subjects. Several other studies have made similar observations, suggesting that the presence of *H. pylori* in the gastric antrum stimulates gastrin release in duodenal ulcer disease [62, 63] and is associated with an exaggerated meal-stimulated gastrin release [64]. Eradication of the organism is associated with a fall in the postprandial gastrin response [62, 63]. How these changes in acid secretion and gastrin release arise as a result of *H. pylori* infection still remains obscure and much further work is required to elucidate the mechanisms involved.

Possible inhibitory effects of infection on gastric secretion in man

The mechanism by which hypochlorhydria occurs remains unclear. In the study reported by Ramsay *et al.* [45], careful histology failed to demonstrate a reduction in parietal cell mass, and, in the case reported by Graham *et al.* [53], parietal cell morphology and numbers appeared normal. Ramsay *et al.* [45] also confirmed that the reduction in gastric acid secretion was real and not the result of an increased rate of hydrogen ion back-diffusion across the damaged gastric mucosa.

Bacterial infections which cause fever have frequently been associated with a marked reduction in acid secretion. Histamine-fast achlorhydria was found in patients suffering from a variety of bacterial infections, including typhoid, paratyphoid, pulmonary tuberculosis, bronchopneumonia and lung abscess [65]. This was reported from a region of China associated with a low natural incidence of achlorhydria.

In 106 febrile patients with infection, body temperature was positively correlated with the degree of suppression of acid secretion [66]. The basal secretion of acid was reduced to approximately one-third of the expected normal, and the prevalence of total achlorhydria was increased eight times. Gastric secretion returned to normal levels in 90% of patients after eradication of the infection.

In a group of 325 patients with pulmonary tuberculosis of varying degrees of severity, there was a steady increase in the prevalence of achlorhydria with advancement of the disease [67].

It is interesting to note that, in 1833, William Beaumont [68] had observed a reduction in the gastric secretion of his gastric fistula patient, Alexis St Martin, during a febrile illness. In the presence of fever, he noted that 'the secretions become greatly vitiated, greatly diminished or entirely suppressed'.

It is possible that fever rather than infection *per se* is responsible for the suppression of acid output. A transient inhibition of gastric secretion has been produced in man by artificially raising body temperature to 38–39 °C in a heating cabinet [69].

There is some evidence that parasitic infections in man cause a reduction in acid secretion. Infection with the fish tapeworm *Diphyllobothrium latum* is more common in association with hypochlorhydria [70], but there is some evidence to suggest that the infection itself may suppress acid output [71] through an unknown mechanism. Infection with *Trypanosoma cruzi*, the causative agent in Chagas' disease, is associated with a reduction in basal and stimulated acid output [72]. This may be because of the gastric parasympathetic denervation caused by the infecting organism, which reduces the responsiveness of the parietal cell to physiological stimuli. Reduced gastric acid secretion has also been documented in patients infected with the hookworm *Ancylostoma duodenale* [73]. The parasite is confined to the small intestine and the mechanism whereby it influences gastric secretion is unknown.

The effects of viral infection on gastric secretion in man have not received much attention, although a virus-derived peptide after vaccinia infection appears to be able to suppress acidity in laboratory animals [74]. As nausea and vomiting are frequent and non-specific symptoms of viral infection in man, it might be expected that certain viruses would produce quantifiable changes in gastric secretion or motility. Ingestion of two strains of parvovirus by human volunteers produced no alteration in either basal or stimulated acid output [75] but markedly slowed gastric emptying. The two viruses used do not cause any inflammation of the gastric mucosa [76], and this situation is quite different from that of epidemic hypochlorhydria, in which there is diffuse gastritis [45, 46].

In the case of *H. pylori*, hypochlorhydria may result from the production of a bacterial toxin acting directly or indirectly on acid secretion. We and others have recently reported the effect of *H. pylori* on acid production, assayed using the ^{14}C-aminopyrine uptake technique in isolated guinea-pig parietal cells [77, 78]. *H. pylori* caused a reduction in basal acid secretion of about 80%, while histamine-stimulated acid secretion was reduced to 50% of maximal stimulation within 15 min of the addition of *H. pylori*. Only a partial return of responsiveness to histamine was seen when *H. pylori* was washed from the preparation. Electron microscopy showed some *H. pylori* remaining attached to parietal cells. It was clear from these studies that, while *H. pylori* does reduce basal and histamine-stimulated acid secretion in this preparation, the effect is only partially reversible. The reduction in acid secretion is therefore unlikely to be solely the result of cytotoxicity or mechanical damage caused by *H. pylori*.

References

1 Howden, C.W. & Hunt, R.H. The relationship between gastric secretion and infection. *Gut* 1987, **28**, 96–107.

2 Cook, G.C. Infective gastroenteritis and its relationship to reduced gastric acidity. *Scand. J. Gastroenterol.* 1985, **20**, suppl. 111, 17–22.

3 Penston, J. & Wormsley, K.G. Achlorhydria: hypergastrinaemia: carcinoids – a flawed hypothesis? *Gut* 1987, **28**, 488–505.

4 Giannella, R.A., Broitman, S.A. & Zamchek, N. Gastric acid barrier to ingested microorganisms in man: studies *in vivo* and *in vitro*. *Gut* 1972, **13**, 251–6.

5 Anonymous. Bacteria in the stomach. *Lancet* 1981, **ii**, 906–7.

6 Milton-Thompson, G.J., Lightfoot, N.F., Ahmet, Z., Hunt, R.H. *et al.* Intragastric acidity, bacteria, nitrite, and *N*-nitroso compounds before, during and after cimetidine treatment. *Lancet* 1982, **i**, 1091–5.

7 Sharma, B.K., Santana, I.A., Wood, E.C. *et al.* Intragastric bacterial activity and nitrosation before, during and after treatment with omeprazole. *Br. Med. J.* 1984, **289**, 717–19.

8 Meyrick Thomas, J., Misiewicz, J.J., Cook, A.R., Hill, M.J. *et al.* Effect of one year's treatment with ranitidine and of truncal vagotomy on gastric contents. *Gut* 1987, **28**, 726–38.

9 Waddell, W.R. & Kunz, L.J. Association of *Salmonella* enteritis with operations on the stomach. *N. Engl. J. Med.* 1956, **255**, 555–9.

10 Grossman, M.I., Kirsner, J.B. & Gillespie, I.E. Basal and histalog-stimulated gastric secretion in control subjects and in patients with peptic ulcer. *Gastroenterology* 1963, **45**, 14–26.

11 Gorbach, S.L. 1983. In Sleisenger, M.H. & Fordran, J.S. (eds) *Gastrointestinal Disease: Pathophysiology, Diagnosis, Management.* W.B. Saunders, Philadelphia, pp. 925–65.

12 Abdou, S. Susceptibility to cholera. *Lancet* 1948, **i**, 903–4.

13 Bhalla, F., Vij, J.C., Anand, B.S. *et al.* Gastric acid secretion in patients with typhoid fever. *Gut* 1985, **26**, 491–4.

14 Howden, C.W. & Hunt, R.H. Gastric secretion in patients with typhoid. *Gut* 1985, **26**, 1387.

15 Mosbech, J. & Vidback, A. Mortality from and risk of gastric carcinoma among patients with pernicious anaemia. *Br. Med. J.* 1950, **2**, 390.

16 Blackburn, E.K., Callender, St., Dacie, J.V. *et al.* Possible association between pernicious anaemia and leukaemia: a prospective study of 1625 patients with a note on the very high incidence of stomach cancer. *Int. J. Cancer* 1963, **3**, 163–70.

17 Caygill, C.P., Hill, M.J., Kirkham, J.S. *et al.* Mortality from gastric cancer following gastric surgery for peptic ulcer. *Lancet* 1986, **i**, 929–31.

18 Correa, P., Haenszel, W., Cuello, C. *et al.* A model for gastric cancer epidemiology. *Lancet* 1975, **ii**, 58–60.

19 Ruddell, W.S.J., Bone, E.S., Hill, M.J. & Walters, C.L. Pathogenesis of gastric cancer in pernicious anaemia. *Lancet* 1978, **i**, 521–3.

20 Hall, C.N., Darkin, D., Brimblecombe, R., Cook, A.J., Kirkham, J.S. & Northfield, T.C. Evaluation of the nitrosamine hypothesis of gastric carcinogenesis in precancerous conditions. *Gut* 1986, **27**, 491–8.

21 Walsh, J.H. & Grossman, M.I. Gastrin. *N. Engl. J. Med.* 1975, **292**, 1324–32.

22 Lanzon-Miller, S., Pounder, R.E., Hamilton, M.R. *et al.* Twenty-four hour intragastric acidity and plasma gastrin concentration in healthy subjects and patients with duodenal or gastric ulcer, or pernicious anaemia. *Aliment. Pharmacol. Ther.* 1987, **1**, 225–37.

23 Lanzon-Miller, S., Pounder, R.E., Hamilton, M.R. *et al.* Twenty-four-hour intragastric acidity and plasma gastrin concentration before and during treatment with either ranitidine or omeprazole. *Aliment. Pharmacol. Ther.* 1987, **1**, 239–51.

24 Yamada, T. Gastric acid suppression: potential long-term consequences. *Postgrad. Med.* 1985, Nov. suppl., 67–75.

25 Dembinski, A.B. & Johnson, L.R. Growth of pancreas and gastrointestinal mucosa in antrectomized and gastrin treated rats. *Endocrinology* 1979, **105**, 769–73.

26 Larsson, H., Carlsson, E., Mattson, H. *et al.* Plasma gastrin and gastric enterochromaffin-like cell activation and proliferation: studies with omeprazole and ranitidine in intact and antrectomized rats. *Gastroenterology* 1986, **90**, 391–9.

27 Ryberg, B., Axelson, J., Hakanson, R. *et al.* Trophic effect of continuous infusion of [Leu¹⁵]-gastrin-17 in the rat. *Gastroenterology* 1990, **98**, 33–8.

28 Ryberg, B., Carlsson, E., Carlsson, K. *et al.* Effects of resection of acid-secreting mucosa on plasma gastrin and enterochromaffin-like cells in the rat stomach. *Digestion* 1990, **45**, 102–8.

29 Ekman, L., Hansson, H., Harvu, N. *et al.* Toxicological

studies on omeprazole. *Scand. J. Gastroenterol.* 1985, **20**, suppl. 108, 53–69.

30 Havu, N., Mattsson, H., Ekman L. & Carlsson, E. Enterochromaffin-like cell carcinoids in the rat gastric mucosa following long-term administration of ranitidine. *Digestion* 1990, **45**, 189–95.

31 Poynter, D., Pick, C.R., Harcourt, R.A. *et al.* Association of long lasting unsurmountable histamine H₂-blockade and gastric carcinoid tumours in the rat. *Gut* 1985, **26**, 1284–95.

32 Eason, C.T., Spencer, A.J., Pattison, A. *et al.* Species variation in gastric toxicity following chronic administration of ciprofibrate to rat, mouse and marmoset. *Toxicol. Appl. Pharmacol.* 1988, **95**, 328–38.

33 Havu, N., Mattsson, H., Carlsson, K. *et al.* Partial fundectomy results in hypergastrinaemia and the development of gastric ECL cell carcinoids in the rat. *Scand. J. Gastroenterol.* 1989, **24**, suppl. 166, 158.

34 Kabori, O., Vuillot, M.T. & Martin, F. Growth responses of rat stomach cancer cells to gastro-entero-pancreatic hormones. *Int. J. Cancer* 1982, **30**, 65–7.

35 Ohkura, H., Hanafusa, K., Maruyama, K. *et al.* Gastrin-enhanced tumor growth of a xenotransplantable human gastric carcinoma in nude mice. *Jap. J. Clin. Oncol.* 1980, **10**, 255–64.

36 Makhlouf, S.M., McManus, J.P.A. & Card, W.I. A comparative study of the effects of gastrin, histamine, histalog and mechothane on the secretory capacity of the human stomach in normal subjects over 20 months. *Gut* 1965, **6**, 525–34.

37 Baron, J.H. Gastric secretion in a healthy man 1949–1969. *Lancet* 1970, **ii**, 547–9.

38 Hirschowitz, B.I., Streeten, D.H.P., London, J.A. *et al.* A steroid-induced gastric ulcer. *Lancet* 1956, **ii**, 1081–3.

39 Spiro, H.M. & Schwartz, R.D.L. superficial gastritis: a cause of temporary achlorhydria and hyperpepsinemia. *N. Engl. J. Med.* 1958, **259**, 682–4.

40 Waterfall, W.E. Spontaneous decrease in gastric secretory response to homoral stimuli. *Br. Med. J.* 1969, **4**, 459–61.

41 Desai, H.G., Zaveri, M.P. & Anita, F.P. Spontaneous and persisting decrease in maximal acid output. *Br. Med. J.* 1971, **2**, 313–15.

42 Lawrie, R.S. & Williamson, A.W.R. Zollinger–Ellison syndrome treated with poldine methyl methosulphate. *Lancet* 1962, **i**, 1002–4.

43 Desai, H.G. & Anita, F.P. Spontaneous achlorhydria with atrophic gastritis in the Zollinger–Ellison syndrome. *Gut* 1969, **10**, 935–9.

44 Wiersinga, W.M. & Tytgat, G.N. Clinical recovery due to target parietal cell failure in a patient with Zollinger–Ellison syndrome. *Gastroenterology* 1977, **73**, 1413–17.

45 Ramsay, E.J., Carey, K.V., Peterson, W.L. *et al.* Epidemic gastritis with hypochlorhydria. *Gastroenterology* 1979, **76**, 1449–57.

46 Gledhill, T., Leicester, R.J., Addis, B., Lightfoot, N., Barnard, J., Viney, N., Karkin, D. & Hunt, R.H. Epidemic hypochlorhydria. *Br. Med. J.* 1985, **289**, 1383–6.

47 Warren, J. Unidentified curved bacilli on gastric epithelium in active chronic gastritis. *Lancet* 1983, **i**, 1273.

48 Marshall, B. Unidentified curved bacilli on gastric epithelium in active chronic gastritis. *Lancet* 1983, **i**, 1273–5.

49 Marshall, B.J., Armstrong, J.A., McGechie, D.B. *et al.* Attempt to fulfil Koch's postulates for pyloric *Campylobacter*. *Med. J. Aust.* 1985, **142**, 436–9.

50 Morris, A. & Nicholson, G. Ingestion of *Campylobacter pylori* causes gastritis and raised fasting gastric pH. *Am. J. Gastroenterol.* 1987, **82**, 192–9.

51 Peterson, W.L., Lee, E. & Skogland, M. The role of *Campylobacter pyloridis* in epidemic gastritis with hypochlorhydria. *Gastroenterology* 1987, **92**, 1575 (abstr.).

52 Peterson, W.L., Lee, E. & Feldman, M. Gastric *Campylobacter* like organisms in healthy humans: correlation with endoscopic appearance and mucosal histology. *Gastroenterology* 1986, **90**, 1585.

53 Graham, D.Y., Alpert, L.C., Smith, J.L. & Yoshimura, H.H. Iatrogenic *Campylobacter pylori* infection is a cause of epidemic achlorhydria. *Am. J. Gastroenterol.* 1988, **83**, 974–80.

54 Sobala, G.M., Crabtree, J., Dixon, M.F. *et al.* Acute *Helicobacter pylori* infection: clinical features, local and systemic immune response, gastric mucosal histology and gastric juice ascorbic acid concentrations. *Gut* 1991 (in press).

55 Mitchell, H.M., Lee, A. & Carrick, J.T.I. Increased incidence of *Campylobacter pylori* infection in gastroenterologists: further evidence to support person to person transmission of *C. pylori*. *Scand. J. Gastroenterol.* 1989, **24**, 396–400.

56 Reif, A., Jacobs, E. & Kist, M. Seroepidemiological study of the immune response to *Campylobacter pylori* in potential risk groups. *Eur. J. Clin. Microbiol. Infect. Dis.* 1989, **8**, 592–6.

57 Unge, P., Gnarpe, H. & Blomquist, C. *Campylobacter pylori*: Swedish experiences. *Scand. J. Gastroenterol.* 1989, **24** suppl. 157, 12–15.

58 Daw, M.A., Deegan, P., Beattie, S. *et al.* Suppression of *Helicobacter pylori* during the clinical use of omeprazole. *Gut* 1990, **31**, A1199.

59 Goldie, J., VanZanten, S.V.J.O., Richardson, H. & Hunt, R.H. Inhibition of *Campylobacter pylori* by ascorbic acid is pH dependent. *Gastroenterology* 1990, **98** (5), A50.

60 Brady, C.E., Hadfield, T.L. & Hyatt, J.R. Acid secretion and serum gastrin levels in individuals with

Campylobacter pylori. Gastroenterology 1988, **94**, 923–7.

61 Smith, J.T.L., Pounder, R.E., Nwokolo, C.U. *et al.* Inappropriate hypergastrinaemia in asymptomatic healthy subjects infected with *Helicobacter pylori. Gut* 1990, **31**, 522–5.

62 Levi, S., Beardshall, K., Swift, I. *et al.* Antral *Helicobacter pylori*, hypergastrinaemia, and duodenal ulcers: effect of eradicating the organism. *Br. Med. J.* 1989, **299**, 1504–5.

63 Levi, S., Beardshall, K., Haddad, G. *et al. Campylobacter pylori* and duodenal ulcers: the gastrin link. *Lancet* 1989, **i**, 1167–8.

64 Graham, D.Y., Opekun, A., Lew, G.M. *et al.* Resolution of exaggerated meal stimulated gastrin release in duodenal ulcer patients after clearance of *Helicobacter pylori* infection. *Am. J. Gastroenterol.* 1990, **4**, 394–8.

65 Berglund, H. & Chang, H.C. Transitory character of the achlorhydria during fever demonstrated by the histamine test. *Proc. R. Soc. Exp. Biol. Med.* 1929, **26**, 422–3.

66 Chang, H.C. Gastric secretion in fever and infectious diseases. *J. Clin. Invest.* 1933, **12**, 155–69.

67 Kruger, A.L. Gastric acidity in pulmonary tuberculosis. *Am. J. Dig. Dis.* 1943, **10**, 111–14.

68 Beaumont, W. 1833. *Experiments and Observations on the Gastric Juice and the Physiology of Digestion.* Harvard University Press, Boston, 1929: 107.

69 Bandes, J., Hollander, F. & Bierman, W. The effect of physically induced pyrexia on gastric acidity. *Gastroenterology* 1948, **10**, 697–707.

70 Giannella, R.A., Broitman, S.A. & Zamchek, N. Influence of gastric acidity on bacterial and parasitic enteric infections. A perspective. *Ann. Intern. Med.* 1973, **78**, 271–6.

71 Salokannell, J. Intrinsic factor in tapeworm anaemia. *Acta Med. Scand.* 1970, **188**, suppl. 517, 1–51.

72 Padovan, W., Godoy, R.A., Meneghelli, U.G. *et al.* Acid and pepsin secretion in chronic 'Chagas' disease patients in response to graded doses of pentagastrin and bethanechol. *Digestion* 1982, **23**, 48–56.

73 Pimparkar, B.D., Sharma, P., Satoskar, R.S. *et al.* Anaemia and gastrointestinal function in ancylostomiasis. *Postgrad. J. Med.* 1982, **28**, 51–63.

74 Aonuma, S., Koihama, Y., Enmi, K. *et al.* Studies on anti-ulcerogenic protein in inflamed rabbit skin tissues. III. Anti-ulcerogenic peptide obtained from tissues infected with vaccinia virus. *Yakugaku Zasshi* 1984, **104**, 362–73.

75 Meeroff, J.C., Schreiber, D.S., Trier, J.S. *et al.* Abnormal gastric motor function in viral gastroenteritis. *Ann. Intern. Med.* 1980, **92**, 370–3.

76 Widerlite, L., Trier, J.S., Blacklow, N.R. *et al.* Structure of the gastric mucosa in acute infectious nonbacterial gastroenteritis. *Gastroenterology* 1975, **68**, 425–30.

77 Defize, J., Goldie, J. & Hunt, R.H. Effect of *Campylobacter pylori* on, and production by, isolated guinea pig parietal cells. *Gut* 1988, **29**, A1435.

78 Cave, D.R. & Vargas, M. Effect of *Campylobacter pylori* protein on acid secretion by parietal cells. *Lancet* 1989, **i**, 187–9.

19 Helicobacter pylori Colonization and Alterations in Gastric Physiology

K.E.L.McCOLL

In contrast to the large literature concerning the histological changes which chronic *Helicobacter pylori* infection induces in the gastric antral mucosa, relatively little is known about its effects on gastric function. The antral region plays an important role in the endocrine and neurocrine regulation of both gastric secretion and gastric motility and in this chapter the effects of chronic *H. pylori* infection on these processes are discussed. It should be emphasized that the disturbances in gastric function associated with acute and chronic *H. pylori* infection differ and only the latter will be discussed here. The effects of acute *H. pylori* infection have been discussed previously.

H. pylori and gastrin

Recently, it has been recognized that patients with chronic *H. pylori* infection of the antral mucosa have increased circulating levels of gastrin. This hormone is mainly synthesized within the G cells of the antral mucosa and plays a major role in the regulation of gastric secretion.

In 1989 Oderda *et al.* [1] observed that eradication of *H. pylori* infection using amoxycillin and tinidazole in children with dyspepsia resulted in a 32% fall in the fasting plasma gastrin concentration. That same year Levi *et al.* [2] reported that basal and meal-stimulated gastrin concentrations were higher in duodenal ulcer (DU) patients with *H. pylori* infection than in such patients who were *H. pylori*-negative. In order to investigate this further, we examined basal and meal-stimulated gastrin concentrations in nine DU subjects before and 1 month after eradicating *H. pylori* infection [3]. Following eradica-

tion, the basal gastrin concentration fell by 27% and the integrated gastrin response to the meal by 50% [3] (Fig. 19.1). We have since reexamined these patients 7 months after eradication and found that the gastrin remains depressed and may be even lower at this later time point [4] (Fig. 19.1). This marked fall in serum gastrin concentrations in DU subjects following eradication of *H. pylori* infection has been confirmed by Levi *et al.* [5] and Graham *et al.* [6].

At present, therefore, there are four separate studies which have reported a marked fall in gastrin concentrations following eradication of *H. pylori* infection in patients with DU disease or other forms of dyspepsia. It is important to be certain that the fall in gastrin is indeed due to the eradication of the bacterial infection and not due to some other factor. None of the above studies included placebo control groups and it might be argued that the fall in gastrin posttreatment was merely due to increased adrenaline levels on the patient's first study day, producing an exaggerated gastrin response on that occasion. Most of the patients in our own eradication study had undergone several previous identical studies of basal and meal-stimulated gastrin and review of these data showed no evidence for a fall in gastrin merely with repeated testing [4]. Another possibility which has to be considered is that the fall in gastrin could be an effect of the drug therapy used to eradicate the infection, rather than related to the infection itself. Bismuth has been a component of the eradication regimen in most studies and it is known to remain in the tissues for some time [7]. However, in the study by Oderda *et al.* [1] in children, bismuth was not

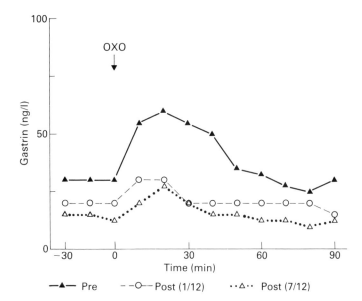

Fig. 19.1 Basal and meal-stimulated plasma gastrin concentrations in nine duodenal ulcer patients before and at 1 and 7 months following eradication of *H. pylori* infection. Reproduced with permission of the publishers of the *Scandinavian Journal of Gastroenterology.*

employed and yet the gastrin still fell following eradication of the infection. Further evidence against the fall in gastrin being merely due to the bismuth is the fact that one patient in our study who received triple eradication therapy including bismuth, but without eradication of the infection, showed no fall in gastrin concentrations [4].

A third possibility is that the fall in gastrin following eradication of *H. pylori* infection in DU patients is due to withdrawal of H_2 receptor antagonist therapy. Most patients entered into studies of the effects on serum gastrin of eradicating *H. pylori* infection have a history of duodenal ulcer disease and may have been taking H_2 receptor antagonist therapy for a considerable time. Following successful eradication, the patients rarely require to continue taking acid-inhibitory drugs. Acid-inhibitory agents are known to raise serum gastrin and it could be argued that the fall in gastrin following eradication of *H. pylori* infection is due to discontinuing these agents. In our own study the patients discontinued any previous acid-inhibitory drugs at least 4 weeks before entering the study and available data indicate that any rise in gastrin due to such therapy has usually worn off by this time [8]. Further evidence against the fall in gastrin being merely due to discontinuing acid-

inhibitory agents is the fact that Graham *et al.* [6] noted that eradication of *H. pylori* infection lowered the gastrin levels in a healthy volunteer, who, presumably, would not have been on acid-inhibitory drugs previously [6]. Smith *et al.* [9] have also reported inappropriately elevated gastrin levels in healthy subjects with *H. pylori* infection.

Critical appraisal of the available data indicates that the fall in gastrin is indeed due to eradication of the *H. pylori* infection. Current evidence also indicates that eradication of *H. pylori* lowers the gastrin concentration not only in patients with DU disease or other forms of dyspepsia but also in healthy volunteers. At present, however, it is not clear whether the gastrin concentration in DU patients with *H. pylori* infection is similar to that in healthy volunteers with the infection. Nor is it clear whether eradication of the infection in DU patients lowers the gastrin level to that in uninfected healthy volunteers.

In contrast to the accumulating data on the effect of *H. pylori* infection on the serum gastrin concentration there is still only very limited information about the effects of the infection on the structure and number of antral G cells. Sankey *et al.* [10] examined gastrin-like immunostaining of endoscopic antral biopsies

H. Pylori and the composition of gastric juice

Urea and ammonium concentrations

Subjects with *P. pylori* infection have a low concentration of urea and high concentration of ammonium in their gastric juice [38]. This can be explained by the organism's high urease activity. We observed that the median gastric juice urea concentration in infected subjects was 0.8 mmol/l (range 0.5–2.9 mmol/l) compared with 2.1 mmol/l (range 1.0–3.7 mmol/l) in those uninfected [39]. Likewise, the ammonium concentration was 3.4 mmol/l (range 1–13 mmol/l) in infected subjects compared with 0.64 mmol/l (range 0.02–1.4 mmol/l) in those uninfected. Though there was an overlap of the two groups with respect to both their urea and their ammonium concentrations, the *H. pylori*-negative and positive subjects could be clearly discriminated by their gastric juice urea/ammonium concentration (Fig. 19.4). This ratio ranged from 0.04 to 0.7 (median 0.26) in infected patients compared with 1.1–113 (median 3.4) in non-infected subjects.

Ascorbic acid

Rathbone *et al.* [40] have reported that patients with *H. pylori* infection and chronic antral gastritis have lowered concentration of ascorbic acid in their gastric juice. Ascorbic acid must be actively secreted into gastric juice as its concentration is higher than that in plasma. However, the concentration achieved in patients with *H. pylori* infection and antral gastritis is only about half that of uninfected subjects with normal histology. In addition, in contrast to uninfected subjects, the ascorbic acid in gastric juice of patients with *H. pylori* infection is predominantly in its biologically inactive, oxidized form. Ascorbic acid is a powerful antioxidant which may prevent the formation of potentially carcinogenic nitrosamines in the stomach.

Conclusions

Over the past few years it has become clear that *H. pylori* infection significantly affects gastric function. However, the relevance of these alterations in gastric function to the pathogenesis of the disease states associated with *H. pylori* infection remains unclear. Much further work is required to fully elucidate the effect of *H. pylori* infection on gastric function and to determine its clinical significance.

The fact that *H. pylori* infection is prevalent in the healthy population means that the vast literature on human gastric physiology must now be interpreted with caution. Many studies of so-called normal gastric physiology will now require to be repeated in subjects confirmed to be free of the infection.

References

1 Oderda, G., Vaira, D., Holton, J., Ainley, C., Altare, F. & Ansaldi, N. Amoxycillin plus tinidazole for *Campylobacter pylori* gastritis in children: assessment by serum IgG antibody, pepsinogen I, and gastrin levels. *Lancet* 1989, **i**, 690–2.

2 Levi, S., Beardshall, K., Haddad, G., Playford, R., Ghosh, P. & Calam, J. *Campylobacter pylori* and duodenal ulcers: the gastrin link. *Lancet* 1989, **i**, 1167–8.

3 McColl, K.E.L., Fullarton, G.M., Nujumi, A.M., Macdonald, A.M., Brown, I.L. & Hilditch, T.E. Lowered gastrin and gastric acidity after eradication of *Campylobacter pylori* in duodenal ulcer, *Lancet* 1989, **ii**, 499–500.

4 McColl, K.E.L., Fullarton, G.M., Chittajallu, R., Nujumi, A.M., Macdonald, A.M., Dahill, S.W. & Hilditch, T.E. Plasma gastrin, daytime intragastric pH and nocturnal acid output before and at one and seven months following eradication of *Helicobacter pylori* in duodenal ulcer subjects. *Scand. J. Gastroenterol.* 1991, **26**, 339–46.

5 Levi, S., Beardshall, K., Swift, I., Foulkes, W., Playford, R., Ghosh, P. & Calam, J. Antral *Helicobacter pylori*, hypergastrinaemia and duodenal ulcers: effect of eradicating the organism. *Br. Med. J.* 1989, **299**, 1504–5.

6 Graham, D.Y., Opekum, A., Lew, G.M., Evans, D.J., Klein, P.D. & Evans, D.G. Ablation of exaggerated meal-stimulated gastrin release in duodenal ulcer patients after clearance of *Helicobacter (Campylobacter) pylori* infection. *Am. J. Gastroenterol.* 1990, **85** (4), 394–8.

7 Gavey, C.J., Szeto, M.L., Nwokolo, C.U., Sercombe, J. & Pounder, R.E. Bismuth accumulates in the body during treatment with tripotassium dicitrato bismuthate. *Aliment. Pharmacol. Ther.* 1989, **3**, 21–8.

8 Karnes, W.E., Berlin, R.G., Maxwell, V., Sytnik, B., Root, J.K. & Walsh, J.H. Prolonged inhibition of acid

secretion causes hypergastrinaemia without altering pH inhibition of gastrin release in humans. *Aliment. Pharmacol. Ther.* 1990, **4**, 443–56.

9 Smith, J.T.L., Pounder, R.E., Nwokolo, C.U., Lanzon-Miller, S., Evans, D.G., Graham, D.Y. & Evans, D.J., Jr. Inappropriate hypergastrinaemia in asymptomatic healthy subjects infected with *Helicobacter pylori*. *Gut* 1990, **31**, 522–5.

10 Sankey, E.A., Helliwell, P.A. & Dhillon, A.P. Immunostaining of antral gastrin cells in quantitatively increased in *Helicobacter pylori* gastritis. *Histopathology* 1990, **16**, 151–5.

11 Wyatt, J.I., Rathbone, B.J., Green, D.M. & Primrose, J. Raised fasting serum gastrin in chronic gastritis in independent of *Campylobacter pylori* status and duodenal ulceration. *Gut* 1989, **30**, A1483.

12 Gedde-Dahl, D. Serum gastrin response to food stimulation and gastric acid secretion in male patients with duodenal ulcer. *Scand. J. Gastroenterol.* 1975, **10**, 187–91.

13 Chittajallu, R.S., Neithercut, W.D., Macdonald, A.M.I. & McColl, K.E.L. Effect of increasing *Helicobacter pylori* ammonia production by urea infusion on plasma gastrin concentrations. *Gut* 1991, **32**, 21–4.

14 Nujumi, A.M.E., Dorrian, C.A., Chittajallu, R.S., Neithercut, W.D. & McColl, K.E.L. Effect of inhibition of *H. pylori* urease activity by acetohydroxamic acid on serum gastrin in duodenal ulcer subjects. *Gut* 1991, **32**, 866–71.

15 Chittajallu, R.S., Dorrian, C.A. & McColl, K.E.L. Is *Helicobacter pylori*-associated hypergastrinaemia due to the bacterium's urease activity or the antral gastritis? *Gut* 1990, **31**, A1175.

16 Yalow, R.S. & Berson, S.A. Radioimmunoassay of gastrin. *Gastroenterology* 1970, **58** (1), 1–14.

17 Walsh, J.H., Richardson, C.T. & Fordtran, J.S. pH dependence of acid secretion and gastrin release in normal and ulcer subjects. *J. Clin. Invest.* 1975, **55**, 462–8.

18 Teichmann, R.K., Pratschke, E., Grab, J., Hammer, C. & Brendel, W. Gastrin release by interleukin-2 and γ-interferon *in vitro*. *Can. J. Physiol. Pharmacol.* 1986, **64**, suppl. 62.

19 Wolfe, M.M., Devendra, K.J., Real, G.M. & McGuigan, J.E. Effects of carbachol on gastrin and somatostatin release in rat antral tissue culture. *Gastroenterology* 1984, **87**, 86–93.

20 Graham, D.Y., Alpert, L.C., Smith, L.J. & Yoshimura, H. Iatrogenic *Campylobacter pylori* infection is a cause of epidemic achlorhydria. *Am. J. Gastroenterology* 1988, **83** (9), 974–80.

21 Cave, D.R., & Vargas, M. Effect of a *Campylobacter pylori* protein on acid secretion by parietal cells. *Lancet* July 1989, 187.

22 Defize, J., Coldie, J. & Hunt, R.H. Inhibition of acid production by *Campylobacter pylori* in isolated guinea pig parietal cells. *Gastroenterology* 1989, **96** (5), part 2, A114.

23 Staub, P., Jost, R., Eberle, C., Stamm, B., Wiist, J. & Hacki, W.H. *Campylobacter-pylori*-Besiedelung des Antrums: Einfluss auf Gastrin, Somatostatin, Pankreatisches Polypeptid und Neurotenson. *Schweiz. Med. Wochenschr.* 1989, **119** (21), 765–7.

24 Wagner, S., Schuler, A., Gebel, M., Freise, J. & Schmidt Werner, F. *Campylobacter pylori* and acid secretion. *Lancet* 1989, **ii**, 562.

25 Montbriand, J.R., Appelman, H.D., Cotner, E.K., Nostrant, T.T. & Elta, G.H. Treatment of *Campylobacter pylori* does not alter gastric acid secretion. *Am. J. Gastroenterol.* 1989, **84** (12), 1513–16.

26 Crean, G.P., Marshall, M.W. & Rumsey, R.D.E. Parietal cell hyperplasia induced by the administration of pentagastrin (ICI 50, 123) to rats. *Gastroenterology* 1969, **57**, 147–55.

27 Ragins, H., Wincze, F., Liu, S.M. & Dittbrenner, M. The origin and survival of gastric parietal cells in the mouse. *Anat. Rec.* 1968, **162**, 99–110.

28 Yokatani, K., DelValle, J., Park, J. & Yamada, T. Dual stimulatory and inhibitory actions of gastrin in isolated canine gastric parietal cells. *Gastroenterology* 1988, **94**, A235.

29 Samloff, I.M. Peptic ulcer: the many proteinases of aggression. *Gastroenterology* 1989, **96**, 586–95.

30 Moore, S.C., Malagalada, J.R., Longstreth, R.G. & Zinsmeister, A.R. Interrelationships among gastric mucosal morphology, secretion and motility in peptic ulcer disease. *Dig. Dis. Sci.* 1986, **31** (7), 673–723.

31 Marzio, L., Di Felice, F., Lacio, M., Celiberti, V., Di Tommasco, C., Dilario, P. *et al.* Gastric and gallbladder emptying in patients affected by idiopathic dyspepsia. *Klin Wochenschr.* 1989, **67**, suppl. SVIII, 44.

32 Wegener, M., Borch, G., Schaffstein, Schulz-Flake, C., Mai, U. & Lewerkus, F. Are dyspeptic symptoms in patients with *Campylobacter pylori*-associated type B gastritis linked to delayed gastric emptying? *Am. J. Gastroenterol.* 1983, **83**, 737–40.

33 Chittajallu, R.S., Dorrian, C.A. & McColl, K.E.L. Serum pepsinogen I in duodenal ulcer – effect of eradication of *H. pylori* and correlation with serum gastrin and antral gastritis. *Gut* 1990, **31**, A1199.

34 Rotter, J.I., Jones, J.Q., Samloff, I.M., Richardson, C.T., Gursky, J.M., Walsh, J.H. *et al.* Duodenal ulcer disease associated with elevated serum pepsinogen I. An inherited autosomal dominant disorder. *N. Engl. J. Med.* 1979, **300**, 53–62.

35 Sumii, K., Inbe, A., Uemura, N., Kimura, M., Haruma, K., Yoshihara, M., Teshima, H., Kajiy, G. & Miyoshi, A. Increased serum pepsinogen I and recurrence of duodenal ulcer. *Scand. J. Gastroenterol.* 1989, **24**, 1200–4.

36 Perasso, A., Testino, G., De Angelis, P., De Grandi, R. & Augeri, C. Chief cell mass in normal gastric mucosa:

relationship with serum pepsinogen I. *Gastroenterol. Clin. Biol.* 1990, **14**, 158–62.

37 Waldum, H.L., Burhol, P.G. & Straume, B.K. Serum group I pepsinogens during prolonged infusion of pentagastrin and secretin in man. *Scand. J. Gastroenterol.* 1979, **14**, 761–8.

38 Marshall, B. & Langton, S. Urea hydrolysis in patients with *Campylobacter pyloridis* infection. *Lancet.* 1986, i, 965–6.

39 Neithercut, W.D., Milne, N., Chittajallu, R.S., Nujumi, A.M., El & McColl, K.E.L. The detection of *Helicobacter pylori* infection of the gastric antrum by measurement of gastric aspirate ammonium and urea concentration. *Gut* 1991, **32**, 973–77.

40 Rathbone, B.J., Johnson, A.W., Wyatt, J.I., Kelleher, J., Heatley, R.V. & Losowsky, M.S. Ascorbic acid: a factor concentrated in human gastric juice. *Clin. Sci.* 1989, **76**, 237–41.

20 Helicobacter pylori: Human Ingestion Studies

A.MORRIS AND G.NICHOLSON

The observation that curved bacilli were almost always present in gastric biopsies showing active chronic gastritis [1] led Australian workers to grow and characterize the organism currently known as *Helicobacter pylori* [2, 3]. Despite their conviction that the organism caused histological gastritis, they were still concerned that the organism could be an opportunistic colonizer of previously abnormal mucosa [4]. In an effort to test the hypothesis of cause and effect, Dr Barry Marshall conducted an ingestion study in July 1984, which was published in 1985 [4].

Marshall ingestion study [4]

At 1 month before challenge, the subject underwent endoscopy and antral, body and duodenal biopsies were taken for histology and culture. Endoscopic findings were normal. No histological abnormalities were present and *H. pylori* was neither seen nor cultured. The same day that the initial biopsies were taken *H. pylori* was isolated from a 66-year-old male with non-ulcer dyspepsia. This isolate had antibiotic susceptibility tests performed before being freeze-dried.

At 3 hours before challenge, gastric acidity was reduced with 600 mg of cimetidine (Smith-Kline & French Laboratories Ltd). The challenge dose was a suspension of a 3-day-culture of *H. pylori*, approximately 10^9 colony-forming units, in 10 ml of alkaline peptone water (pH 8.0).

Apart from borborygmi in the 24 hours following ingestion, the subject was asymptomatic for 1 week. On day 7 epigastric fullness was felt after the evening meal. The following day early-morning hunger occurred and a small amount of mucus was vomited. There was no fever or diarrhoea but headaches, irritability and 'putrid' breath were experienced.

Endoscopy was repeated on day 10, when antral biopsies were obtained for culture and histology. Histological gastritis was present and was characterized by neutrophils within the lamina propria and on the mucosal surface. A reduction in the amount of intracellular mucus was noted. Organisms were seen adhering to the epithelial surface in silver-stained and electron microscopic sections. *H. pylori* was recovered.

Early-morning hunger continued and on day 14 endoscopy was repeated. Biopsies were taken and evidence of persisting infection was expected. However, the histological gastritis had diminished, no neutrophils were present and only a mild accumulation of mononuclear cells remained. The mucus content of the epithelial cells had increased. No organisms were seen in any biopsy. Tinidazole (500 mg b.d. for 7 days) was begun on day 14 and symptoms completely resolved within 24 hours of therapy. No seroconversion was detected when sera were tested in a passive haemagglutination assay [4]. Long-term follow-up has been performed by this volunteer and no evidence of infection has been found on endoscopy and biopsy and he remains seronegative (B.Marshall, personal communication).

This experiment was the first direct evidence that *H. pylori* could colonize normal gastric mucosa. More importantly, colonization was associated with the histological changes typically seen in infected patients. It supported the hypothesis that *H. pylori* is a cause of superficial active chronic gastritis.

positive 'fuzzy' layer stains the epithelial cell brush border as well as the extraneous coat of the bacteria, suggesting the involvement of a negatively charged polysaccharide in connecting the bacteria glycocalyx with that of the epithelial cell [3]. A number of groups have reported cell surface haemagglutinins. A sialic acid-specific haemagglutinin has been described [4, 5] and a Canadian group has defined a surface component of *H. pylori* interacting with a glycolipid from human erythrocyte membranes [6]. A fibrillar N-acetylneuraminyl-lactose-binding haemagglutinin has been described which covers the entire bacterial surface [7]. Recently it has reported that some strains of *H. pylori* bind an epithelial basal membrane component of lamanin [8, 9].

It would appear likely that a number of adhesins may be important in *H. pylori* adherence and tissue damage, and it may be that different strains vary in their adhesins and hence their capacity to adhere and cause damage.

Biochemical factors

Bacterial enzyme activity

Enzymatically, *H. pylori* has a wide range of enzymes [10], a number of which may play a role in pathogenesis. The most notable is urease, the activity of which is so marked that colonization may be diagnosed by a urea breath test or a biopsy urease test. It has been postulated that the ammonia produced envelops the bacteria, protecting it from acidic damage. Ammonia is certainly toxic to cells in tissue culture, and recent animal studies have shown ammonia to cause a dose-dependent decrease in gastric mucosal potential difference, together with increasing gastric epithelial damage [11, 12].

Hazell & Lee [13] have postulated that the urease activity at the epithelial surface is a major factor in pathogenesis, with the rapid hydrolysis of urea creating a mucosal urea gradient and a transmucous ammonia gradient, resulting in an increase of epithelial surface pH. This in turn, they suggest, might affect mucosal

charge gradient, paracellular permeability and epithelial cell Na^+/K^+ adenosine triphosphatase (ATPase), leading to back-diffusion of H^+ ions and concomitant hypochlorhydria. This may then in extreme circumstances result in gastric ulcer formation. There is little direct evidence to support this hypothesis, and the finding of gastric urease-positive spirals in other animals without inflammation [14] is against the urease being of prime pathogenic importance. As this enzyme is seen in all the spirals colonizing mammalian upper gastrointestinal mucus-secreting epithelia, it would appear to play an important role in bacterial colonization or survival. Studies using urease blockers may help define the role of this enzyme.

As yet, little work has been directed to the effects of ammonia production on the mucus–bicarbonate barrier and epithelial and parietal cell metabolism. Attempts to measure epithelial pH have, however, been carried out and demonstrate a reduced epithelial pH in gastritis, which suggests that the mucus–bicarbonate barrier is being compromised.

One important mechanism by which *H. pylori* might be pathogenic is by direct alteration of the gastric mucus gel. Increased cell turnover and epithelial cell mucus depletion are well recognized features of chronic gastritis. *In vitro* studies of gastric mucus glycoprotein synthesis and secretion suggest an increased turnover of mucus glycoprotein in *H. pylori*-associated chronic gastritis [15]. Whether this is purely secondary to the increased epithelial cell turnover found in chronic gastritis is unclear. *H. pylori* has been demonstrated to have proteolytic enzymes capable of degrading porcine gastric mucus [16]. Interestingly, the optimum pH for this reaction is pH 7. The same group has also reported that the mucus in peptic ulcer patients is less viscous than in normals, has a higher proportion of low-molecular-weight mucin, less mucin polymer and a diminished ability to retard H^+ diffusion [17, 18].

If, as appears possible, *H. pylori* compromises the mucus–bicarbonate barrier, the gastric epithelium would then become exposed to the conventional aggressive lumenal factors — acid, pepsin, bile and perhaps various drugs. These agents, singly or in combination, may then be the factors resulting in mucosal damage.

Toxins

One well-recognized method for gut bacteria to exert a cytopathic effect is via toxin production.

Mattsby-Baltzer & Goodwin [19] have presented data showing that the *H. pylori* lipopolysaccharide contained lipid A, a class of substance responsible for the endotoxic properties of a wide range of Gram-negative bacteria.

Leunk *et al.* [20], studying *H. pylori* strains from different parts of the world, reported that 55% of 201 isolates produced a substance in broth culture which caused intracellular vacuolization in a range of cell lines. This cytotoxic activity was heat-labile and protease-sensitive and appeared to have a molecular weight of greater than 100 kD. Studies by Figura *et al.* [21] have confirmed the presence of cytotoxin activity in broth supernatants and have reported that, unlike isolates from patients without ulcers, those from subjects with ulceration produced toxin significantly more frequently. Systemic antibodies to the vacuolating toxin have been identified [22, 23] and are also found more commonly in *H. pylori*-positive patients with ulceration, again suggesting that this vacuolating cytotoxin may be particularly important in the pathogenesis of duodenal ulceration.

Immunological factors

Non-autoimmune chronic gastritis (type B gastritis) is essentially a chronic inflammatory response, with or without polymorph infiltration and architectural damage. The very strong association between *H. pylori* and chronic gastritis in the absence of any other bacteria raised the possibility that the inflammatory response seen in chronic gastritis is a response to *H. pylori* antigens.

In the initial report documenting the association between *H. pylori* and chronic gastritis, it was noted that the organism was particularly associated with a polymorph response (active gastritis) [24]. Most workers have confirmed this association and in active gastritis the neutrophils appear predominantly between epithelial cells, being most numerous in the deep portion of the gastric pit [25]. Relatively few neutrophils are seen in the gastric gland lumen, and the finding of phagocytosed *H. pylori* has been documented [26]. It is currently unclear whether the polymorph response is elicited by the organisms, or whether the environment of an actively inflamed mucosa is more favourable for the growth of *H. pylori*.

Humoral responses

Soon after the original *H. pylori* isolation, it was recognized that there was a systemic immunoglobulin G (IgG) and IgA antibody response. This systemic response can be used to diagnose *H. pylori* colonization and is particularly useful in population studies [27]. Following clearance of the organisms, the antibody titres decrease [28].

Studies on local gastric humoral responses prior to the isolation of *H. pylori* demonstrated that, with the development of histological gastritis, plasma cells increase in number and the epithelium of the isthmic zone shows secretion of IgA, together with lysozyme [29] and lactoferrin [30].

Initial studies on local *H. pylori* humoral responses concentrated on identifying organism-specific antibodies in gastric juice. Measurable titres of *H. pylori*-specific IgA and IgM were demonstrated in a proportion of subjects with *H. pylori*-associated chronic gastritis [31]. The absence of a demonstrable gastric juice IgG response was expected, as this antibody would be rapidly broken down in the acidic gastric juice. No specific IgA, IgM or IgG antibodies were found in the gastric juice of *H. pylori*-negative, histologically normal patients.

Proof that gastric juice immunoglobulins are gastric in origin has been provided by short-term organ culture studies, where only *H. pylori*-positive biopsies produced high titres of *H. pylori*-specific antibodies [32]. Plasma cell counts were assessed in the same patients and the density of the plasma cell infiltrate was found to correlate with the specific immunoglobulin titre [33]. The data thus suggest that a proportion of the plasma cell infiltrate, which characterizes chronic gastritis, is responsible for the humoral response to *H. pylori* antigens.

Similar organ culture studies have been carried out using duodenal tissue and demonstrate a duodenal humoral response in *H. pylori*-positive patients [34]. The duodenal response was most marked in those patients with active duodenitis, and such patients have previously been shown to have duodenal *H. pylori* colonization on areas of gastric metaplasia [35, 36].

Antibody coating of *H. pylori* in tissue secretions from patients with chronic gastritis has been investigated, using an immunoperoxidase technique [25]. IgG, IgA and IgM coating has been demonstrated. However, it is unclear whether this coating is by specific or non-specific immunoglobulins. An interesting finding in this study was the failure of bacteria deep in the gastric pits to be coated, despite being in a location where a high concentration of IgA might be expected.

In vitro studies have demonstrated *H. pylori* to be sensitive to antibody-dependent, complement-mediated bactericidal activity of serum [37]. In the presence of serum opsonins the bacteria were phagocytosed and efficiently killed by polymorphs. The relevance of these studies to the situation at the mucosal surface, where the concentration of complement is unknown and IgA is the major antibody class, is unclear. There is the possibility that the bacterial coating is protective to the organism or that *H. pylori* has the ability to produce an IgA protease.

The antigen specificity of the local immune response has been studied by immunoblotting gastric organ culture supernatants [38]. This has demonstrated the tremendous heterogeneity in the local antigen recognition. The systemic response tends to mirror the local response in terms of antigen specificity. Of considerable interest was the finding that isolates from patients with peptic ulcer disease were more likely to have an anti-120 kD protein response than those from patients without ulceration. Those patients with a 120 kD response tended to

have a more severe histological surface degeneration. This strongly suggests virulence differences between different isolates and also raises the possibility that the 120 kD protein seen on gel electrophoresis may be important in ulcerogenesis. One possibility is that the 120 kD protein represents the cytotoxin isolated from broth culture supernatants, which has also been found more commonly with isolates from peptic ulcer patients. Another possibility is that the 120 kD protein is a marker of bacteria that are better able to colonize the duodenum.

The immune response associated with *H. pylori* remains for as long as the bacteria colonize the stomach, which in the majority of cases means for many years. In such a situation, with long-term inflammation and damage, gastric autoantibodies could develop. Gastric autoantibodies have been recognized for many years, particularly in association with pernicious anaemia. In type B chronic gastritis, IgG autoantibodies to gastrin cells have been demonstrated in a small proportion of patients [39]. In relation to *H. pylori*, the only data suggesting possible autoimmune mechanisms come from the raising of monoclonal antibodies. At least one monoclonal antibody to *H. pylori* cross-reacts with healthy gastric epithelium, suggesting that autoimmunity may be a possibility [40].

Cytokines and cell-mediated immunity

Our knowledge of the cell-mediated immune response and gastric cytokine response to *H. pylori* is limited. The inflammatory response seen in *H. pylori*-associated gastritis is marked and it appears likely that locally produced cytokines would be expected to be involved in modulating the immune response. Crabtree *et al.* [41] investigated the local gastric production of interleukin-6 and tumour necrosis factor (TNF) in *H. pylori*-positive and negative patients. Colonization was associated with significantly greater levels of both cytokines. In the case of TNF-α, the response was associated with the degree of neutrophil response.

Previous work on gastric cell-mediated immunity has concentrated on type A autoimmune chronic gastritis, where T cell subset and functional studies have given conflicting results [42, 43]. Studies on type B gastritis have demonstrated that the inflamed mucosa, unlike normal gastric mucosa, is human leucocyte antigen (HLA)-DR positive and thus theoretically may be capable of antigen presentation [44].

In type B gastritis, T cells are increased in both the epithelial compartment and the lamina propria. Studies on T cell subsets give no consistent picture, with some workers reporting the majority of epithelial T cells to be of the suppressor/cytotoxic phenotype [45]. Others have, however, reported an increase in the T-helper phenotype [46]. In this latter study, the T-helper cells from patients with gastritis showed increased expression of CD7, a T cell stimulation market. Although of unknown function there has been considerable interest in δT cell receptor-postive (TCR+) cells in the gut. In coeliac disease δTCR+ intraepithelial lymphocytes are significantly increased, but recent studies of other inflammatory conditions of the bowel, including *H. pylori* gastritis, show no significant changes [47].

One particularly interesting group of gastritic patients from an immunological point of view are those with lymphocytic gastritis. This is a histologically identifiable condition where the epithelial compartment has a great excess of T cells. In one study *H. pylori* was histologically detected in less than half of the cases [48]. A serological response to *H. pylori* was, however, demonstrable in four out of six patients who were histologically negative. This suggests either that the organism was present in small numbers and not detected, or that there had been a recent infection by *H. pylori*. Lymphocytic gastritis may thus represent an effective immune response to *H. pylori* which is capable of clearing the organism.

Conclusions

The mechanisms by which bacteria colonize and damage the host are often complex and multiple. In the case of *H. pylori* the organism has to gain access to the stomach and then survive the potentially hostile gastric mileau. Once in contact with the mucus gel, it must penetrate this barrier and move to the deeper levels of the mucus gel and epithelial surface where it may adhere to the epithelium. Adherence could be damaging in its own right, but it also creates a situation where the organism is in very close proximity to host tissue and thus any cytotoxins will exert a maximal effect and soluble bacterial antigens may be absorbed and stimulate the local immune response. This response fails to clear the infection, at least in some, and becomes chronic, with a continuous antigen drive. Such an immune response will be damaging in its own right and thus an important factor in pathogenesis. Why the immune response is not always totally effective may be due to any one of a number of bacterial or host factors. Identification of these may be important in developing new approaches to treatment and vital if vaccination is ever to be considered.

The question why only some patients with *H. pylori* gastritis are prone to develop ulcers is clearly complex. Adequate acid secretion, *H. pylori* colonization of the antrum and the presence of gastric metaplasia in the duodenum all seem to be important, even necessary, factors for duodenal ulceration to develop. Increasingly, it appears that there are also virulence differences between *H. pylori* strains which may determine the severity of the mucosal damage and also those subjects at high risk of developing ulceration. Clearly this is an important and exciting area for future research.

References

1 Old, D.C. Bacterial adherence. *Med. Lab. Sci.* 1985, 42, 78–85.

2 Goodwin, C.S., Armstrong, J.A. & Marshall, B.J. *Campylobacter pyloridis*, gastritis and peptic ulceration. *J. Clin. Pathol.* 1986, 39, 353–65.

3 Hessey, S.J., Spencer, J., Wyatt, J.I., Sobala, G., Rathbone, B.J., Axon, A.T.R. & Dixon, M.F. Bacterial adhesion and disease activity in *Helicobacter* associated chronic gastritis. *Gut* 1990, 31, 134–8.

4 Emody, L., Carlsson, A. & Wadstrom, T. Mannose-resistant haemagglutination by *Campylobacter pylori*. *Scand. J. Infect. Dis.* 1988, 20, 253–4.

5 Carlsson, A., Aleljung, P., Emody, L., Ljungh, A. &

Wadstrom, T. Carbohydrate receptor specificity of hemagglutination of *Campylobacter pylori*. In Mégraud, F. & Lamouliatte, H. (eds) *Gastroduodenal Pathology and Campylobacter pylori*. Excerpta Medica, Amsterdam, pp. 375–8.

6 Lingwood, C.A., Law, H., Pellizzari, A., Sherman, P. & Drumm, B. Gastric glycerolipid as a receptor for *Campylobacter pylori*. *Lancet* 1989, ii, 238–41.

7 Evans, D.G., Evans D.J., Moulds, J.J. & Graham, D.Y. N-acetylneuraminyllactose-binding fibrillar hemagglutinin of *Campylobacter pylori*: a putative colonization factor antigen. *Infect. Immun.* 1988, 56, 2898–906.

8 Slomiany, B.L., Piotrowski, J., Sengupta, S. & Slomiany, A. Inhibition of gastric mucosal laminin receptor by *Helicobacter pylori* lipopolysaccharide. *Biochem. Biophys. Res. Commun.* 1991, 175, 963–70.

9 Trust, T.J., Doig, P., Emody, L. Kienle, Z., Wadstrom, T. & O'Toole, P. High affinity binding of the basement membrane proteins collagen type IV and laminin to the gastric pathogen *Helicobacter pylori*. *Infect. Immun.* 1991 (in press).

10 Mégraud, F., Bonnet, M., Garnier, M. & Lomouliatte, H. Characterization of *Campylobacter pyloridis* by culture, enzymatic profile, and protein content. *J. Clin. Microbiol.* 1985, 22, 1007–10.

11 Murakami, M., Yoo, J.K., Mizuno, M., Saita, H., Inada, M. & Miyake, T. Effects of ammonia, urea, and urease on the rat gastric mucosa. *Gastroenterology* 1987, 92, 1544.

12 Murakami, M., Yoo, J.K., Mizuno, M., Saita, H., Inada, M. & Miyake, T. Role of gastric ammonia, urea and urease in gastric mucosal lesions in azotemia. *Gastroenterology* 1987, 92, 1545.

13 Hazell, S.L. & Lee, A. *Campylobacter pyloridis*, urease, hydrogen ion back diffusion, and gastric ulcers. *Lancet* 1986, ii, 15–17.

14 Tompkins, D.S., Wyatt, J.I., Rathbone, B.J. & West, A.P. The characterization and pathological significance of gastric *Campylobacter*-like organisms in the ferret: a model for chronic gastritis? *Epidem. Inf.* 1988, 101, 269–78.

15 Crabtree, J.E., Rathbone, B.J., Wyatt, J.I., Heatley, R.V. & Losowsky, M.S. *In vitro* mucus glycoprotein synthesis and secretion by gastric mucosa colonized with *Campylobacter pyloridis*. *Gut* 1987, 28, A1409.

16 Slomiany, B.L., Bilski, J., Sarosiek, J., Murty, V.L.N., Dworkin, B., Van Horn, K., Zielenski, J. & Slomiany, A. *Campylobacter pyloridis* degrades mucin and undermines gastric mucosal integrity. *Biochem. Biophys. Res. Commun.* 1987, 144, 307–14.

17 Slomiany, B.L., Bilski, J., Murty, V.L.N., Sarosiek, J., Dworkin, B., Van Horn, K. & Slomiany, A. *Campylobacter pyloridis* degrades mucin and undermines gastric mucosal integrity. *Gastroenterology* 1987, 92, 1645.

18 Sarosiek, I., Gabryelewicz, A. & Slomiany, B.L. Changes in the macromolecular organization and physical properties of gastric mucus with peptic ulcer. *Gastroenterology* 1987, 92, 1615.

19 Mattsby-Baltzer, I. & Goodwin, C.S. 1988. Lipid A in *C. pylori*. In Kaijser, B. & Falsen, E. (eds) *Campylobacter IV*, University of Göteborg, Göteborg, abstr. No. 232.

20 Leunk, R.D., Johnson, P.T., David, B.D., Kraft, W.G. & Morgan, D.R. 1988. Identification of cytotoxic activity produced by *Campylobacter pyloridis*. In Kaijser, B. & Falsen, E. (eds) *Campylobacter IV*. University of Göteborg, Göteborg, abstr. No. 97.

21 Figura, N., Guglielmetti, A., Rossolini, A., Barber, A., Cusi, G., Musmanno, R.A., Russi, M. & Quaranta, S. Cytotoxin production by *Campylobacter pylori* strains isolated from patients with peptic ulcers and from patients with chronic gastritis only. *J. Clin. Microbiol.* 1989, 27, 225–6.

22 Cover, T.L., Dooley, C.P. & Blaser, M.J. Characterisation of and human serological response to proteins in *Helicobacter pylori* broth culture supernatants with vacuolising cytotoxin activity. *Infect. Immum.* 1990, 58, 603–10.

23 Figura, N., Bugnoli, M., Guglielmetti, P., Musmanno, R.A., Russi, M. & Quaranta, S. Antibodies to vacuolating toxin of *Helicobacter pylori* in dyspeptic patients. *Rev. Esp. Enf. Dig.* 1990, 78, suppl. 1, 7.

24 Warren, J.R. Unidentified curved bacilli on gastric epithelium in active chronic gastritis. *Lancet* 1983, i, 1273.

25 Wyatt, J.I., Rathbone, B.J. & Heatley, R.V. Local immune response to gastric *Campylobacter* in non-ulcer dyspepsia. *J. Clin. Pathol.* 1987, 39, 863–70.

26 Shousha, S., Bull, T.B. & Parkins, R.A. Gastric spiral bacteria. *Lancet* 1984, ii, 101.

27 Newell, D.G. & Rathbone, B.J. The serodiagnosis of *Campylobacter pylori* infection. *Serodiagnosis Immunother.* 1989, 3, 1–6.

28 Vaira, D., Holton, J., Cairns, S.R., Falzon, M., Polydorou, A., Dowsett, J.F. & Salmon, P.R. Antibody titre to *Campylobacter pylori* after treatment for gastritis. *Br. Med. J.* 1988, 297, 397.

29 Isaacson, P. Immunoperoxidase study of the secretory immunoglobulin system and lysozyme in normal and diseased gastric mucosa. *Gut* 1982, 23, 578–88.

30 Valnes, K., Brandtzaeg, P., Elgjo, K. & Stave, R. Specific and non-specific humoral factors in the epithelium of normal and inflamed gastric mucosa. *Gastroenterology* 1984, 86, 402–12.

31 Rathbone, B.J., Wyatt, J.L., Worsley, B.W., Shires, S.E., Trejdosiewicz, L.K., Heatley, R.V. & Losowsky, M.S. Systemic and local antibody responses to gastric *Campylobacter pyloridis* in non-ulcer dyspepsia. *Gut* 1986, 27, 642–7.

32 Rathbone, B.J., Wyatt, J.I., Tompkins, D. & Heatley, R.V. *In vitro* production of *Campylobacter pyloridis*

specific antibodies by gastric mucosal biopsies. *Gut* 1986, **27**, A607.

33 Wyatt, J.I. & Rathbone, B.J. Immune response of the gastric mucosa to *Campylobacter pylori*. *Scand. J. Gastroenterol.* 1988, **23**, suppl. 142, 44–9.

34 Crabtree, J.E., Rathbone, B.J., Shallcross, T.M., Wyatt, J.I., Heatley, R.V. & Losowsky, M.S. Duodenal secretion of *Campylobacter pylori* specific antibodies in patients with gastritis and duodenitis. *Gut* 1988, **29**, A1438.

35 Wyatt, J.I., Rathbone, B.J., Dixon, M.F. & Heatley, R.V. *Campylobacter pyloridis* and acid induced gastric metaplasia in the pathogenesis of duodenitis. *J. Clin. Pathol.* 1987, **40**, 841–8.

36 Johnson, B.J., Reed, P.I. & Ali, M.H. *Campylobacter* like organisms in duodenal and antral endoscopic biopsies: relationship to inflammation. *Gut* 1987, **27**, 1132–7.

37 Pruul, H., Lee, P.C., Goodwin, C.S. & McDonald, P.J. Interaction of *Campylobacter pyloridis* with human immune defence mechanisms. *J. Med. Microbiol.* 1987, **23**, 233–8.

38 Crabtree, J.E., Taylor, J.D., Wyatt, J.I., Heatley, R.V., Shallcross, T.M., Tomkins, D.S. & Rathbone, B.J. Mucosal IgA recognition of *Helicobacter pylori* 120 kDa protein, peptic ulceration, and gastric pathology. *Lancet* 1991, **338**, 332–5.

39 Vandelli, C., Bottazzo, G.F., Doniach, D. & Franceshi, F. Auto-antibodies to gastrin-producing cells in antral (type B) chronic gastritis. *N. Engl. J. Med.* 1979, **300**, 1406–10.

40 Rathbone, B.J. & Trejdosiewicz, L.K. 1988. A strain-restricted monoclonal antibody to *Campylobacter pyloridis*. In Kaijser, B. & Falsen, E. (eds) *Campylobacter IV*. University of Göteborg, Göteborg, abstr. no. 137.

41 Crabtree, J.E., Shallcross, T.M. Heatley, R.V. & Wyatt, J.I. Mucosal tumour necrosis factor alpha and interleukin-6 in patients with *Helicobacter pylori*-associated gastritis. *Gut* 1991, **44**, 768–71.

42 Rathbone, B.J. & Heatley, R.V. 1986. Gastritis. In Losowsky, M.S. & Heatley, R.V. (eds) *Gut Defences in Clinical Practice*. Churchill Livingstone, Edinburgh, pp. 228–42.

43 Wright, R. 1988. Role of autoimmunity in disease of the gastrointestinal tract and liver. In Heyworth, M.F. & Jones, A.L. (eds) *Immunology of the Gastrointestinal Tract and Liver*, Raven Press, New York, pp. 193–217.

44 Engstrand, L., Scheynius, A., Grimelius, L., Schwan, A. & Gustavsson, L. Induced expression of class II transplantation antigens on gastric epithelial cells in patients with *Campylobacter pylori* positive gastric biopsies. *Gastroenterology* 1988, **94**, A115.

45 Papadimitriou. C.S., Ioachim-Velogianni, E.E., Tsianos, E.B. & Moutsopoulos, H.M. Epithelial HLADR expression and lymphocyte subsets in gastric mucosa in type B chronic gastritis. *Virchows Arch. (A) Pathol. Anat.* 1988, **413**, 197–204.

46 Rathbone, B.J., Wyatt, J.I., Trejdosiewicz, L.K., Heatley, R.V. & Losowsky, M.S. Mucosal T cell subsets in normal gastric antrum and *C. pylori* associated chronic gastritis. *Gut* 1988, **29**, A1438.

47 Trejdosiewicz, L.K., Calabrese, A., Smart, C.J., Oakes, D.J., Howdle, P.D., Crabtree, J.E., Losowsky, M.S., Lancaster, F. & Boylston, A.W. $\gamma\delta$ T cell receptor-positive cells of the human gastrointestinal mucosa: occurrence and V region gene expression in *Helicobacter pylori*-associated gastritis, coeliac disease and inflammatory bowel disease. *Clin. Exp. Immunol.* 1991, **84**, 440–4.

48 Dixon, M.F., Wyatt, J.I., Burke, D.A. & Rathbone, B.J. Lymphocytic gastritis — relationship to *Campylobacter pylori* infection. *J. Pathol.* 1988, **154**, 125–32.

and gastric cancer mortality in rural China. *Int. J. Cancer* 1990, **46**, 608–11.

4 Scott, N., Landsdown, M., Diament, R. *et al.* Helicobacter gastritis and intestinal metaplasia in a gastric cancer family. *Lancet* 1990, **335**, 728.

5 Bayerdorffer, E. & Ottenjann, R. The role of antibiotics in *Campylobacter pylori* associated peptic ulcer disease. *Scand. J. Gastroenterol.* 1988, **23**, suppl. 142, 93–100.

6 Goodwin, C.S., Armstrong, J.A., Chilvers, T., Peters, M. *et al.* Transfer of *Campylobacter pylori* and *Campylobacter mustelae* to Helicobacter gen. nov. as *Helicobacter pylori* comb. nov. and *Helicobacter mustelae* comb. nov., respectively. *Int. J. Systematic Bacteriol.* 1989, **39**, 397–405.

7 Goodwin, C.S., Blake, P. & Blincow, E. The minimum inhibitory and bactericidal concentrations of antibiotics and anti-ulcer agents, against *Campylobacter pyloridis*. *J. Antimicrob. Chemother.* 1986, **17**, 309–14.

8 McNulty, C.A.M., Dent, J.C. & Wise, R. Susceptibility of clinical isolates of *Campylobacter pyloridis* to 11 antimicrobial agents. *Antimicrob. Agents Chemother.* 1985, **28**, 837–8.

9 McNulty, C.A.M. & Dent, J.C. Susceptibility of *Campylobacter pylori* to twenty-one antimicrobial agents. *Eur. J. Clin. Microbiol. Infect. Dis.* 1988, **7**, 566–9.

10 Hardy, D.J., Hanson, C.W., Hensey, D.M., Beyers, J.M. & Fernades, P.B. Susceptibility of *Campylobacter pylori* to macrolides and fluoroquinolones. *J. Antimicrob. Chemother.* 1988, **22**, 631–6.

11 Glupczynski, Y., Burette, A., DeKoster, E. *et al.* Metronidazole resistance in *Helicobacter pylori*. *Lancet* 1990, **335**, 976–7.

12 Andreasen, J.J. & Andersen, L.P. *In vitro* susceptibility of *Campylobacter pyloridis* to cimetidine, sucralfate, bismuth and sixteen antibiotics. *Acta Pathol. Immunol. Scand.* 1987, **95**, 147–9.

13 Shungu, K.L., Nalin, D.R., Gilman, R.H. *et al.* Comparative susceptibilities of *Campylobacter pylori* to norfloxacin and other agents. *Antimicrob. Agents Chemother.* 1987, **31**, 949–50.

14 Marshall, B.J., Armstrong, J.A., Francis, G.I. *et al.* The antibacterial action of bismuth in relation to *Campylobacter pyloridis* colonisation and gastritis. *Digestion* 1987, **37**, Suppl. 2, 16–30.

15 Armstrong, J.A., Wee, S.H., Goodwin, C.S. & Wilson, D.H. Response of *Campylobacter pyloridis* to antibiotics, bismuth and an acid-reducing agent *in vitro*. An ultrastructural study. *J. Med. Microbiol.* 1987, **24**, 343–50.

16 Armstrong, J.A. Cooper, M., Goodwin, C.S. *et al.* Influence of soluble haemagglutinins on adherence of *Helicobacter pylori* to Hep-2 cells. *J. Med. Microbiol.* 1991, **34**, 181–7.

17 Kondo, I., Nagate, T., Adaski, S., Kaneda, Y. & Suwa, A. *In vitro* suspectibility of *Campylobacter pylori* to anti-ulcer drug, sofalcone, and other agents. In Takemonto, T., Kawai, K. & Shimoyama, T. (eds) *Campylobacter pylori and Gastroduodenal Diseases. Second Tokyo International Symposium on Campylobacter pylori.* Tokyo, Taisho, pp. 286–97.

18 Wang, C. Mutagenicity of hydroxamic acids for *Salmonella typhimurium*. *Mutation Res.* 1977, **56**, 7–12.

19 Rauws, E.A.J., Langenberg, W., Houthoff, H.J., Zanen, H.C. & Tytgat, G.N.J. *Campylobacter pyloridis* associated chronic active antral gastritis. A prospective study of its prevalence and the effects of antibacterial and antiulcer treatment. *Gastroenterology* 1988, **94**, 33–40.

20 Gilman, R., Leon-Barua, R., Ramirez-Ramos, A. *et al.* Efficacy of nitrofurantoin in the treatment of antral gastritis associated with *Campylobacter pyloridis*. *Gastroenterology* 1986, **92**, 1405.

21 McNulty, C.A.M., Gearty, J.C., Crump, B. *et al.* *Campylobacter pyloridis* and associated gastritis: investigator blind, placebo controlled trial of bismuth salicylate and erythromycin ethylsuccinate. *Br. Med. J.* 1986, **293**, 645–9.

22 Glupczynski, Y., Labbe, M., Burette, A., Delmee, M., Avesani, V. & Bruck, C. Treatment failure of ofloxacin in *Campylobacter pylori* infection. *Lancet* 1987, **i**, 1096.

23 Stone, J.W., Wise, R., Donovan, I.A. & Gearty, J. Failure of ciprofloxacin to eradicate *Campylobacter pylori* from the stomach. *J. Antimicrob. Chemother.* 1988, **22**, 92–3.

24 McNulty, C.A.M., Dent, J.C., Ford, G.A. & Wilkinson, S.P. Inhibitory antimicrobial concentrations against *Campylobacter pylori* in gastric mucosa. *J. Antimicrob. Chemother.* 1988, **22**, 729–38.

25 Quigley, E.M.M. & Turnberg, L.A. pH of the microclimate lining human gastric and duodenal mucosa *in vivo*. *Gastroenterology* 1987, **92**, 1876–84.

26 Goodwin, C.S., Armstrong, J.A. & Marshall, B.J. *Campylobacter pyloridis*, gastritis and peptic ulceration. *J. Clin. Pathol.* 1986, **39**, 353–65.

27 Nelson, L.A. Physicochemical factors influencing the absorption of erythromycin and its esters. *Chem. Pharm. Bull. (Tokyo)* 1962, **10**, 1099–101.

28 Bayerdorffer, E., Kasper, G., Sommer, A. & Ottenjann, R. 1988. Ofloxacin therapy of *Campylobacter pylori* positive ulcers. In Kaijser, B. & Falson, E. (eds) *Campylobacter IV.* University of Gothenburg, Sweden, pp. 372–3.

29 Goodwin, C.S., Marshall, B.J., Blincow, E.D., Wilson, D.H., Blackbourn, S. & Phillips, M. Prevention of nitroimidazole resistance in *Campylobacter pylori* by coadministration of colloidal bismuth subcitrate: clinical and *in vitro* studies. *J. Clin. Pathol.* 1988, **41**, 207–10.

30 Hirschi, A.M., Hentschel, E., Schutze, K. *et al.* The

efficacy of antimicrobial treatment in *Campylobacter pylori*-associated gastritis and duodenal ulcer. *Scand. J. Gastroenterol.* 1988, **23**, suppl. 142, 76–81.

31 Graham, D.Y., Klein, P.D. & Opekun, A.R. *In vivo* susceptibility of *Campylobacter pylori. Am. J. Gastroenterol.* 1989, **84**, 233–8.

32 Kristiansen, J.E., Justesen, T., Hvidberg, E.F. & Andersen, L.P. Trimipramine and other antipsychotics inhibit *Campylobacter pylori in vitro. Pharmacol. Toxicol.* 1989, **64**, 386–8.

33 Hey, H., Matzen, P., Thorup Andersen, J., Didriksen, E. & Nielsen, B. A gastroscopic and pharmacological study of the disintegration time and absorption of pivampicillin capsules and tablets. *Br. J. Clin. Pharmacol.* 1979, **8**, 237–42.

34 Gorbach, S.L. Bismuth therapy in gastrointestinal diseases. *Gastroenterology* 1990, **99**, 863–75.

35 Goodwin, C.S. & Carrick, J. Peptic ulcer disease and *Helicobacter (Campylobacter) pylori* infection. *Curr. Opinion Gastroenterol.* 1990, **6**, 72–8.

36 Fleming, L.W., Moreland, T.A., Stewart, W.K. & Scott, A.C. Ciprofloxacin and antacids. *Lancet* 1986, **ii**, 294.

37 Caekenberghe, D.L. & Breyssens, V.J. *In vitro* synergistic activity between bismuth subcitrate and various antimicrobial agents against *Campylobacter pyloridis (C. pylori). Antimicrob. Agents Chemother.* 1987, **31**, 1429–30.

38 Borsch, G., Mai, U. & Opferkuch, W. Oral triple therapy (OTT) may effectively eradicate *Campylobacter pylori* in man: a pilot study. *Gastroenterology* 1988, **94** (5), A44.

39 Lambert, J.R., Way, D.J., King, R.G., Wan, A. & McLean, A.J. Bismuth pharmacokinetics in human gastric mucosa. *Gastroenterology* 1988, **94** (5), A248.

40 Lambert, J.R., Borromeo, M., Eaves, E.R., Hansky, J. & Korman, M. Efficacy of different dosage regimes of bismuth in eradicating *Campylobacter pylori. Gastroenterology* 1988, **94** (5), A248.

the ^{14}C-urea breath test after 6 months' treatment (unpublished observation). In the antral biopsies, heavier colonization with *H. pylori* after treatment with omeprazole could not be detected compared with the pre-therapy colonization density. Unfortunately we took no biopsies from the corpus–fundic area where more extensive colonization might have occurred.

Mucosal protective agents

Neither sucralfate [11, 13] nor prostaglandins [28] have any effect on *H. pylori* colonization in the stomach. Unge *et al.* [29] treated 24 patients with active duodenal ulcer or reflux oesophagitis with positive culture for *H. pylori* with 35 or 75 μg enprostil for 4–8 weeks (11 patients), or 300 μg rioprostil for 4 weeks (13 patients). No clearance of *H. pylori* was observed in any patient in these open pilot studies. There were no biopsies taken for histological examination.

In contrast, bismuth-containing preparations (CBS, BSS) are clearly effective in suppressing or clearing *H. pylori* from the stomach [9–11]. This may be due to bismuth's antimicrobial activity, its cytoprotective effects or both. *In vitro* CBS inhibits the growth of *H. pylori* at concentrations in the range of 4–32 mg/l [13, 30]. Marshall *et al.* [9] were the first to report on the *in vivo* bactericidal effect of CBS on *H. pylori*. Clearance of *H. pylori* with CBS monotherapy has now been observed by many investigators, as has been demonstrated in a controlled study using BSS (PeptoBismol) [10]. Clearance of *H. pylori* using bismuth preparations was exciting, but permanent eradication using bismuth monotherapy was rather disappointing (Table 23.1) [9, 31–35]. The overall results of many studies demonstrated clearance of *H. pylori* while using bismuth monotherapy in about 45–100%, but long-term eradication was only achieved in 6–43%. The mechanisms underlying the observed antibacterial effect of bismuth compounds have to be clarified. Administration of CBS leads to rapid onset of lytic changes and disappearance of the micro-organisms within 24 hours, suggesting a direct bactericidal effect, possibly by inactivating bacterial enzyme systems. In antral

mucosal biopsies obtained a few hours after ingestion of CBS tablets, strong accumulation of bismuth particles along the bacterial membranes may be readily observed [36, 37].

It is unclear how the apparent preferential accumulation of bismuth is to be explained. The selective precipitation of bismuth along the outer membrane of the micro-organisms may perhaps be explained by alteration of pH immediately adjacent to the bacteria. *H. pylori* produces large amounts of urease [38] and in the presence of urea can be expected to generate ammonium ions. High alkalinity would increase the solubility of CBS. Sudden reversion from an alkaline to acid milieu after *H. pylori* becomes metabolically inactivated by bismuth could explain the selective precipitation of the bismuth complex along the micro-organisms. An alternative hypothesis could be selective absorption of bismuth particles along the lipopolysaccharide (LPS) layer of the bacterial outer membrane. A few hours after administration of CBS, many bacteria show structural disintegration, especially the bacteria present at the lumenal surface, but not those living deep in the foveolae.

This may suggest that the micro-organisms deep in the gastric pits survive the bactericidal effects of CBS and recolonize the gastric mucosa after discontinuation of this drug. The clinical inefficacy might thus be caused by the inability of bismuth compounds to reach all micro-organisms in sufficient concentration. This question has been addressed by Lambert *et al.* [39] and Skoglund & Watters [40]. They measured bismuth concentrations in mucosal biopsies. Lambert *et al.* found bismuth concentrations above minimum inhibitory concentration (MIC) for 3 hours after ingestion of two tablets of CBS (= 240 mg Bi_2O_3). Skoglund measured bismuth concentrations above MIC_{90} in dogs for 3 hours after a single dose of BSS liquid (30 ml containing 525 mg BSS) and for 6 hours with four-times-daily dosing. This might explain why continuous exposure (four times daily) revealed better clearance and eradication rates compared with twice-daily dosing (Table 23.2) [32, 41, 42]. A prolonged treatment period and even a double dose (four times daily)

Table 23.1 Influence of treatment with bismuth compounds on *H. pylori* status immediately after treatment (= clearance) and during further follow-up (= eradication).

Investigator	n	Drug[a] (28 days)	Clearance (%)	Eradication[b] % (n)
Marsall *et al.* [9]	6	CBS	100	ND
Börsch *et al.* [31]	17	BSS	47	6 (1)
Rauws & Tytgat [32]	151	CBS	33	7 (10)
Wagner *et al.* [33]	35	BSS	ND	23 (8)
Lambert *et al.* [34]	20	CBS	ND	25 (5)
O'Riordan *et al.* [35]	43	CBS	ND	32 (14)

[a] CBS = colloidal bismuth subcitrate (tablet containing 120 mg as Bi_2O_3); BSS = bismuth subsalicylate (tablet containing 140 mg as Bi_2O_3).
[b] ND = not done.

are not superior to the standard dose regimen. No comparative studies are available, comparing CBS four times daily and BSS four times daily in eradicating *H. pylori*.

Antibiotics (monotherapy)

Many antimicrobial agents with *in vitro* activity have now been tried *in vivo* in clinical studies. The efficacy of most of these agents *in vivo* is rather poor. The results of these studies are summarized in Table 23.3 [10, 11, 21, 31, 32, 43–49]. The best results with antibiotics as monotherapy in eradicating *H. pylori* are obtained with amoxicillin (30%), nitrofurantoin (22%) and ofloxacin (20%). These results, mostly

from small pilot studies, are rather disappointing. As antibiotics can have serious side-effects and especially as monotherapy may induce acquired resistance to antimicrobial agents [50, 51], these should no longer be studied *in vivo* as monotherapy.

Bismuth–antibiotic combinations

Combination therapy of bismuth salts and various antibiotics has been tried to improve the long-term eradication of *H. pylori* [11, 52]. Triple therapy using two antibiotics has been used and the results obtained are superior to the eradication rates obtained with dual therapy alone [53, 54]. The success might be explained

Table 23.2 Efficacy of different dosage regimens of bismuth compounds in clearing and eradicating *H. pylori*.

Investigator	Disease[a]	n	Drug[b]	Clearance[a] (%)	Eradication[a] (%)
Coghlan (unpublished)	DU	30	CBS 2 × 2 tablets	32	ND
		30	CBS 4 × 1 tablet	64	ND
Menge *et al.* [41]	NUD	24	BSS 3 × 3 tablets (5 days)	83	ND
Lambert *et al.* [42]	NUD/DU	20	CBS 4 × 1 tablet (4 weeks)	65	N.D.
		20	CBS 4 × 1 tablet (8 weeks)	70	30 (6 months)
		20	CBS 2 × 2 tablets (8 weeks)	30	15 (6 months)
Rauws & Tytgat [32]	NUD	115	CBS 4 × 1 tablet (4 weeks)	31	10 (24 months)
		16	CBS 4 × 1 tablet (8 weeks)	31	ND
		17	CBS 4 × 2 tablets (4 weeks)	ND	6 (> 1 year)
		13	CBS 2 × 2 tablets (4 weeks)	15	0 (1 month)
		9	CBS 1 × 4 tablets (4 weeks)	11	0 (1 month)

[a] ND = not done; DU = duodenal ulcer; NUD = non-ulcer dyspepsia.
[b] Daily divided doses. CBS = colloidal bismuth subcitrate; BSS = bismuth subsalicylate.

organisms in the stomach of patients and healthy individuals. *Lancet* 1984, **i**, 1348.

39 Lambert, J.R., Way, D.J., Kings, R.S., Eaves, E.A. & Hansky, J. Bismuth pharmacokinetics in the human gastric mucosa. *Gastroenterology* 1988, **94**, A248.

40 Skoglund, M.L. & Watters, K. Bismuth concentration at the site of *Campylobacter pylori* colonization. *Gastroenterology* 1988, **94**, A430.

41 Menge, H., Hofmann, J. & Gregor, M. Dosis-Wirkungs-Studien mit Wismutsalzen zur Elimination von *Campylobacter pylori*. *Z. Gastroenterol.* 1987, **25**, suppl. 4, 44–6.

42 Lambert, J.R., Borromeo, M., Eaves, E.A., Hansky, J. & Korman, M. Efficacy of different dosage regimes of bismuth in eradicating *Campylobacter pylori*. *Gastroenterology* 1988, **94**, A248.

43 Burette, A., Glupczynski, Y., Dereuck, M. *et al.* 1987. *Campylobacter pyloridis* associated gastritis investigator blind, placebo controlled trial with amoxicillin. In *Proceedings Göteborg*.

44 Oderda, G., Dell'Olio, D., Morro, J. & Ansaldi, N. *Campylobacter pylori* gastritis: long-term results of treatment with amoxicillin. *Arch. Dis. Child* 1989, **64**, 326–9.

45 Glupczynski, Y., Burette, A., Duprez, C. *et al.* Evaluation of clindamycin in patients with non-ulcer dyspepsia and *Campylobacter pylori*-associated gastritis. *Klin. Wochenschr.* 1989, **67**, suppl. XVIII, 24.

46 Schaub, N., Stalder, H., Vischer, W. *et al.* Versagen von Doxycyclin bei *Campylobacter pylori*-positiver Gastritis. *Dtsch. Med. Wochenschr.* 1987, **112**, 117–18.

47 Morgan, D., Kragt, W., Bender, M. & Pearson, A. Nitrofurans in the treatment of gastritis associated with *Campylobacter pylori*. *Gastroenterology* 1988, **95**, 1178–84.

48 Gilman, R., Leon-Brava, R., Ramirez-Ramos, A. *et al.* Efficacy of nitrofurans in the treatment of antral gastritis with *Campylobacter pyloridis*. *Gastroenterology* 1987, **92**, 1405.

49 Glupczynski, Y., Labbe, M., Burette, A. *et al.* Treatment failure of ofloxacin in *Campylobacter pylori* infection. *Lancet* 1987, **i**, 1006.

50 Bayerdorffer, E., Simon, T.H., Bastlein, C.H., Ottenjuan, R. & Kasper, G. Bismuth/ofloxacin combination for duodenal ulcer. *Lancet* 1987, **ii**, 1467–8.

51 Goodwin, C.S., Marshall, B.J., Blincow, E.D. *et al.* Prevention of nitroimidazole resistance in *C. pylori* by coadministration of colloidal bismuth subcitrate: clinical and *in vitro* studies. *J. Clin. Pathol.* 1988, **41**, 207–10.

52 Marshall, B.J., Goodwin, C.S., Warren, J.R. *et al.* Longterm healing of gastritis and low duodenal ulcer relapse after eradication of *Campylobacter pyloridis*: a prospective double blind study. *Gastroenterology* 1987, **92**, 1518.

53 Börsch, G., Mai, U. & Opferkuch, W. Oral triple therapy may effectively eradicate *Campylobacter pylori* in man: a pilot study. *Gastroenterology* 1988, **94**, A44.

54 Borody, T., Cole, P., Noonan, S. *et al.* Long term *Campylobacter pylori* recurrence post-eradication. *Gastroenterology* 1988, **94**, A43.

55 Boero, M., Ponzetto, A., Rosina, F. *et al.* Rate of eradication of *Campylobacter pylori* with different drug schedules. *Klin. Wochenschr* 1989, **67**, suppl. XVIII, 5–6.

56 Sabbatini, F., D'Arienzo, Piai, G. *et al.* Influence of blood group and secretor status on *Campylobacter pylori* infection. *Gastroenterology* 1989, **96**, A433.

57 Mathai, E., O'Riordan, T., Tobin, A. *et al.* Drug resistance in *Campylobacter pylori*. *Klin. Wochenschr.* 1989, **67**, suppl. XVIII, 46.

58 Marshall, B.J., Goodwin, C.S., Warren, J.R. *et al.* Prospective double-blind trial of duodenal ulcer relapse after eradication of *Campylobacter pylori*. *Lancet* 1988, **ii**, 1437–42.

59 Mannes, G.A., Bayerdörffer, E., Höchter, W. *et al.* Early relapse after healing of *Campylobacter pylori*-positive duodenal ulcers. *Klin Wochenschr.* 1989, **67**, suppl. XVIII, 44.

60 Marshall, B.J., Dye, K.R., Plankey, M. *et al.* Eradication of *Campylobacter pylori* infection with bismuth subsalicylate and antibiotic combinations. *Am. J. Gastroenterol.* 1988, **83**, 1035.

61 Bayerdörffer, E., Simon, T., Bästlein, C., Ottenjann, R., Kasper, G. *et al.* Bismuth/ofloxacin combination for duodenal ulcer. *Lancet* 1987, **ii**, 1467–8.

62 Burette, A., Glupczynski, Y., Thibaumont, F. & Deprez, C. Evaluation of short-term amoxicillin/tinidazole combination in the treatment of *Campylobacter pylori* infection. *Klin. Wochenschr.* 1989, **67**, suppl. XVIII, 7–8.

63 Oderda, G., Vaira, D., Holton, J. *et al.* Amoxycillin plus tinidazole for *Campylobacter pylori* gastritis in children: assessment by serum IgG antibody, pepsinogen I, and gastrin levels. *Lancet* 1989, **i**, 690–2.

64 Hentschel, E., Hirschl, A.M., Schütze, K. & Dufer, W. Amoxicillin and metronidazol in the eradication of *Campylobacter pylori*. *Klin. Wochenschr.* 1989, **67**, suppl. XVIII, 29.

65 Burette, A., Glupczynski, Y. & Deprez, C. Combined therapy with ofloxacin and amoxicillin on the eradication of *Helicobacter pylori*. *Gastroenterology* 1990, **98**, A26.

66 De Koster, E., Nyst, J.F., Glupczynski, Y. *et al.* Short term double drug *Helicobacter pylori* treatment: one week amoxicillin + tinidazole vs amoxicillin + nitrofurantoin. *Gastroenterology* 1990, **98**, A35.

67 Lamouliatte, H., Mascarel, de, A., Mégraud, F. *et al.* Omeprazole improves amoxicillin therapy directed towards *Helicobacter pylori* associated chronic gastritis. *Gastroenterology* 1990, **98**, A75.

68 Glupczynski, Y., Bourdeaux, L., Verhas, M. *et al.*

Short-term double or triple oral drug treatment of *Helicobacter pylori* (Hp) in Central Africa. *Gastroenterology* 1990, **98**, A48.

69 Coelho, L.G.V., Passos, M.C.F., Quelroz, D.M.M. *et al.* Five days triple therapy and 15 days double therapy on *C. pylori* eradication. *Klin. Wochenschr.* 1989, **67**, suppl. XVIII, 11.

70 Borody, T., Hennesey, W., Daskalopoulos, G., Garrick, J. & Hazell, S. Double-blind trial of De-Nol in non-ulcer dyspepsia associated with *Campylobacter pyloridis* gastritis. *Gastroenterology* 1987, **92**, 1324.

71 Burette, A. & Glupczynski, Y. 1990. Evaluation of four short-term amoxicillin/tinidazole regimens for eradication of *Helicobacter pylori*. In *Rev. Esp. Enf. Dig. Third Workshop of the European Helicobacter pylori Study Group*. Toledo vol. 78, suppl. I, part 201, pp. 94–5.

72 Burette, A., Glupczynski, Y. & Deprez, C. Combined therapy with ofloxacin and amoxycillin in the eradication of *Helicobacter pylori*. *Gastroenterology* 1990, **98**, A26.

73 Lambert, J.R., Lin, S.K., Schembri, M., Nicholson, L. & Korman, M.G. 1990. *Helicobacter pylori* therapy randomized study of De-Nol/antibiotic combinations. In *Rev. Esp. Enf. Dig. Third Workshop of the European Helicobacter pylori Study Group*. Toledo, part 251, pp. 115–16.

74 Rokkas, T., Pursey, C., Simmons, N.A., Filipe, M.I. & Sladen, G.E. Non-ulcer dyspepsia and colloidal bismuth subcitrate therapy: the role of *Campylobacter pyloridis*. *Gastroenterology* 1987, **92**, 1599.

75 Lambert, J.R., Borromeo, M., Korman, M.G. & Hansky, J. Role of *Campylobacter pyloridis* in non-ulcer dyspepsia. A randomised controlled trial. *Gastroenterology* 1987, **91**, 1488.

76 Loffeld, R.J.L.F., Potters, H.V.J.P., Stobberingh, E., Flendrig, J.A., Spreeuwel, J.P.V. & Arends, J.W. *Campylobacter* associated gastritis in patients with non-ulcer dyspepsia: a double blind placebo controlled trial with colloidal bismuth subcitrate. *Gut* 1989, **30**, 1206–12.

77 Kang, J.Y., Tay, H.H., Wee, A., Guan, R., Math, M.V. & Yap. I. Effect of colloidal bismuth subcitrate on symptoms and gastric histology in non-ulcer dyspepsia. A double blind placebo controlled study. *Gut* 1990, **31**, 476–80.

78 Veldhuyzen van Zanten, S.J.O., Tytgat, K.M.A.J., Jalali, S., Goodoere, R.L. & Hunt, R.H. Can gastritis symptoms be evaluated in clinical trials? An overview of treatment of gastritis, non-ulcer dyspepsia and *Campylobacter*-associated gastritis. *J. Clin. Gastroenterol.* 1990, **11** (5), 496–501.

79 Halley, F.J. & Newson, J.H. Evaluation of bismuth subsalicylate in relieving symptoms of ingestion. *Arch. Intern. Med.* 1984, **144**, 269–72.

80 Nyren, O., Adami, H.O., Bates, S. *et al.* Absence of therapeutic benefit from antacids or cimetidine in non-ulcer dyspepsia. *N. Engl. J. Med.* 1986, **314**, 339–43.

81 Thomson, W.G. Non-ulcer dyspepsia. *Can. Med. Assoc. J.* 1984, **130**, 565–9.

likely, therefore, that *H. pylori* infection precedes ulcer recurrence.

Further studies are necessary. This initial evidence, however, strongly suggests that agents which efficiently eradicate *H. pylori* infection will significantly reduce DU relapse, at least in the year after treatment, and may fundamentally alter the natural history of the disease.

Mechanism of action

The bactericidal action of bismuth on *H. pylori* is clearly an important factor in the healing of gastritis [34], ulcers [60], and in the prevention of ulcer relapse in humans. However, the correlation between post-treatment *H. pylori* status and ulcer healing or gastritis is far from absolute. Bismuth has multiple biochemical cytoprotective actions on the gastric and duodenal mucosae which are independent of *H. pylori*.

CBS binds to gastric mucin, forming a glycoprotein–bismuth complex which adheres to the ulcer crater and retards hydrogen ion diffusion [70]. It also increases local prostaglandin (PGE$_2$) [71] and bicarbonate concentrations [72], while reducing the concentrations of local aggressive factors such as leucotriene C$_4$ [73] and pepsin [74].

CBS has been shown to protect against gastric damage due to ethanol and stress in rats [72]. Rats are not naturally colonized by *H. pylori*.

It is therefore important not simply to equate bismuth compound-induced ulcer healing with *H. pylori* eradication and consequent protection against ulcer relapse.

Formulation and damage

CBS is available in liquid form, as chewable tablets and as coated 'swallow tablets'. There is no evidence that any of these particular formulations is superior in respect of ulcer healing efficacy. Three blind studies have compared liquid with chewable tablets and have shown equal efficacy in healing DUs [75–77]. A single-blind study of 189 patients revealed no difference between chewable and coated tablets [78]. In respect of *H. pylori* suppression we have found coated tablets to be at least as effective as liquid, although no direct comparative study was undertaken. A reduction in culture positivity of 42% was achieved in 26 patients after 6 weeks' treatment with coated tablets versus a 42% reduction in 32 patients treated with liquid CBS in sequential studies.

Frequency of administration is important in the treatment of *H. pylori*, but not in respect of ulcer healing. Four studies have shown indistinguishable ulcer healing rates with twice-daily or four-times-daily CBS [79–82]. However, two blind studies have recently demonstrated that a 240 mg twice-daily dosage is ineffective in suppressing the organism [79, 83]. It is believed to be due to the inability of 12-hourly doses to maintain cytotoxic concentrations of bismuth within the gastric mucin [84].

Duration of therapy may be more important in respect of ulcer healing than *H. pylori* suppression. From Table 24.3 it is apparent that 10–20% more ulcers are healed after 6 or 8 weeks of CBS therapy than after 4 weeks. However, Lambert *et al.* [83] found no major change in *H. pylori* status between 4 (65% *H. pylori*-negative) and 8 (70% *H. pylori*-negative) weeks' treatment.

Safety profile

while bismuth compounds are effectively topical agents, acting at a local level to heal ulcers and histological gastritis and also eradicate *H. pylori*, some of the drug is absorbed and may accumulate, particulary in renal, hepatic and neural tissues. Our experience and that of other workers has been that bismuth is well tolerated with few side-effects which only cause a nuisance, darkening of the stool and blackening of teeth and tongue with liquid preparations and chewable tablets, other effects being rare. Possible drug toxicity has, however, been a major source of concern with regard to bismuth therapy, since nearly 200 cases of bismuth encephalopathy were recorded in France. These cases occurred as a result of prolonged high-dose treatment and were almost invariably associated with blood bismuth levels in excess of

100 μg/l. Gavey *et al.* [85] demonstrated that bismuth accumulates in the body during a 6-week course of treatment with De-Noltab 240 mg b.d., with urine excretion of bismuth persisting for 12 weeks after cessation of therapy. Median plasma bismuth concentrations after the morning dose increase to maximum levels in the sixth week of treatment [85]. However, further work [86] showed that plasma bismuth levels peaked 30 min after taking De-Noltab 240 mg when fasting, and in 10% of patients neurotoxic levels (by definition > 50 ng/ml) [87] were found. All patients remained asymptomatic and the plasma bismuth levels dropped below 50 ng/ml within 100 min in most cases. As suggested, it may be that toxic levels of blood bismuth causing symptoms may relate to trough rather than peak values. Bismuth toxicity is also less likely with a q.d.s. regimen, as is currently recommended [82].

To date, there is no record of serious side-effects with the recommended dosage of 480 mg/day for a maximum of 2 months, with at least 2 months between courses. Minor side-effects of mild dizziness and headache have been noted on a few occasions [11]. However, as excretion is almost completely renal, caution is advised in patients with significant renal impairment. Finally, in the absence of proof that bismuth is not toxic to the fetus, these compounds should clearly be avoided in pregnancy.

Therapeutic indications

Despite limits to our knowledge, the benefits of CBS therapy in the long-term healing of histological gastritis and the reduction of DU recurrences are well documented. This therapy can be recommended for these reasons alone. For the purpose of eradicating *H. pylori*, bismuth compounds should not be used without adjuvant therapy, as their efficacy in this regard is inadequate.

Antibiotics

Two studies comparing furazolidone with cimetidine [8, 9] and one with metronidazole versus cimetidine [10] have shown similar healing rates with the antibiotics and the H$_2$ antagonists. As none of these agents has known anti-ulcer actions, these results are compatible with an infective pathogenesis for peptic ulcer disease, and suggest a possible role for antibiotic therapy in peptic ulceration.

Marshall *et al.* [88] demonstrated that *H. pylori* is sensitive to a wide range of antibiotics. Several studies of the *in vitro* sensitivities of this organism have since been completed. These have recently been reviewed [89] and the review shows that *H. pylori* is highly sensitive to all macrolides, tetracyclines, most β-lactams, aminoglycosides (neomycin not studied) and the older quinolone, ofloxacin. Moderate sensitivity is found with nitroimidazoles, nitrofurans and the newer quinolones. Resistance to sulphonamides, trimethoprim, vancomycin and amphotericin B is almost invariable. Given the above evidence, it was clearly imperative to study clinically the effects of antibiotic therapy on *H. pylori* and DU.

Studies of antibiotic therapy *in vivo* have shown that many are indeed active against *H. pylori*, although there is a surprising discrepancy between *in vitro* and *in vivo* activity in some cases, e.g. erythromycin ethylsuccinate is inactivated by the acidic stomach pH. However, antibiotic therapy used alone is not superior to CBS monotherapy and the organism readily develops resistance to most antimicrobials. The ideal antibiotic, therefore, is stable in the acidic environment of the stomach, is capable of penetrating the gastric mucus layer and has both local and systemic activity without developing resistance. Synergy between CBS and many of the antibiotic groups has been demonstrated, significantly increasing the number of patients rendered *H. pylori*-negative and reducing the likelihood of bacterial resistance. It is therefore suggested that, in treating DUs, antibiotic therapy should only be used in combination with bismuth compounds.

Furthermore, studies of antibiotic adjuvant therapy (detailed below) show that, despite improved *H. pylori* eradication, the ulcer-healing efficacy of combination therapy is the same as CBS monotherapy. Thus, the sole aim of combination therapy is the eradication of *H. pylori* and consequently reducing the ulcer relapse rate.

Beta lactams

The β-lactam group of antibiotics has been extensively studied with respect to *in vivo* activity against *H. pylori* and in ulcer healing. Penicillin, becampicillin and amoxycillin have each been investigated. Interestingly, neither penicillin nor becampicillin [90] appears to eradicate *H. pylori* *in vivo*. This is despite very low MIC_{90}s (0.03–0.225 μg/ml) and the failure of treated organisms to develop resistance during treatment. It has been postulated that this failure has been partially due to the fact that penicillins only destroy replicating organisms [90]. This explanation is not the complete answer, since amoxycillin is moderately active *in vivo* and benzylpenicillin rapidly destroys *H. pylori in vitro* [91]. It may be of relevance that Hollingsworth *et al.* [92] have shown that ampicillin is not effectively secreted into the gastric pits. McNulty *et al.* [93] found that amoxycillin attains high gastric mucosal concentrations and is stable at acidic pH. Local and systemic absorption contributes to crypt and mucus concentrations and to date no acquired resistance to either ampicillin or amoxycillin has been documented [93].

Amoxycillin monotherapy has been found to be as effective as CBS in respect of *H. pylori* suppression and eradication. Rauws *et al.* [94] and Tytgat *et al.* [95] respectively have found 68% and 64% of patients culture-negative immediately after treatment with amoxycillin 375 mg three times daily (the duration of therapy was not specified) and 1 month later 23% and 31% remained culture-negative.

Van Ceakenberg & Breyssens [53] have demonstrated *in vitro* synergy between ampicillin and CBS. Therefore it might be expected that *in vivo* the combination of amoxycillin and CBS would produce dramatic results, in terms of both *H. pylori* eradication and ulcer healing. Indeed, two studies have produced impressive initial

suppression rates of 85% (in 23 patients) and 90% (in 20 patients) with combination therapy. Unfortunately, 1 month later only 35% and 40% respectively of patients remained *H. pylori*-negative [94, 95], not dissimilar to CBS alone. In our comparative study (50 patients) of CBS alone versus CBS (for 6 weeks) and amoxycillin (250 mg three times daily for the first week), only 42% were rendered culture-negative by either treatment [96]. This study also revealed identical healing rates of DUs with CBS used alone or in combined therapy.

Duration of amoxycillin therapy would not appear to be critical in respect of either *H. pylori* suppression or ulcer healing. One open study found 87% ulcer healing and 47% *H. pylori* eradication in 15 patients receiving amoxycillin (500 mg four times daily) for 7 days plus CBS for 14 days. When both agents were taken for 14 days, 68% ulcer healing with 44% *H. pylori* eradication was achieved [60].

Thus, the β-lactams studied to date are not superior to CBS as a monotherapy and confer little advantage over CBS alone when used in combination with CBS. Therefore on present data β-lactams cannot be recommended as ideal adjuvant agents to CBS.

Nitroimidazoles

Theoretically, tinidazole and metronidazole should not contribute significantly to the eradication of *H. pylori* in the setting of DU. They are only moderately active against *H. pylori in vitro*, with an MIC_{90} of 8–16 μg/ml. Naturally occurring resistance has been documented [60] and, as a monotherapy, the number of resistant strains has been shown to increase dramatically, with virtually no eradication [60, 90]. These agents are notorious for causing abdominal upset when used to treat other infections. However, metronidazole is known to be an effective ulcer-healing agent [10], the mechanism of which is difficult to explain unless metronidazole is active against *H. pylori in vivo*.

Although synergy between CBS and metronidazole was found in only 4/12 strains tested [53], the nitroimidazoles have, to date, proved the most successful adjuvant to CBS in ulcer healing and *H. pylori* eradication. Comparing 8 weeks' CBS treatment alone with CBS plus 10 days of tinidazole, Goodwin *et al.* [60] showed that the combination therapy did not improve the rate of DU healing but significantly increased the anti-*H. pylori* action. Eradication occurred in 7/22 in the CBS group versus 20/27 in the latter group. Furthermore, there was little change in the resistance profile, since virtually no strains remained to develop resistance. Not surprisingly, the relapse rate in the combination treatment group was considerably less than in the CBS group [60].

In our unit we also compared CBS alone with CBS plus 7 days of metronidazole [97]. Again, DU healing rates were similar in both groups and *H. pylori* eradication was significantly improved with combination therapy (32% vs. 73%). However, resistance to metronidazole was not prevented by the addition of CBS. Our results correlate closely with those of Weil *et al.* [98], who used a 2-week course of metronidazole. This implies that a 1-week course of metronidazole is sufficient and may reduce side-effects.

Disappointing results were obtained with short-term combination therapy of amoxycillin and tinidazole. Despite eradiction rates of 65% there was a high incidence of acquired resistance (30%) which accounted for nearly all treatment failures. [99].

Therefore it appears that acquired nitroimidazole resistance is more of a problem than pretreatment resistance, and this now represents the major obstacle to achieving 100% eradication of *H. pylori*.

Other antibiotics

While numbers are as yet small, antibiotic monotherapy (with/without another inactive agent) has yielded disappointing results. With the exception of furazolidone (which has only moderate *in vitro* activity), none of the antibiotics has achieved eradication rates comparable to CBS [89].

Both of the quinolones tested were ineffective,

but ofloxacin and ciprofloxacin also readily induced the development of resistance in most strains tested [90].

Even fewer studies have, to date, addressed bismuth adjuvant chemotherapy with these antibiotics.

Nitrofurantoin combined with bismuth in one small study (six patients) yielded an unimpressive eradication rate 0/6 [100]. Bismuth plus ofloxacin in 14 patients was no more effective than could be expected of CBS alone [89]. Ofloxacin is relatively inactive, however, at a low pH and, unlike at least one of the newer quinolones (norfloxacin), exhibits no synergism with CBS *in vitro* [53].

Oral triple therapy

Oral triple therapy is a possible means of overcoming the problem of *H. pylori* resistance to antibiotics. However, there is an increased likelihood of side-effects [59, 101], and there is the problem of poor compliance with taking so many tablets. Therefore, the length of treatment is an important consideration.

Borody *et al.* [59] treated 100 patients with CBS and amoxycillin for 4 weeks and metronidazole for the first 2 weeks. Minor side-effects occurred in over 30 patients and potentially lethal side-effects (*Clostridium difficile*-positive diarrhoea) in one patient [59]. In our unit, using CBS therapy for 4 weeks, with metronidazole and tetracycline during the first week only, *H. pylori* was eradicated in 90% (27/30). It is of note that there were no reports of any side-effects and, equally, there was no emergence of resistant *H. pylori* strains during therapy [102].

In the light of these findings, CBS triple therapy appears to be the current optimum regimen for treating DU and eradicating *H. pylori*.

Omeprazole

This drug, which suppresses gastric acid secretion by parietal cell proton pump inhibition, has also been shown to inhibit *H. pylori in vitro* [103]. Recent work suggests that profound gastric acid suppression by omeprazole potentiates the local effects of antibiotics. Labenz et al. [104] achieved H. pylori eradication in 65% of patients treated with omeprazole and amoxicillin. Acid suppression by H_2 antagonists may also achieve similar results, as Westblom & Duriex [105] have shown that, with concurrent administration of cimetidine, the gastric mucosal concentration of clinelamycin is five times greater than the concentration found under physiological conditions.

Omeprazole triple therapy has also been advocated. However, results of H. pylori eradication to date are not as good as those achieved with CBS triple therapy, though DU healing rates are satisfactory. Further long-term follow-up studies are required.

Antacids

Berstad et al. [106] detailed their findings on the effects of a magnesium–aluminium antacid, pirenzepine, and placebo on H. pylori and gastric histology in patients with non-ulcer dyspepsia. Of 88 patients studied, 47% had histological gastritis before treatment but only 20 were H. pylori-positive at that time. Antacid treatment, but not pirenzepine or placebo therapy, reduced H. pylori infection (H. pylori not detected in 5/10 post-treatment specimens) but increased histological gastritis. It is speculated that, far from being cytoprotective, this antacid is a chemical irritant.

This paper raises two important points: firstly, do antacids, often allowed liberally to DU patients during studies of H. pylori and healing agents, significantly bias results? and, secondly, why was there no reduction in histological gastritis in parallel with the reduction of H. pylori infection?

The effect of antacids on H. pylori has not been the subject of detailed study to date. However, available data suggest that aluminium-based antacids are inactive against H. pylori. The MIC_{90} of $Al(OH)_3$ in one in vitro study was $> 3200 \, \mu g/ml$ [107], and in one clinical study involving 10 patients aluminium phosphate was found to be ineffective against H. pylori [96].

'Various' antacids have been found to have MIC_{90}s ranging between 40 and $1280 \, \mu g/ml$ [107], the lower levels of which are certainly achievable for a short period in vivo. Studies must now be undertaken to ascertain the MIC_{90} for magnesium-based antacids and their in vivo activity. Until the result of these are available, magnesium-based antacids should be specifically avoided during studies of the effects of other agents of H. pylori.

Despite this, it is unlikely that incidental antacid consumption has undermined the results of previous studies on H. pylori eradication, as CBS has been consistently shown to be superior to cimetidine in this regard and antacid consumption is always lower in the groups receiving CBS.

Conclusions

The treatment of DU has entered a new and exciting phase. While the presence of 'acid' remains a prerequisite for ulcer development, it is clear that a relative acid excess is not the sole aetiological agent in DU disease. Cytoprotective bismuth compounds provide an alternative mode of therapy know to be as effective as H_2 antagonists in initial healing but with reduced relapse rates. Finally, H. pylori may well be of aetiological significance in DU disease and would thus provide a rational basis for treatment, with the possible elimination of DU relapse.

Acknowledgement

We are grateful to Mrs Betty Turner for her assistance in the preparation of this chapter.

References

1 Boyd, E.J.S., Wilson, J.A. & Wormsley, K.G. 1984. Recurrent ulcer disease. In Misiewicz, J.J. & Woods, J.R. (eds) *Ranitidine Therapeutic Advances*. Excerpta Medica, Amsterdam, pp. 14–42.

2 Feston, H.P. Lamers, C.B., Tangerman, A. & Van Tongeran, J.H.M. Effect of treatment with cimetidine for one year on gastrin cell and parietal cell function and sensitivity to cimetidine in patients with duodenal or gastric ulcers. *Postgrad. Med. J.* 1980, **56**, 698–701.

3 Armstrong, C.P. & Blower, A.L. Non-steroidal anti-inflammatory drugs and life threatening complications of peptic ulcer disease. *Gut* 1987, **28** (5), 527–32.

4 Welch, C.E., Rodkey, G.V. & von Ryll Grysku, P. A thousand operations for ulcer disease. *Ann. Surg.* 1986, **204** (4), 454–67.

5 Flemstrom, G. & Turnberg, L.A. Gastroduodenal defence mechanisms. *Clin. Gastroenterol.* 1984, **13** (2), 327–54.

6 Ippoliti, A., Elashoff, J., Valenzuela, J., Cano, R., Frankl, H., Samloff, M. & Koretz, R. Recurrent ulcer after successful treatment with cimetidine or antacid. *Gastroenterology* 1983, **85**, 875–80.

7 Freedberg, A.S. & Barron, L.E. The presence of spirochetes in human gastric mucosa. *Am. J. Dig. Dis.* 1940, **7**, 433–45.

8 Zheng, Z.T., Wang, Z.Y., Chu, Y.X., Li, Y.N., Li, Q.F., Lin, S.R. & Xu, Z.M. Double blind short-term trial of furazolidone in peptic ulcer. *Lancet* 1985, **i**, 1048–9 (letter).

9 Zhao, H.Y., Li, G., Guo, J., Yan, Z., Sun, S., Li, L., Duan, Y. & Yue, F. Furazolidone in peptic ulcer. *Lancet* 1985, **ii**, 276–7, (letter).

10 Quintero Diaz, M. & Sotto Eschobar, A. Metronidazole versus cimetidine in the treatment of gastroduodenal disease. *Lancet* 1986, **i**, 907.

11 Bader, J.P. The safety profile of De-Nol. *Digestion* 1987, **37**, suppl. 2, 53–9.

12 Salmon, P.R., Brown, P., Williams, R. & Read, A.E. Evaluation of colloidal bismuth (De-Nol) in the treatment of duodenal ulcer employing endoscopic selection and follow-up. *Gut* 1974, **15**, 189–93.

13 Moshal, M.G. The treatment of duodenal ulcers with TDB: a duodenoscopic double blind cross-over investigation. *Postgrad. Med. J.* 1975, **51**, suppl. 5, 36–40.

14 Shreeve, D.R. A double blind study of tripotassium dicitrato bismuthate in duodenal ulcer. *Postgrad. Med. J.* 1975, **51**, suppl. 5, 33–6.

15 Vissoulis, C., Vissoulis, G., Golfis, G. & Psimenos, G. Endoscopic evaluation of TDB in the treatment of duodenal ulceration. *Iatrica Chronica* 1977, **17**, 157–64.

16 Coughlin, G.P., Kupa, A. & Alp, M.H. The effect of tripotassium dicitrato bismuthate (De-Nol) on the healing of chronic duodenal ulcer. *Med. J. Aust.* 1977, **1**, 294–8.

17 Cannon, J.J. De-Nol, an effective drug in the therapy of duodenal ulceration. *J. Ir. Med. Assoc.* 1977, **70** (6), 206–7.

18 Lee, S.P. & Nicholson, G.I. Increased healing of gastric and duodenal ulcers in a controlled trial using tripotassium dicitrato bismuthate. *Med. J. Aust.* 1977, **1**, 808–12.

19 Poulantzas, J., Polymeropoulos, P.S. & Papasomatious, A. A double blind evaluation of the effect of tripotassium dicitrato bismuthate in peptic ulcer. *Br. J. Clin. Pract.* 1978, **32**, 147–8.

20 Dekker, W. & Reisma, K. Double blind controlled trial with colloidal bismuth subcitrate in the treatment of symptomatic duodenal ulcers with special reference to blood and urine levels. *Ann. Clin. Res.* 1979, **11**, 94–7.

21 Bank, S., Marks, I.N., Novis, B.H. & Barbezat, G.O. Colloidal bismuth tablets (tripotassium dicitrato bismuth) in the treatment of peptic ulceration. *Gastroenterology* 1979, **76**, 1093.

22 Wilson, P. & Alp, M.H. Colloidal bismuth subcitrate tablets and placebo in chronic duodenal ulceration: a double blind randomised trial. *Med. J. Aust.* 1982, **1**, 222–3.

23 Tytgat, G.T.N. Colloidal bismuth subcitrate in peptic ulcer disease – a review. *Digestion* 1987, **37**, suppl. 2, 31–41.

24 Bianchi Porro, G., Petrillo, M., De Nichola, C. & Lazzaroni, M. A double blind endoscopic study with De-Nol tablets and cimetidine for duodenal ulcer. *Scand. J. Gastroenterol.* 1984, **19**, 905–8.

25 Kang, J.Y. & Piper, D.W. Cimetidine and colloidal bismuth subcitrate in the treatment of chronic duodenal ulcer, comparison of initial healing and recurrence after healing. *Digestion* 1982, **23**, 73–9.

26 Martin, D.F., Hollanders, D., May, S.J., Ravenscroft, M.M., Tweedle, D.E.F. & Miller, J.P. Difference in relapse rates of duodenal ulcer after healing with cimetidine or tripotassium dicitrato bismuthate. *Lancet* 1981, **i**, 7–10.

27 Moshal, M.G., Spitaels, J.M. & Khan, F. Tripotassium dicitrato bismuthate chewing tablets and cimetidine tablets in the treatment of duodenal ulcers – a double-blind double-dummy comparative study. *S. African Med. J.* 1981, **60**, 420–3.

28 Ward, M., Pollard, E.J. & Cowen, A. A double-blind trial of cimetidine versus tripotassium dicitrato bismuthate in chronic duodenal ulceration. *Med. J. Aust.* 1981, **1**, 363–4.

29 Bianchi Porro, G., Barbara, L., Cheli, R., Dal Monte, P.R. & Mazzacca, G. Comparison of tripotassium dicitrato bismuthate (TDB) and ranitidine in healing and relapse of duodenal ulcers. *Gut* 1984, **25**, A565.

30 Ward, M., Halliday, C. & Cowen, A.E. A comparison of colloidal bismuth subcitrate tablets and ranitidine in the treatment of chronic duodenal ulcers. *Digestion* 1986, **34**, 173–7.

31 Lee, F.I., Samlof, I.M. & Hardman, M. Comparison of tripotassium dicitrato bismuthate tablets with ranitidine in healing and relapse of duodenal ulcers. *Lancet* 1985, **i**, 1299–301.

32 Lam, S.K., Lee, N., Koo, J., Hui, W., Fok, K. & Ng, M. Randomised cross-over trial of tripotassium dicitrato bismuthate versus high dose cimetidine for

85 Gavey, C.J., Szeto, M.-L., Nwokolo, C.U., Sercombe, J. & Pounder, R.E. Bismuth accumulates in the body during treatment with tripotassium dicitrato bismuthate. *Aliment. Pharmacol. Ther.* 1989, **1**, 21–8.

86 Nwokolo, C.U., Gavey, C.J., Smith, J.T.L. & Pounder, R.E. The absorption of bismuth from oral doses of tripotassium dicitrato bismuthate. *Aliment. Pharmacol. Ther.* 1989, **1**, 29–39.

87 Lock, M., Nichol, H. & Ketola-Pirie, C. Binding of bismuth to cell components: due to mode of action and side effects. *Can. Med. Assoc. J.* 1987, **137**, 991–2.

88 Marshall, B., McGechie, D., Rogers, P. & Glancy, R. Pyloric *Campylobacter* infection and gastroduodenal disease. *Med. J. Aust.* 1985, **142**, 439–44.

89 Bayerdoffer, E. & Ottenjann, R. The role of antibiotics in *Campylobacter pylori* associated peptic ulcer disease. *Scand. J. Gastroenterol.* 1988, **22** suppl. 142, 93–100.

90 Hirshl, A.M., Hentschel, E., Schutze, K., Nemec, H., Potzi, R., Gangl, A., Weiss, W., Pletschette, M., Stanek, G. & Rotter, M.L. The efficacy of antimicrobial treatment in *Campylobacter pylori* associated gastritis and duodenal ulcer. *Scand. J. Gastroenterol.* 1988, **23** suppl. 142, 76–81.

91 Armstrong, J.A., Wee, S.H., Goodwin, C.S. & Wilson, D.H. Response of *Campylobacter pyloridis* to antibiotics, bismuth and acid reducing agents *in vitro* – an ultrastructural study. *J. Med. Microbiol.* 1987, **24**, 343–50.

92 Hollingsworth, J.A., Goldie, J., Silletti Li, Y., Richardson, H. & Hunt, R.H. Gastric secretion of antibiotics used for *Campylobacter pyloridis*. *Gut* 1987, **28**, A1409.

93 McNulty, C.A., Dent, J.C., Ford, G.A. & Wilkinson, S.P. Inhibitory antimicrobial concentrations against *Campylobacter pylori* in gastric mucosa. *J. Antimicrob. Chemother.* 1988, **5**, 729–38.

94 Rauws, E.A., Langenberg, W., Houtoff, H., Zanen, H. & Tytgat, G.N.T. *Campylobacter pyloridis* associated chronic active gastritis. *Gastroenterology* 1988, **94**, 33–41.

95 Tytgat, G.N.T., Rauws, E.A., Langenberg, W. & Houtoff, H. Long term follow-up of *Campylobacter pylori* associated gastritis after treatment with colloidal bismuth subcitrate and/or amoxycillin. *Gastroenterology* 1988, **94** (5), part 2, A469.

96 O'Morain, C., Coghlan, G., Tobin, A., Casey, E., Hutchinson, L., Gilligan, D., McKenna, D., Sweeney, E. & Keane, C. Adjuvant antibiotic therapy and colloidal bismuth subcitrate in duodenal ulcer healing and the eradication of *Campylobacter pylori*. *Gastroenterology* 1988, **94** (5), part 2, A334.

97 O'Riordan, T., Mathai, E., Tobin, A., McKenna, D. *et al.* Adjuvant antibiotic therapy in duodenal ulcers treated with colloidal bismuth subcitrate. *Gut* 1990, **31**, 999–1002.

98 Weil, J., Bell, G.D., Powell, K., Morden, A. *et al.* *Helicobacter pylori* infection treated with a tripotassium dicitrato bismuthate and metronidazole combination. *Aliment. Pharmacol. Ther.* 1990, **6**, 651–7.

99 Burette, A. & Glupczynski, Y. Evaluation of four short-term amoxycillin/tinidazole regimens for eradication of *Helicobacter pylori*. *Rev. Esp. Enf. Dig.* 1990, p-201 (abstr.)

100 Borsch, G., Mai, U. & Muller, K.M. Monotherapy or polychemotherapy in the treatment of *Campylobacter* related gastroduodenal disease. *Scand. J. Gastroenterol.* 1988, **23** suppl. 142, 101–6.

101 Rauws, E.A. & Tytgat, G.N. Cure of duodenal ulcer associated with eradication of *Helicobacter pylori*. *Lancet* 1990, **335** (8700), 1233–5.

102 Patchett, S., Beattie, S., Keane, C. & O'Morain, C. Treatment of *H. pylori*-associated PUD. A safe and effective regimen. *Rev. Esp. Enf. Dig.* 1990, p-268 (abstr.)

103 Paradis, A., Goldie, J., Veldhuyzen van Zanten, S.J.O., Richardson, H. & Hunt, R.H. The *in vitro* inhibitory effect of omeprazole on *Helicobacter pylori*: a biochemical distribution? *Rev. Esp. Enf. Dig.* 1990, p-207 (abstr.)

104 Labenz, J., Gyenes, E., Ruhl, G.H. & Borsch, G. Amoxycillin–omeprazole treatment for eradication of *Helicobacter pylori*. *Rev. Esp. Enf. Dig.* 1990, p-204 (abstr.)

105 Westblom, T.U. & Duriex, D.E. H_2 blockers increase antibiotic concentrations in gastric mucosa. *Rev. Esp. Enf. Dig.* 1990, p-262 (abstr.)

106 Berstad, A., Alexander, B. & Hirschowitz, B.I. Antacids reduce *Campylobacter pylori* colonisation without healing the gastritis in patients with non-ulcer dyspepsia and erosive prepyloric changes. *Gastroenterology* 1988, **95**, 619–24.

107 Anderson, L.P. Cytoprotective agents and *c. pylori* associated acid peptic disease. *Scand. J. Gastroenterol.* 1988, **23** suppl. 142, 110–13.

25 Helicobacter pylori and Helicobacter-like Organisms in Animals: Overview of Mucus-colonizing Organisms

A.LEE

Intestinal mucus as an ecological niche

To the microbial ecologist there is no more satisfying and challenging ecosystem than the gastrointestinal tract. The contents of the human large bowel contain more than 10^{11} bacteria per gram with over 200 different species living in homoeostatic balance. Over the period of evolution these organisms have adapted to the many ecological niches that are present in the gut [1]. The stomach has not featured strongly in discussions on intestinal ecology as it was always assumed to be mostly barren due to the antibacterial effects of gastric acidity. Some populations of gastric bacteria have been described – for example, the acid-tolerant lactobacilli and the yeast *Torulopsis* in the rodent stomach [2]. The isolation of *Helicobacter pylori* and the subsequent debate as to its role in gastroduodenal disease has focused interest on the stomach as a bacterial habitat. Close examination of gastric biopsies [3] revealed that *H. pylori* was inhabiting a niche that was well protected from stomach acid, i.e. the organism colonizes the gastric mucus.

As the mucus lining the intestinal tract of all animals studied contains large numbers of highly specialized bacteria, it is not really surprising that stomach mucus provides a haven for similar bacteria. The difference with *H. pylori* is that the bacterium causes a change in histopathology in all persons colonized, albeit mild; this is not the case with the normal mucus-associated bacteria in other areas of the intestine. There are other pathogens belonging to this broad group of mucus-associated bacteria; for example, *Campylobacter jejuni* colonizes intestinal mucus [4], as does the pig pathogen, *Treponema hyodysenteriae* [5].

Spiral/helical-shaped bacteria in the stomachs of animals other than humans

Even though the focus of this book is *H. pylori*-associated disease in humans, it is appropriate to consider the inhabitants of the same ecological niche in other animal species. Spiral-shaped bacteria were seen in the stomach of animals late last century. Rappin [6] is credited with the first observation, followed by Bizzozero in 1893 [7] and Salomon in 1896 [8].

A collage of the diagrams from some of these early papers on gastric bacteria in animals is shown in Fig. 25.1. It is clear from the pictures that the organisms, even though they had a spiral morphology, were very different from *H. pylori*. They tended to be longer, consisted of a number of very tight spirals and were more helical than spiral. Even though many of the bacteria discussed in this chapter are more helical in shape than spiral, the term spiral has been used throughout to describe both spiral and helical-shaped organisms, as this is the description most commonly found in the literature.

Salomon's early study was the most extensive investigation of spiral-shaped bacteria in the stomach of animals; he saw large numbers in dogs, cats and the brown Norway rat but failed to find them in humans, apes, monkeys, cattle, pigs, mice, pigeons, crows and even owls! Dubosq & Lebailly [9] in 1912 found them in a fox.

The most studied animals have been the cat and dog. Weber *et al.* [10, 11] examined the

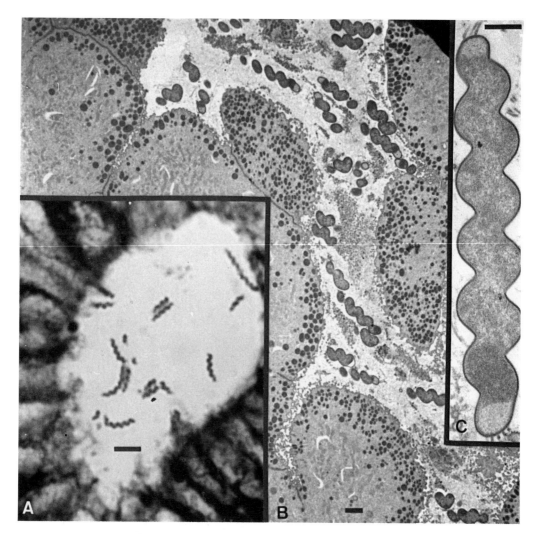

Fig. 25.7 Non-*H. pylori* spiral-shaped bacteria from the antrum of a human patient colonizing the stomach of a laboratory mouse. A, Light micrograph of the spiral bacteria seen in a biopsy from a 32-year-old Indonesian male (bar = 5 μm). B, Transmission electron micrograph showing the same bacteria colonizing the glandular epithelium of a mouse stomach following orogastric administration of a homogenate of the human antral biopsy (bar = 1 μm). C, High-magnification view of a single organism originating from the human in the mouse stomach showing the insertion sites of the bipolar flagella and the regular spiral morphology (bar = 0.5 μm).

colonized with the organism from the patient (Fig. 25.7B and C).

The second patient, who presented to Dr John Mitchell, Sydney, was especially interesting because she was only 2 years old. We were unable to culture the organism from the child and there was not enough material to inoculate a mouse. However, the family had two pet cats, which had recently been put down for independent reasons.

Spiral organisms seen in gastric sections taken from these animals have not as yet been cultured but mice have been colonized with them. Photographs of gastric mucosa from this patient and the organism in one of her cats are shown in Fig. 25.8.

ELISAs on the sera from the Indonesian and the child above showed the same results as patients 2 and 3 in the Dent study, i.e. the organisms infecting the patients were more

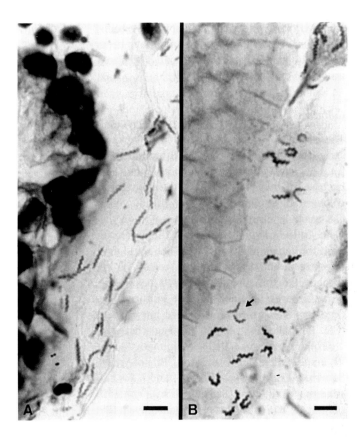

Fig. 25.8 A, Light micrograph of the surface mucus of the antral biopsy of a 2-year-old girl showing numerous non-*H. pylori* spiral bacteria (bar = 5 μm). B, Light micrograph of the surface mucus of the gastric mucus of the girl's cat showing spiral bacteria. Some of the organisms appear more darkly staining than the others, suggesting two types. The organisms shown by the arrow have the same morphology as the spirals in the girl's stomach (bar = 5 μm).

closely related to our cat isolate than to *H. pylori* but were not the same organism.

All the patients with '*Gastrospirillum*' infection share features with the above cases. The presence of the organism was associated with gastritis of varying severity and the patients had all been endoscoped for gastric symptoms. However, like *H. pylori*, the case for organisms causing dyspeptic symptoms is 'not proven'. Infection and gastritis were resolved in a number of these cases with anti-*H. pylori* therapy and it was claimed that symptoms cleared in some.

Further evidence as to the source of these bacteria is likely to emerge as the incidence of infection amongst different groups is reported. There is a distinct possibility that the incidence of these organisms will be higher in groups that come into very close contact with domestic animals such as cats and dogs, i.e. children, or persons from cultures where family members live in very close contact with animals. The observation of

Craige [28] that spirilla are present in the vomitus of cats and dogs with signs of gastritis is obviously relevant to the mode of transmission of these bacteria. Both of the cases of Dye *et al* [21] had a clear long-standing history of close contact with pets. In the first case a 36-year-old female presenting with nausea, bloating and chronic epigastric pain was fond of animals and as a child her family owned 14 cats! Their cats were cuddled and kissed on many occasions. Her symptoms of dyspepsia had been present since childhood. The other case involved a 77-year-old male who had two Irish setters as house pets and related having dogs living in the house for most of his adult life.

Culture of spiral-shaped bacteria from animal stomach mucosae

To date, very few of the non-*H. pylori* spiral bacteria from the stomachs of animals have been cultured. Fox *et al* [29] have cultured an organism from the gastric mucosa of ferrets and

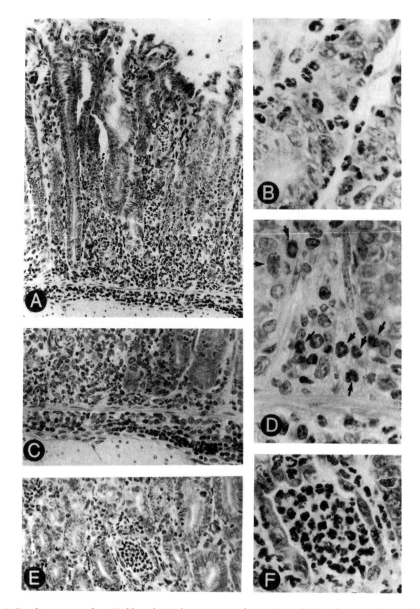

Fig. 25.9 A, Fundic mucosa of an *H. felis*-colonized mouse 4 weeks post-inoculation, demonstrating an increase in the magnitude of the cell infiltrate in the mucosa and the presence of microabscesses and hyperplastic changes in the glandular epithelium. Haematoxylin and eosin (H&E); original magnification × 30. B, High magnification of an area illustrating the migration of polymorphonuclear leucocytes from the lamina propria into the cytoplasm of glandular epithelial cells. H&E; original magnification × 160. C, High magnification of an area showing that the mucosal infiltrate is predominantly composed of polymorphonuclear leucocytes with an influx of mononuclear leucocytes into the submucosa. H&E; original magnification × 65. D, High magnification of an area illustrating the large numbers of eosinophils present in the inflammatory infiltrate (arrows). H&E; original magnification × 65. E, High magnification of a microabscess. H&E; original magnification × 65. F, High magnification of a microabscess. H&E; original magnification × 60. Lee *et al.* 1990 [37].

The literature is confused as to how many different types there are, either in the one animal or in the different animal species. Thus, even though in any one animal up to three different morphologies are seen, the authors talk about 'the' organism in the cat or 'the' organism in the dog. Fig. 25.2 shows the morphologies seen by Lockard & Boler [12], who hypothesize that the three forms are all of the same organism and represent stages in the mechanism of movement, which is accomplished by the organism changing the length of its body rather than by expansion and contraction of the filament. Recent success in our laboratory in growing animal spirals on laboratory media and in the mouse stomach has helped to clarify the situation [18]. The morphology of the spiral organism, H. felis, isolated from the cat stomach in vitro is shown in Fig. 25.5. It appears identical to Lockard & Boler's organism 2A [12] and to the picture of an organism seen in the Beagle dog in Henry et al. [14]. When H. felis is fed to mice, it establishes in the stomach and is seen in electron micrographs to have the identical morphology with the easily recognizable periplasmic fibrils (Fig. 25.6B). We have observed a second spiral organism in sections of the cat stomach viewed by electron microscopy and this is seen in Fig. 25.3. This appears to be identical to Lockard & Boler's 3A (Fig. 25.2) [12]. Attempts to culture the organism have been unsuccessful. However, we can maintain this organism in the laboratory by feeding cat mucus, in which it is dominant, to mice, where it establishes in the stomach and is seen to have the same morphology. This organism is clearly 'Gastrospirillum'-like and if the suggestions on transmission mentioned above are correct it is probably 'G. hominis'. The conclusion from this work with mice is that the cat, dog and primate can be colonized with a variety of spirals, often more than one species being present at any one time. The species seen in the different animals may vary.

Determinants of colonization in bacteria adapted to mucus-secreting intestinal mucosa

The bowel is inhabited by a large variety of bacterial species but the number colonizing the mucosae is relatively few. These bacteria must share common properties that allow them to selectively colonize mucus-covered surfaces rather than living in the lumen. Some are likely to be general properties common to colonizers of all mucus environments, while others are likely to determine the colonization of a particular location in the gut, e.g. stomach compared with small bowel. As factors influencing colonization are better understood the more likely it becomes that rational intervention steps can be developed. As H. pylori can, at this time, only be studied in primates, gnotobiotic piglets or gnotobiotic dogs [35, 36, 39–41], it is useful to study closely related organisms that do grown in convenient laboratory animal models and study the factors which influence their colonization, because information relevant to one mucus-associated bacterium could be relevant to all.

Colonizing factors shared by all organisms colonizing intestinal mucus

Spiral morphology. The one distinctive feature of all these bacteria, be they isolated from mouse colon, rat ileum, cat stomach or human stomach, is their spiral morphology. We have proposed that this gives the organisms an increased ability to move in the viscous environment of mucus [4, 42]. In vitro experiments with C. jejuni [43], the rodent ileal isolate and H. felis (Danon & A. Lee, unpublished results) and H. pylori [3] show that they cope with viscous environments very well. The exception is H. mustelae, which is a rod-shaped bacterium. Although not proved, we feel that its unusual flagella configuration may give it a specialized form of motility equivalent to the gastric spirals.

Colonizing factors of organisms preferentially colonizing stomach and small bowel mucus

Microaerophilism. The intestinal lumen is not oxygenated, unlike the tissues that line it. Therefore, at the interface, i.e. the intestinal

these infections in humans. *H. pylori* and closely related organisms appear to cause chronic gastritis in non-human primates [20–22]. These infections most clearly resemble *H. pylori* infection in humans, but non-human primates are not suitable for intensive study because of their cost and lack of wide availability.

We now know that *H. pylori* was the first recognized organism in the rapidly expanding genus, *Helicobacter*. *H. pylori* appears well adapted to humans and other primates since, on the one hand, infection is so common in humans and primates [21, 22] and, on the other hand, it is so difficult to establish infection in any animals other than primates. One exception to this observation is that gnotobiotic animals may be susceptible to *H. pylori* infection [23, 24]. However, along with primates, such animals are also not a practical option for most investigators. Nevertheless, by use of gnotobiotic piglets investigators have been able to establish infection with *H. pylori* that is localized to the stomach and produces both an inflammatory response and a host immune response [23]. Although this model differs from human infection in a number of ways, including lack of a neutrophilic inflammatory response, it has been possible to assess the relative virulence of strains and responses to antimicrobial therapy, among other phenomena [23, 25, 26].

Many other mammalian species harbour members of the genus *Helicobacter* or other *Helicobacter*-like organisms, including *H. mustelae* in ferrets [27–29], *H. felis* in dogs and cats [30], *H. acinonyx* in cheetahs [31], and related organisms in swine [32]. It is likely that many other mammalian species will be found to harbour their own gastric microbes resembling *H. pylori* [33]. These natural infections are potentially a good way of studying *H. pylori* infection, but none of the described models appears to be exactly analogous to *H. pylori* in humans.

Human models?

Paradoxically, the best 'animal' model may be *H. pylori* infections in humans because infection is so common, clinical specimens are so readily

available and clinically indicated treatments may provide interventions that can be used to answer particular questions. Nevertheless, models of *H. pylori* infection in other animals have important advantages as well. These include the ability to initiate infection with strains having defined properties and the opportunity for intensive sampling and follow-up, and also there are economic and ethical considerations.

It is also worthwhile to attempt to find other microbial analogies for *H. pylori* infections in humans. In general, *H. pylori* infections can be considered as chronic mucosal infections in immunocompetent hosts in which recognition of the organisms is present. As far as I can determine, no other infectious disease is exactly analogous, although several other conditions have a few similar characteristics. These include chronic periodontal disease and *Pseudomonas aeruginosa* infection in patients with cystic fibrosis. Each of these represents a chronic bacterial process, causing inflammation at a mucosal surface, from which the host is unable to eliminate the offending organisms. Leprosy is another chronic bacterial infection in which the host recognizes the invader (with cellular immunity in the tuberculoid form and humoral immunity in the lepromatous form), although it does not principally involve a mucosal surface. Schistosomiasis is another analogue, in which the parasite survives within the host for years or decades. Interestingly, it is chiefly the intensity of the host response to the organisms and their products (ova) that determines the pathological responses and clinical outcome [34].

Conclusions

An important question that will need to be addressed in animal or human studies is how the host response modulates *Helicobacter* infection [35]. The host recognizes *H. pylori* during its long tenure in the stomach, as evidenced by the nearly universal humoral immune response [4, 36, 37]. With suppression of the organism by antimicrobial therapy antibody levels fall, but with recurrence there is new antibody production [2]. Thus, no absolute tolerance for the organism is seen. However, at present the cellular component of the immune response to *H. pylori* remains largely unexplored. It is likely that the interrelation between the bacterial pro-inflammatory activities [38, 39] and the host's immune reactivity and perhaps immune suppression [35] will be an important determinant of infection outcome. In any event, it is clear that investigations of *H. pylori* infections in humans will break new ground in understanding mucosal infections and defences and immune responses in chronic active infections and in neoplastic processes as well. *H. pylori* is both an important pathogen of humans and an important probe for our normal gastric metabolic and immune physiology.

References

1 Taylor, D.N. & Blaser, M.J. The epidemiology of *Helicobacter pylori* infections. *Epidemiol. Rev.* 1991, **13**, 42–9.

2 Morris, A.J., Ali, M.R., Nicholson, G.I., Perez-Perez, G.I. & Blaser, M.J. Long term follow-up of voluntary ingestion of *Helicobacter pylori*. *Ann. Intern. Med.* 1991, **114**, 662–3.

3 Siurala, M., Varis, K. & Wiljasalo, M. Studies of patients with atrophic gastritis: a 10–15 year follow-up. *Scand. J. Gastroenterol.* 1966, **1**, 40–8.

4 Dooley, C.P., Fitzgibbons, P.L., Cohen, H., Appleman, M.D., Perez-Perez, G.I. & Blaser, M.J. Prevalence of *Helicobacter pylori* infection and histologic gastritis in asymptomatic persons. *N. Engl. J. Med.* 1989, **321**, 1562–6.

5 Rauws, E.A.J., Langenberg, W., Houthoff, H.J., Zanen, H.C. & Tytgat, G.N.J. *Campylobacter pyloridis*-associated chronic active antral gastritis. A prospective study of its prevalence and the effects of antibacterial and anti-ulcer treatment. *Gastroenterology* 1988, **94**, 33–40.

6 Blaser, M.J. *Helicobacter pylori* and the pathogenesis of gastroduodenal inflammation. *J. Infect. Dis.* 1990, **161**, 626–33.

7 Rauws, E.A.J. & Tytgat, G.N.J. Eradication of *Helicobacter pylori* cures duodenal ulcer. *Lancet* 1990, **i**, 1233–5.

8 Daskopoulos, G., Carrick, J., Lian, J.X. & Lee, A. Comparison of risk factors in duodenal and gastric ulcers. *Microb. Ecol. Health Dis.* 1991, **4**, S112.

9 Sipponen, P., Seppala, K., Aarynen, M., Helske, T. & Kettunen, P. Chronic gastritis and gastroduodenal ulcer: a case control study on risk of coexisting duodenal or gastric ulcer in patients with gastritis. *Gut* 1989, **30**, 922–9.

10 Rokkas, T., Pursey, C., Uzoochina, E. *et al.* Non-ulcer dyspepsia and short-term De-Nol therapy: a placebo-controlled trial with particular reference to the role of *Campylobacter pylori*. *Gut* 1988, **29**, 1386–91.

11 Kang, J.Y., Tay, H.H., Wee, A., Gvan, R., Math, M.V. & Yap, I. Effect of colloidal bismuth subcitrate on symptoms and gastric histology in non-ulcer dyspepsia. A double-blind placebo-controlled study, *Gut* 1990, **31**, 476–80.

12 Karnes, W.E., Samloff, I.M., Siurala, M., Kekki, M., Sipponen, P., Kim, S.W.R. & Walsh, J.H. Positive serum antibody and negative tissue staining for *Helicobacter pylori* in subjects with atrophic body gastritis. *Gastroenterology* 1991, **101**, 167–74.

13 Nomura, A., Stemmerman, G.N., Chyou, P.-H., Kato, I., Perez-Perez, G.I. & Blaser, M.J. *Helicobacter pylori* infection and gastric carcinoma in a population of Japanese-Americans in Hawaii. *N. Engl. J. Med.* 1991, **325**, 1132–6.

14 Parsonnet, J., Friedman, G.D., Vandersteen, D.P. *et al. Helicobacter pylori* infection and the risk of gastric carcinoma. *N. Engl. J. Med.* 1991, **325**, 1127–31.

15 Coghlan, J.G., Gilligan, D., Humphreys, H. *et al. Campylobacter pylori* and recurrence of duodenal ulcers – a 12-month follow-up study. *Lancet* 1987, **ii**, 1109–11.

16 Wyatt, J.I., Rathbone, B.J., Dixon, M.F. & Heatley, R.V. *Campylobacter pyloridis* and acid-induced gastric metaplasia in the pathogenesis of duodenitis. *J. Clin. Pathol.* 1987, **40**, 841–8.

17 Crabtree, J.R., Taylor, J.D., Wyatt, J.I. *et al.* Mucosal IgA recognition of *Helicobacter pylori* 120 kDa protein, peptic ulceration, and gastric pathology. *Lancet* 1991, **338**, 332–5.

18 Figura, N., Guglielmetti, P., Rossolini, A. *et al.* Cytotoxin production by *Campylobacter pylori* strains isolated from patients with peptic ulcers and from patients with chronic gastritis only. *J. Clin. Microbiol.* 1989, **27**, 225–6.

19 Cover, T.L., Dooley, C.P. & Blaser, M.J. Characterization and human serologic response to proteins in *Helicobacter pylori* broth culture supernatants with vacuolizing cytotoxin activity. *Infect. Immun.* 1990, **58**, 603–10.

20 Bronsdon, M.A., Bowman, J.P., Stackebrandt, E. & Sly, L.I. The systematics and phylogeny of *Helicobacter nemestrinae* isolated from the stomach of a pigtailed macaque (*Macaca nemestrina*). *Microb. Ecol. Health Dis.* 1991, **4**, S106.

21 Newell, D.G., Hudson, M.J. & Baskerville, A. Isolation of a gastric *Campylobacter*-like organism from the stomach of four rhesus monkeys, and identification as *Campylobacter pylori*. *J. Med. Microbiol.* 1988, **27**, 41–4.

22 Euler, A.R., Zurenko, G.E., Moe, J.B., Ulrich, R.G. & Yagi, Y. Evaluation of two monkey species (*Macaca mulatta* and *Macaca fascicularis*) as possible models for

human *Helicobacter pylori* disease. *J. Clin. Microbiol.* 1990, **28**, 2285–90.

23 Krakowka, B., Morgan, D.R., Kraft, W.G. *et al.* Establishment of gastric *Campylobacter pylori* infection in the neonatal gnotobiotic piglet. *Infect. Immun.* 1987, **55**, 2789–96.

24 Fox, J.G., Lee, A., Otto, G., Taylor, N.S. & Murphy, J.C. *Helicobacter felis* gastritis in gnotobiotic rats: an animal model of *Helicobacter pylori* gastritis. *Infect. Immun.* 1991, **59**, 785–91.

25 Eaton, K.A., Morgan, D.R. & Krakowka, S. *Campylobacter pylori* virulence factors in gnotobiotic piglets. *Infect. Immun.* 1989, **57**, 1119–25.

26 Eaton, K.A., Morgan, D.R. & Krakowka, S. Persistence of *Helicobacter pylori* in conventionalized piglets. *J. Infect. Dis.* 1990, **161**, 1299–301.

27 Fox, J.G., Correa, P., Taylor, N.S., Lee, A., Otto, G., Murphy, J.C. & Rose, R. *Helicobacter mustelae*-associated gastritis in ferrets. An animal model of *Helicobacter pylori* gastritis in humans. *Gastroenterology* 1990, **99**, 352–61.

28 Fox, J.G., Otto, G., Murphy, J.C., Taylor, N.S. & Lee, A. Gastric colonization of the ferret with *Helicobacter* species: natural and experimental infections. *Rev. Infect. Dis.* 1991, **13**, suppl. 8, S671–S680.

29 Fox, J.G., Otto, G., Taylor, N.S., Rosenblad, W. & Murphy, J.C. *Helicobacter mustelae*-induced gastritis and evaluated gastric pH in the ferret (*Mustela putorius furo*). *Infect. Immun.* 1991, **59**, 1875–80.

30 Lee, A., Fox, J.G., Otto, G. & Murphy, J. A small animal model of human *Helicobacter pylori* active chronic gastritis. *Gastroenterology* 1990, **99**, 1315–23.

31 Eaton, K.A., Radin, M.J., Fox, J.G. *et al. Helicobacter acinonyx*, a new species of *Helicobacter* isolated from cheetahs with gastritis. *Microb. Ecol. Health Dis.* 1991, **4**, S104.

32 Jones, D.M. & Curry, A. 1989. The ultrastructure of *Campylobacter pylori*. In Rathbone, B.J. & Heatley, R.V. (eds) *Campylobacter pylori and Gastroduodenal Disease*. Blackwell Scientific Publications, Oxford, pp. 48–62.

33 Paster, B.J., Lee, A., Fox, J.G. *et al.* Phylogeny of *Helicobacter felis* sp. nov., *Helicobacter mustelae*, and related bacteria. *Int. J. Systematic Bacteriol.* 1991, **41**, 31–8.

34 Colley, D.G. Dynamics of the human immune response to schistosomes. *Baillière's Clin. Trop. Med. Commun. Dis.* 1987, **2**, 315–32.

35 Blaser, M.J. Hypotheses on the pathogenesis and natural history of *Helicobacter pylori*-induced inflammation: a 'slow' bacterial infection. *Gastroenterology* 1992, **102**, 720–7.

36 Rathbone, B.J., Wyatt, J.I., Worsley, B.W. *et al.* Systemic and local antibody responses to gastric *Campylobacter pyloridis* in non-ulcer dyspepsia. *Gut* 1986, **27**, 642–7.

37 Drumm, B., Perez-Perez, G.I., Blaser, M.J. & Sherman, P. Intrafamilial clustering of *Helicobacter pylori* infection. *N. Engl. J. Med.* 1990, **322**, 359–63.

38 Mai, U.E.H., Perez-Perez, G.I., Wahl, L.M., Wahl, S.M., Blaser, M.J. & Smith, P.D. Soluble surface proteins from *Helicobacter pylori* activate monocytes/macrophages by lipopolysaccharide-independent mechanism. *J. Clin. Invest.* 1991, **87**, 894–900.

39 Mai, U.E., Perez-Perez, G.I., Allen, J.B., Wahl, S.M., Blaser, M.J. & Smith, P.D. Surface proteins from *Helicobacter pylori* exhibit chemotactic activity for human leukocytes and are present in gastric mucosa. *J. Exp. Med.* 1992, **175**, 517–25.

27 Is Helicobacter pylori a Significant Pathogen?

E.J.S.BOYD AND K.G.WORMSLEY

Introduction

There are well-documented associations between infection with *Helicobacter pylori* and a range of upper gastrointestinal disorders, including chronic antral gastritis, chronic fundic gastritis, chronic duodenitis, duodenal ulceration, gastric ulceration and gastric cancer. The purpose of the present chapter is to evaluate whether these associations imply causality or coincidence.

As is commonly the case with diseases of interest to epidemiologists, each of the above disorders associated with colonization by *H. pylori* may have a multifactorial aetiology. That is, each disorder may have more than one sufficient cause (a sufficient cause is one which, when present, inevitably results in the development of the clinical disorder) [1]. However, a sufficient cause may not be a single aetiological factor, but may comprise a range of component factors, which may be either necessary (that is, a component of all sufficient causes) or not (that is, a component of some, but not all, constellations of factors which constitute a sufficient cause). These concepts are represented diagramatically in Fig. 27.1. Thus, taking duodenal ulcer disease as an example, gastric secretion of acid and pepsin (A) appears to be a necessary causal factor (although probably not by itself a sufficient causal factor), while ingestion of nonsteroidal anti-inflammatory drugs (B) or cigarette smoking (C) is not a necessary cause.

To assess the causal significance of associations in multifactorial diseases, criteria are employed which differ from Koch's original postulates [2]. These criteria are summarized in Table 27.1. In a multifactorial disease, these criteria cannot provide absolute proof of causality, but permit an assessment of the probability of a causal relationship between individual factors and a disease. As far as is possible, given the current state of knowledge, we shall use these criteria to evaluate the significance of the role of *H. pylori* as a pathogen in the upper gastrointestinal tract.

Chronic gastritis

Chronic gastritis is characterized histologically by the presence of an infiltrate containing plasma cells and lymphocytes. Superficial chronic gastritis involves only the upper third of the mucosa, while in chronic atrophic gastritis inflammatory changes extend down through the full thickness of the mucosa and there is loss of gastric glands. Often, chronic gastritis is patchy in distribution, and areas of superficial gastritis and atrophic gastritis may coexist in the same patient. Activity of chronic gastritis is characterized by the presence of a polymorphonuclear leucocyte (PMN) infiltrate, mucus depletion and evidence of damage to surface epithelial cells. Chronic gastritis may involve the gastric antrum, the gastric fundus, or both – pan-gastritis.

Chronic antral gastritis

When the appearance of active chronic antral gastritis are present on histological examination, antral colonization by *H. pylori* is also detectable in up to 100% of patients studied [3–6]. Only rarely is activity of chronic antral gastritis present in the absence of *H. pylori* [7].

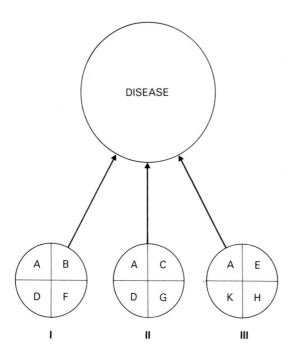

Fig. 27.1 Causation. I–III are each sufficient causes of the disease. A–K are component causes: A is a necessary component cause; B–K are non-necessary component causes.

The strength of this association appears to be consistent in all studied populations, and is present whatever method is used to establish colonization by *H. pylori* (microscopy, culture, serology or urea breath testing). In the absence of histological evidence of activity, the rate of

Table 27.1 Surgeon General's Advisory Committee criteria for causation.

1 Specificity	The distinctiveness of the association of the aetiological agent with the disease
2 Strength	The magnitude of the association, and in particular a positive dose–effect relationship, and the effect of removal of the aetiological agent
3 Consistency	The replication of results when the causal relationship is studied in different localities and by different techniques
4 Timing	Exposure to the aetiological factor should precede the effect
5 Coherence	The association should be plausible in the context of the known facts of the natural history and biology of the disease

detection of *H. pylori* in the presence of chronic antral gastritis falls to approximately 80% [6].

A positive dose–response relationship has been reported between the numbers of *H. pylori* colonizing the antrum and the severity of the chronic antral gastritis [8–10]. Correlation appears to be limited solely to the degree of PMN infiltrate, and such a dose–response association has also been denied [11, 12].

The specificity of the association between *H. pylori* and chronic antral gastritis is not total, since *H. pylori* is present on the antral mucosa in up to 24% of patients in whom no histological abnormality is demonstrable [6]. In one study *H. pylori* has been detected in 75% of patients presenting with non-ulcer dyspepsia with histologically normal gastric antral mucosa [13].

Causality has been inferred from the results of therapeutic intervention, since active chronic superficial antral gastritis improves or resolves completely during treatment with agents that kill *H. pylori in vitro* [14–18]. In patients in whom *H. pylori* was successfully eradicated histological improvement was maintained, while failure to eradicate *H. pylori* was associated with recrudescence of the gastritis.

These data must be interpreted with caution. Firstly, the drugs used to treat *H. pylori*-associated chronic antral gastritis may have effects other than antibacterial ones which may be responsible for the histological improvement of the gastritis. For example, metronidazole protects against experimental ulceration in animals [19], and heals peptic ulcers in man by mechanisms which are probably independent of any effect on *H. pylori*. During treatment with metronidazole alone, 70% of patients may be expected to become colonized with metronidazole-resistant *H. pylori* [20], yet ulcers heal in approximately 80% of patients [21]. Other antibiotics have cytoprotective effects in experimental gastric ulceration in rats [22]. Bismuth-containing preparations inactivate pepsin and increase mucosal concentrations of cytoprotective prostaglandins [23, 24], and are effective in the treatment of chronic gastritis not associated with colonization by *H. pylori* [25]. It is therefore possible that the therapeutic effects depend on normalization of the gastric mucosa making it uninhabitable by *H. pylori*, rather than directly on the effect of the drugs on *H. pylori* with secondary healing of the antral mucosal disease.

Secondly, the claim that ulcer-healing agents which are devoid of activity against *H. pylori* do not improve the chronic antral gastritis which accompanies ulcer disease [26] has been refuted. Several studies show that treatment with H_2-receptor antagonists [19, 27], prostaglandins [28], antacids [18] or sucralfate [18, 29] results in improvement in the antral gastritis. This improvement is apparently not as marked as that observed in patients receiving treatment which kills *H. pylori*, but no comparative studies have been performed within individuals. The converse is also true – although histological evidence of activity usually disappears after successful eradication of *H. pylori*, chronic gastritis may persist [14–16, 30], possibly indicating the presence of a primary mucosal abnormality which predisposes to infection with *H. pylori*. Treatment with antacids reduces the numbers of *H. pylori* colonizing the antrum in patients with active chronic antral gastritis and erosions, but this was not accompanied by improvement in

the mucosal disease [31]. Thus, dissociation between the effects of therapy on *H. pylori* and the effects on the associated chronic antral gastritis weakens a possible causal relationship.

A crucial problem in attributing a causal relationship to *H. pylori* in the genesis of chronic antral gastritis relates to the lack of data concerning the temporal relationship between infection and the occurrence of antral gastritis. There have been no prospective studies of the development of *H. pylori* infection and the subsequent occurrence of chronic antral gastritis in patients previously demonstrated to have normal gastric morphology and function. Thus, it is not possible to define the risk of developing antral gastritis after being infected with *H. pylori* or to exclude the converse possibility that a pre-existing gastric mucosal abnormality is necessary for, or predisposes to, colonization with *H. pylori*.

Oral self-infection studies performed by two subjects have been cited as evidence that *H. pylori* colonizes normal gastric mucosa and causes active chronic superficial antral gastritis, since both subjects had normal antral histology and no evidence of previous infection with *H. pylori* shortly before ingesting the organism [30, 32]. However, this evidence is inconclusive, since infection only occurred after the administration of doses of H_2-receptor antagonists, which abolished normal gastric secretion and therefore permitted colonization with other organisms, the presence of which was not sought. In one subject, an attempt to cause infection in the presence of normal gastric acid secretion was unsuccessful despite a large inoculum of *H. pylori*, suggesting that a healthy stomach which secretes normal gastric juice is not susceptible to infection with *H. pylori*. These studies cannot, therefore, be taken as evidence that the acute type of gastric illness suffered by both subjects bears any relationship to the usual manifestation of clinical infection with *H. pylori*. Indeed, one of the subjects spontaneously cleared the organism (while failing to develop an antibody response), a sequence which is reported not to occur in patients colonized by *H. pylori* [33].

26 McIntyre, R.L.E., Piris, J. & Truelove, S.C. Effect of cimetidine on chronic gastritis in gastric ulcer patients. *Aust. NZ J. Med.* 1982, **12**, 106.

27 Hui, W.-M., Lam, S.-K., Chau, P.-Y. *et al.* Persistence of *Campylobacter pyloridis* despite healing of duodenal ulcer and healing of accompanying duodenitis and gastritis. *Dig. Dis. Sci.* 1987, **32**, 1255–60.

28 Hui, W.-M., Lam, S.-K., Ho, J. *et al.* Chronic antral gastritis in duodenal ulcer. Natural history and treatment with protaglandin E₁. *Gastroenterology* 1986, **91**, 1095–101.

29 Hui, W.-M., Lam, S.-K., Ho, J. *et al.* Effect of sucralfate and cimetidine on duodenal ulcer-associated antral gastritis and *Campylobacter pylori*. *Am. J. Med.* 1989, **86**, suppl. 6A, 60–4.

30 Morris, A.M. & Nicholson, G. Ingestion of *Campylobacter pyloridis* causes gastritis and raised fasting pH. *Am. J. Gastroenterol.* 1987, **83**, 192–9.

31 Berstad, A., Alexander, B., Weberg, R. *et al.* Antacids reduce *Campylobacter pylori* colonisation without healing the gastritis in patients with non-ulcer dyspepsia and erosive pre-pyloric changes. *Gastroenterology* 1988, **95**, 619–25.

32 Marshall, B.J., Armstrong, J.A., McGechie, D.B. & Glancy, R.J. Attempts to fulfil Koch's postulates for pyloric *Campylobacter*. *Med. J. Aust.* 1985, **142**, 436–9.

33 Tytgat, G.N.J. *Campylobacter pyloridis*. *Acta Clin. Belg.* 1987, **42**, 146–52.

34 Ramsey, E.J., Carey, K.V., Peterson, W.L. *et al.* Epidemic gastritis with hypochlorhydria. *Gastroenterology* 1979, **76**, 1449–57.

35 Peterson, W.L., Lee, E. & Skoglund, M. The role of *Campylobacter pyloridis* in epidemic gastritis with hypochlorhydria. *Gastroenterology* 1987, **92**, 1575.

36 Gledhill, T., Leicester, R.J., Addis, B. *et al.* Epidemic hypochlorhydria. *Br. Med. J.* 1985, **290**, 1383–6.

37 Graham, D.Y., Alpert, L.C., Smith, J.L. *et al.* Iatrogenic *Campylobacter pylori* infection is a cause of epidemic achlorhydria. *Am. J. Gastroenterol.* 1988, **83**, 974–80.

38 Peterson, W.L., Lee, E. & Feldman, M. Relationship between *Campylobacter pylori* and gastritis in healthy humans after administration of placebo or indomethacin. *Gastroenterology* 1988, **95**, 619–25.

39 Cave, D.R. & Vargas, M. Effect of *Campylobacter pylori* protein on acid secretion by parietal cells. *Lancet* 1989, **ii**, 187–9.

40 Borody, T., Noonan, S., Cole, P. *et al.* Triple therapy of *C. pylori* can reverse hypochlorhydria. *Gastroenterology* 1989, **95**, A53.

41 Bode, G., Malfertheiner, P. & Ditschuneit, H. Pathogenetic implications of ultrastructural findings in *Campylobacter pylori* related gastroduodenal disease. *Scand. J. Gastroenterol.* 1988, **23**, suppl. 142, 25–39.

42 Lawson, H.H. Definition of gastroduodenal junction in health subjects. *J. Clin. Pathol.* 1988, **41**, 393–6.

43 Wyatt, J.I., Rathbone, B.J., Dixon, M.F. & Heatley, R.V. *Campylobacter pyloridis* and acid-induced gastric metaplasia in the pathogenesis of duodenitis. *J. Clin. Pathol.* 1987, **40**, 841–8.

44 Kreuning, J., Bosman, F.T., Kuiper, G. *et al.* Gastric and duodenal mucosa in 'healthy' individuals. *J. Clin. Pathol.* 1978, **31**, 69–77.

45 Johansen, A.A. & Hansen, O.H. Heterotopic gastric epithelium in the duodenum and its correlation to gastric disease and acid level. *Acta Pathol. Microbiol. Scand.* 1973, **A81**, 676–80.

46 Tominaga, K. Distribution of parietal cells in the antral mucosa of human stomachs. *Gastroenterology*, 1975, **69**, 1201–7.

47 Andersen, L.P., Holck, S., Poulsen, C.O., Elsborg, L. & Justesen, T. *Campylobacter pyloridis* in peptic ulcer disease. 1. Gastric and duodenal infection caused by *C. pyloridis*: histopathologic and microbiologic findings. *Scand. J. Gastroenterol.* 1987, **22** 219–24.

48 Levi, S., Beardshall, K., Haddad, G., Playford, R., Ghosh, P. & Calam, J. *Campylobacter pylori* and duodenal ulcers: the gastrin link. *Lancet* 1989, **i**, 1167–9.

49 Goodwin, C.S. Duodenal ulcer, *Campylobacter pylori*, and the 'leaking roof' concept. *Lancet* 1988, **ii**, 1467–9.

50 Bendtsen, F., Rosenkilde-Gram, B., Tage-Jensen, U. *et al.* Duodenal bulb acidity in patients with duodenal ulcer. *Gastroenterology* 1987, **93**, 1263–9.

51 El Nujumi, A.M., Dorian, C.A. & McColl, K.E.L. Effect of inhibition of *Helicobacter pylori* urease activity with acetohydroxamic acid on plasma gastrin in subjects with duodenal ulcer. *Gut* 1990, **31**, A117.

52 Brady, C.E., Hadfield, T.L., Hyatt, J.R. *et al.* Acid secretion and serum gastrin levels in individuals with *Campylobacter pylori*. *Gastroenterology* 1988, **94**, 923–7.

53 Staub, P., Jost, R., Eberle, C. *et al. Campylobacter pylori* Besiedlung des Antrums: Einfluß auf Gastrin, Somatostatin, pankreatisches Polypeptid und Neurotensin. *Schweiz. Med. Wochenschr.* 1989, **119**, 765–7.

54 Karttunen, T., Niemelä, S., Lehtola, J., Heikkilä, J., Mäntausa, O. & Räsänen, O. *Campylobacter*-like organisms and gastritis: histopathology, bile reflux and gastric fluid composition. *Scand. J. Gastroenterol.* 1987, **22**, 478–86.

55 Malfertheiner, P., Stanescu, A., Bode, G., Baczako, K., Kühl, P. & Ditschuneit, H. 1990. Gastric metaplasia in duodenal mucosa – key factor for *H. pylori* colonization and duodenal ulcer pathogenesis? In Malfertheiner, P. & Ditschuneit, H. (eds) *Helicobacter pylori, Gastritis and Peptic Ulcer*. Springer-Verlag, Berlin, pp. 292–301.

56 Mobius, G. & Tungler, D. Zur Intensität und Lokalisation entzündlicher Magenschleimhautveränderungen bei Ulcus ventriculi, Ulcus duodeni und

Magenkarzinom. Untersuchungen an Magenresek-
tionspräparaten. *Dtsch. Z. Verdau. Stoffwechselkr.*
1975, **35**, 113–22.

57 Cheli, R. & Aste, H. 1976. *Duodenitis*. George Thieme,
Stuttgart, pp. 72–5.

58 Blanco, M., Pajares, J.M., Jiminez, M.L. & Lopez-Brea,
M. Effect of acid inhibition on *Campylobacter pylori*.
Scand. J. Gastroenterol. 1988, **23**, suppl. 142, 107–9.

59 Gad, A., Hradsky, M., Furugard, K. & Malmodin, B.
Campylobacter pylori and gastroduodenal ulcer
disease: a prospective study in a Swedish population.
Scand. J. Gastroenterol. 1989, **24**, suppl. 167, 81–5.

60 Rauws, E.A.J., Langenberg, W., Houthoff, H.I. &
Tytgat, G.N.J. 1988. Attempts to eradicate *Campylobacter* – Dutch experiences. In Menge, H., Gregor,
M., Tytgat, G.N.J. & Marshall, B.M. (eds) *Campylobacter pylori*. Springer-Verlag, Berlin, pp. 215–18.

61 Sipponen, P., Seppälä, K., Ääyrnen, M. & Kettunen,
P. Chronic gastritis and gastroduodenal ulcer: a case-
control study on risk of co-existing duodenal or gastric ulcer in patients with gastritis. *Gut* 1989, **30**,
922–9.

62 Mégraud, F., Brassens-Rabbe, M., Denis, F., Belbouri,
A. & Hoa, D.Q. Seroepidemiology of *Campylobacter
pylori* infection in various populations. *J. Clin. Microbiol.* 1989, **27**, 1870–3.

63 Blaser, M. Epidemiology and pathophysiology of
Campylobacter pylori infections. *Rev. Infect. Dis.* 1990,
12, suppl. 1, S99–S106.

64 Boyd, E.J.S. & Wormsley, K.G. 1985. Epidemiology
and pathophysiology of peptic ulcer. In Berk, J.E. (ed.)
Bockus Gastroenterology. W.B. Saunders, Philadelphia, pp. 1013–59.

65 Coghlan, J.G., Gilligan, D., Humphries, H. *et al.*
Campylobacter pylori and recurrence of duodenal
ulcers – a 12 month follow-up study. *Lancet* 1987, **ii**,
1109–11.

66 Marshall, B.J., Warren, R.J., Blincow, E.D. *et al.* Prospective double-blind trial of duodenal ulcer relapse
after eradication of *Campylobacter pylori*. *Lancet* 1988,
ii, 1437–42.

67 Rauws, E.A.J. & Tytgat, G.N.J. Cure of duodenal ulcer
associated with eradication of *Helicobacter pylori*.
Lancet 1990, **i**, 1233–5.

68 Anand, B.S., Kumar, N. & Nanda, R. *Campylobacter
pyloridis* is not responsible for duodenal ulcer formation: results of a controlled therapeutic trial. *Dig. Dis.
Sci.* 1986, **31**, 151S.

69 Hirschl, A.M., Hentschel, E., Schutze, K. *et al.* The
efficacy of antimicrobial treatment of *C. pylori* associated gastritis and duodenal ulcer. *Scand. J. Gastroenterol.* 1988, **23**, suppl. 142, 76–81.

70 Bianchi Porro, G. & Lazzaroni, M. *Campylobacter
pylori* and ulcer recurrence. *Lancet* 1988, **i**, 593.

71 Mannes, G.A., Bayerdörffer, E., Höchter, W. *et al.*
1990. Early relapse rate after healing of *Helicobacter
pylori* positive duodenal ulcers. Munich duodenal
ulcer trial. In Malfertheiner, P. & Ditschuneit, H. (eds)
Helicobacter pylori, Gastritis and Peptic Ulcer. Springer-
Verlag, Berlin, pp. 327–34.

72 Sariosek, J., Slomiany, A. & Slomiany, B.L. Evidence
for weakening of gastric mucus integrity by *Campylobacter pylori*. *Scand. J. Gastroenterol.* 1988, **23**,
585–90.

73 Slomiany, B.L., Kasinathan, C. & Slomiany, A. Lip-
olytic activity of *Campylobacter pylori*: effect of colloidal bismuth subcitrate (De Nol). *Am. J. Gastroenterol.* 1989, **84**, 1273–7.

74 Yeomans, N.D. Bacteria in ulcer pathogenesis. *Baillière's Clin. Gastroenterol.* 1988, **2**, 573–91.

75 Pym, B.M., Eckstein, R.P., Piper, D.W. & Stiel, D.
Campylobacter-like organisms and gastric ulcer. *Med.
J. Aust.* 1986, **144**, 387–8.

76 Ihamäki, T., Saukkonen, M. & Siurala, M. Long-term
observation of subjects with normal mucosa and
with superficial gastritis: results of 23–27 years' follow-up examinations. *Scand. J. Gastroenterol.* 1978,
13, 771–5.

77 Jaskiewicz, K., Ouwrens, H.D., Woodruff, C.W., Van
Wyk, M.J. & Price, S.K. The association of *Campylobacter pylori* with mucosal pathological changes
in a population at risk for gastric cancer. *S. African
Med. J.* 1989, **75**, 417–19.

78 Correa, P., Cuello, C., Duque, E. *et al.* Gastric cancer
in Colombia. III. Natural history of precursor lesions.
J. Nat. Cancer. Inst. 1976, **57**, 1207–235.

79 Howson, C.P., Hiyama, T. & Wynder, E.L. The decline
in gastric cancer: epidemiology of an unplanned
triumph. *Epidemiol. Rev.* 1986, **8**, 1–27.

80 Hole, D.J., Quigley, E.M.M., Gillis, C.R. & Watkinson,
G. Peptic ulcer and cancer: an examination of the
relationship between chronic peptic ulcer and gastric
carcinoma. *Scand. J. Gastroenterol.* 1987, **22**, 17–23.

81 Hansen, O.H., Johansen, A., Larsen, J.K., Pedersen, T.
& Svendsen, L.B. Relationship between gastric acid
secretion, histopathology, and cell proliferation
kinetics in human gastric mucosa. *Gastroenterology*
1977, **73**, 453–6.

82 Raedsch, R., Stiehl, A., Waldherr, R., Pasch, B.,
Plachky, J. & Kommerell, B. Intragastrale Gallen-
säuren und Lyzolezithin bei Gastritis-Patienten mit
und ohne *Campylobacter pylori* Besiedlung des
Magens. *Inn. Med.* 1988, **15**, 40–5.

Index

Page references in *italics* refer to figures, and those in **bold** refer to tables.